Towards adulthood: exploring the sexual and reproductive health of adolescents in South Asia

Edited by

Sarah Bott

Shireen Jejeebhoy

Iqbal Shah

Chander Puri

World Health Organization

Department of Reproductive Health and Research

WHO Library Cataloguing-in-Publication Data

Towards adulthood : exploring the sexual and reproductive health of adolescents in South Asia / edited by Sarah Bott ... [et al.]

1.Adolescent behavior 2.Sex behavior 3.Risk-taking 4.Knowledge, attitudes, practice 5.Reproductive health services 6.Adolescent health services 7.Asia I.International Conference on Reproductive Health (2000 : Mumbai, India) II.Bott, Sarah.

ISBN 92 4 156250 1 (NLM classification: WS 462)

Credits

Cover design: Máire Ní Mhearáin
Cover photo: POPULATION COUNCIL/BONNIE HAZURIA
Back cover photo: CENTER FOR COMMUNICATION PROGRAMS, JOHNS HOPKINS UNIVERSITY

Printed in Switzerland

CONTENTS

Acknowledgements vii

I. INTRODUCTION

Adolescent sexual and reproductive health in South Asia: an overview of findings from the 2000 Mumbai Conference
Sarah Bott and Shireen J. Jejeebhoy 3

II. INAUGURAL PRESENTATIONS

On being an adolescent in the 21st century
Paul F.A. Van Look 31

Addressing the reproductive health needs of adolescents in India: directions for programmes
A.R. Nanda 43

Adolescent reproductive health in South Asia: key issues and priorities for action
Ena Singh 48

III. SEXUAL AND REPRODUCTIVE HEALTH OF MARRIED ADOLESCENTS

The reproductive health status of married adolescents as assessed by NFHS-2, India
Sumati Kulkarni 55

Pregnancy and postpartum experience among first time young parents in Bangladesh: preliminary observations
Syeda Nahid M. Chowdhury 59

Early marriage and childbearing: risks and consequences
Ramesh K. Adhikari 62

Newly married adolescent women: experiences from case studies in urban India
Annie George 67

IV. SEXUAL RISK BEHAVIOURS, PERCEPTIONS AND NORMS AMONG UNMARRIED ADOLESCENTS: EVIDENCE FROM CASE STUDIES

Risk behaviour and misperceptions among low-income college students of Mumbai
Leena Abraham 73

Adolescent reproductive health in Pakistan
Yasmeen Sabeeh Qazi 78

The influence of gender norms on the reproductive health of adolescents in Nepal—perspectives of youth
Cynthia Waszak, Shyam Thapa and Jessica Davey 81

Differences in male and female attitudes towards premarital sex in a sample of Sri Lankan youth
Kalinga Tudor Silva and Stephen Schensul 86

V. UNWANTED SEX: SEXUAL VIOLENCE AND COERCION

Sexual coercion among unmarried adolescents of an urban slum in India
Geeta Sodhi and Manish Verma 91

Experiences of sexual coercion among street boys in Bangalore, India
Jayashree Ramakrishna, Mani Karott and Radha Srinivasa Murthy 95

Gender, sexual abuse and risk behaviours in adolescents: a cross-sectional survey in schools in Goa, India
Vikram Patel, Gracy Andrews, Tereze Pierre and Nimisha Kamat 99

VI. MEETING ADOLESCENTS' NEEDS FOR CONTRACEPTION

Adolescence and safety of contraceptives
Olav Meirik 105

Contraceptive behaviours of adolescents in Asia: issues and challenges
Saroj Pachauri and K.G. Santhya 108

Constraints on condom use among young men in border towns of Nepal
Anand Tamang and Binod Nepal 114

Situation analysis of emergency contraceptive use among young people in Thailand
Wanapa Naravage and Siriporn Yongpanichkul 116

VII. THE CONTEXT OF ABORTION AMONG ADOLESCENTS

Menstrual regulation among adolescents in Bangladesh: risks and experiences
Halida Hanum Akhter 123

Induced abortions: decision-making, provider choice and morbidity experience among rural adolescents in India
Bela Ganatra and S.S. Hirve 127

VIII. REPRODUCTIVE TRACT AND SEXUALLY TRANSMITTED INFECTIONS

Impact of sexually transmitted infections including AIDS on adolescents: a global perspective
Purnima Mane and Ann P. McCauley 133

Gynaecological problems among young married women in Tamil Nadu, India
Abraham Joseph, Jasmin Prasad and Sulochana Abraham 138

Developing an interactive STI-prevention programme for youth: lessons from a north Indian slum
Shally Awasthi, Mark Nichter and V.K. Pande 142

Sexual health services for adolescents at sex clinics in Rawalpindi, Pakistan
Shahid Maqsood Ranjha and Anusheh Hussain 148

IX. COMMUNICATION BETWEEN ADOLESCENTS AND ADULTS ABOUT SEXUAL AND REPRODUCTIVE HEALTH

Access to reproductive health information in Punjab and Sindh, Pakistan: the perspectives of adolescents and parents
Minhaj ul Haque and Azeema Faizunnisa 153

Building a supportive environment for adolescent reproductive health programmes in India: essential programme components
Rekha Masilamani 156

Experience of family violence: reflections from adolescents in Uttar Pradesh, India
Bella Patel Uttekar, M.E. Khan, Nayan Kumar, Sandhya Barge and Hemlata Sadhwani 159

X. FAMILY LIFE AND SEX EDUCATION

Population education in formal and non-formal sectors in India
Vandana Chakrabarti 165

Communicating with rural adolescents about sex education: experiences from BRAC, Bangladesh
Sabina Faiz Rashid 168

Reproductive health education: experiences of Parivar Seva Sanstha in communicating with youth in India
Sudha Tewari and Sumita Taneja 174

Counselling young people on sexual and reproductive health: individual and peer programmes
Raj Brahmbhatt 178

The Healthy Adolescent Project in India (HAPI)
Matthew Tiedemann and Shakuntala DasGupta 181

XI. BUILDING SELF-EFFICACY AMONG ADOLESCENTS

Adolescent girls in India choose a better future: an impact assessment of an educational programme
Marta Levitt-Dayal, Renuka Motihar, Shubhada Kanani and Arundhati Mishra 187

Training school teachers to pass on life skills to adolescents
Mridula Seth 190

XII. ACCESS TO AND QUALITY OF REPRODUCTIVE HEALTH SERVICES

Adolescent-friendly health services
V. Chandra Mouli 195

Making nongovernmental organization initiatives "youth friendly"
Sharon Epstein 199

Reproductive health services for adolescents: recent experiences from a pilot project in Bangladesh
Ismat Bhuiya, Ubaidur Rob, M.E. Khan and Ahmed Al Kabir 203

Attitudes of family planning workers towards providing contraceptive services for unmarried young adults in eight centres in China
Gao Ersheng, Tu Xiaowen and Lou Chaohua 207

Providing adolescent-friendly reproductive health services: the Thai experience
Yupa Poonkhum 210

Establishing adolescent health services in a general health facility
Rajesh Mehta 213

XIII. PANEL DISCUSSIONS: VIEWS OF YOUNG PEOPLE, GOVERNMENTS AND INTERESTED AGENCIES

Putting reproductive health within the wider context of adolescent lives: challenges and experiences 219

Enhancing adolescents' reproductive health: strategies and challenges 223

XIV. LOOKING FORWARD: RECOMMENDATIONS OF THE CONFERENCE

Looking forward: recommendations for policies, programmes and research
Sarah Bott, Iqbal Shah and Shireen J. Jejeebhoy 229

ANNEX 1

International Conference on Adolescent Reproductive Health: Evidence and Programme Implications for South Asia
Conference agenda 239

Acknowledgments

The International Conference on Adolescent Reproductive Health: Evidence and Programme Implications for South Asia was organized jointly by the Institute for Research in Reproduction, Mumbai, the Indian Society for the Study of Reproduction and Fertility, and the UNDP/UNFPA/WHO/World Bank Special Programme of Research, Development and Research Training in Human Reproduction (HRP) of WHO's Department of Reproductive Health and Research. The Conference was held in Mumbai, India, in November 2000 and was attended by some 400 participants.

The rationale for this Conference is self-evident. Despite the fact that adolescents aged 10–19 and young people aged 10–24 constitute a significant proportion of the population of the region, their reproductive and sexual health needs are poorly understood and ill-served. This neglect has major implications, since reproductive and sexual behaviours formed in adolescence have far-reaching consequences for the lives of young people as they develop into adulthood, and later on, as adults. The central theme of the Conference was to respond to this need. Objectives were to review the evidence on adolescent sexual and reproductive health, with particular reference to the situation in South Asia; and to draw lessons from the evidence for programming for adolescents in this region.

By bringing together policy-makers, programme managers, service providers and researchers, the International Conference on Adolescent Reproductive Health provided a unique opportunity to amass the most recent evidence assessing the situation, needs and perspectives of adolescents, to learn from successes and failures, and to assess programmes that respond to their unique needs. The Conference generated a great deal of interest in the sexual and reproductive health situation of young people in the region.

This volume documents the diversity of presentations made at the Conference. Presented in the form of detailed summaries of almost all presentations, the volume provides a succinct overview of the available evidence from research and programmes.

Preparation of this volume would have been impossible without the insights, cooperation and support of many. Paul Van Look, Director, Department of Reproductive Health and Research, World Health Organization (Geneva) responded enthusiastically to the idea of assembling a volume of this nature. We owe him a special debt of gratitude for this and for his valuable guidance and insights in shaping the volume both in terms of its content and its form.

The success of a Conference depends to a considerable extent on the input of its local organizers. Staff of the Institute for Research in Reproduction, Mumbai, and members of the Indian Society for the Study of Reproduction and Fertility have excelled in this respect. Their efficiency and attentiveness went a long way in enabling thought provoking discussion, and in maintaining a record of the proceedings.

The administrative requirements attached to the production of a volume with 42 summaries and a host of contributors cannot be underestimated, and the assistance of Nicky Sabatini-Fox in facilitating this is much appreciated. We gratefully acknowledge her role in the administrative arrangements relating to both the organization of the Conference and the preparation of this volume.

The Conference could not have taken place without generous financial support from many organizations, including the Wellcome Trust (London), the Ford Foundation (New Delhi), the MacArthur Foundation (Chicago) and the UNDP/UNFPA/WHO/World Bank Special Programme of Research, Development and Research Training in Human Reproduction (HRP), Department of Reproductive Health and Research, World Health Organization. The support of these organizations is gratefully acknowledged.

Finally, we thank the authors themselves for agreeing to take on this ambitious project. Not only did they present their valuable insights and findings at the Conference, but they also readily agreed to contribute summaries of their presentations for inclusion in this volume. We are grateful to them for responding so amiably to a host of requests from peer reviewers and editors. Their insights and comments have enriched what is known about the sexual and reproductive health of adolescents in the region.

Sarah Bott
Shireen Jejeebhoy
Iqbal Shah
Chander Puri

I

Introduction

Adolescent sexual and reproductive health in South Asia: an overview of findings from the 2000 Mumbai conference

Sarah Bott and Shireen J. Jejeebhoy

Conference background

The World Health Organization (WHO) defines adolescents as the age group 10–19, a definition used throughout this volume. The meaning of adolescence as a cultural construct has been understood in many different ways throughout the world, however. In general terms, it is considered a time of transition from childhood to adulthood, during which young people experience changes following puberty, but do not immediately assume the roles, privileges and responsibilities of adulthood. The nature of adolescence varies tremendously by age, sex, marital status, class, region and cultural context. As a group, however, adolescents have sexual and reproductive health needs that differ from those of adults in important ways and which remain poorly understood or served in much of the world.

Moreover, social, economic and political forces are rapidly changing the ways that young people must prepare for adult life. These changes have enormous implications for adolescents' education, employment, marriage, childbearing and health. Adolescents are increasingly spending more time in school, experiencing puberty at younger ages, marrying and having children later than in the past. Neglect of this population has major implications for the future, since reproductive and sexual behaviours during adolescence have far-reaching consequences for people's lives as they develop into adulthood.

In South Asia, by the end of the 1990s, both researchers and governments had begun to shed their traditional ambivalence towards young people's sexual and reproductive health, and a growing body of empirical evidence and government interest provided an opportunity to take stock of the sexual and reproductive health situation of youth in the region. In response, HRP[1], ISRRF[2] and IRR[3] jointly organized an international conference in November 2000 entitled: "Adolescent Reproductive Health: Evidence and Programme Implications for South Asia", held in Mumbai, India. Although international organizations subdivide Asia in different ways, this conference focused on five South Asian countries, namely, Bangladesh, India, Nepal, Pakistan and Sri Lanka. Insights from other Asian settings were also presented, notably from China and Thailand.

1 HRP stands for the UNDP/UNFPA/WHO/World Bank Special Programme of Research, Development and Research Training in Human Reproduction.

2 ISRRF stands for the Indian Society for Research on Reproduction and Fertility.

3 IRR stands for the Institute for Research in Reproduction.

The conference aimed to review the evidence on adolescents' sexual and reproductive health situation, needs and perspectives in South Asia, to learn from programme successes and failures in the region, and to identify acceptable yet effective ways to respond to adolescents' unique needs. The conference addressed a number of central questions, including: What are adolescents' needs in regards to sexual and reproductive health? How can we increase their ability to make informed reproductive choices? How do we enhance their access to reproductive health services that are acceptable, unthreatening, and affordable? What kind of information do they need in order to exercise these choices and access services? How can we tailor programmes to deliver information and services? And, how can programmes improve communication between adolescents and adults?

This conference brought together researchers from different disciplines, as well as service providers, programme managers, government representatives, policy-makers, representatives from international and donor agencies and, most importantly, young people themselves. Participants came from more than 13 countries, including South Asia, other Asian countries such as China, Indonesia, and Thailand, and countries beyond the region such as Chile, Colombia, several European countries and the United States of America. The agenda included 42 full presentations, 12 brief abstract presentations, comments from nine discussants and 72 poster presentations, supplemented by panel discussions among young people themselves and policy-makers.

In an attempt to record the evidence and insights that emerged from the conference, organizers asked the conference participants to write summaries of their presentations. As a result, this volume contains summaries of 40 of the 42 major presentations and two of the three panel sessions. This overview chapter provides a brief social and demographic profile of adolescents in South Asia, together, where possible, with information on other Asian countries—China, Indonesia, the Philippines, Thailand and Viet Nam—to enable readers to place South Asia within the larger Asian context. This is followed by a review of the entire collection of papers contained in this volume.

Profile of adolescents in South Asia

Of the estimated 1.2 billion adolescents in the world today, nearly half live in Asia, and nearly one in

Table 1. Demographic profile of adolescents in South Asia and other selected Asian countries

Country	Estimated population aged 15–19 circa 2000 (thousands)	Estimated population aged 10–19 circa 2000 (thousands)	Adolescents aged 15–19 (% of total population)	Adolescents aged 10–19 (% of total population)
South Asia	**135 163**	**281 840**	**10**	**21**
Bangladesh	15 089	31 816	11	23
India	100 963	209 148	10	21
Nepal	2 373	5 116	10	22
Pakistan	14 841	32 117	11	23
Sri Lanka	1 897	3 643	10	19
Other Asian Countries				
China*	100 760	218 497	8	17
Indonesia	21 564	43 355	10	20
Philippines	8 145	17 087	11	23
Thailand	5 807	11 345	9	18
Viet Nam	8 275	1 784	11	22

*Note: Not including data for Hong Kong Special Administrative Region of China.

Source: United Nations (2001) *World Population Prospects: The 2000 Revision. Volume II. The sex and age distribution of the world population.* New York, United Nations.

four (282 million) live in South Asia. Adolescents aged 10–19 comprise over one-fifth of South Asia's population (Table 1). Within the region, Bangladesh and Pakistan have the greatest proportion of adolescents, while India has the greatest absolute number.

Though the situation of adolescents varies widely within the region and within individual countries, literacy and school enrolment rates among adolescents have risen in all South Asian countries over the past couple of decades. In Bangladesh, India and Pakistan, for example, the proportion of women aged 20–24 who report seven or more years of education is dramatically higher than the proportion of older women aged 40–44 who do so, as illustrated by Figure 1.

Nevertheless, according to United Nations estimates, secondary school enrolment ratios remain low in most South Asian countries, except Sri Lanka, and large proportions of teenage girls aged 15–19 remain illiterate. It is important to note that geographic disparities are wide within individual countries. Differences between the sexes are also wide, particularly in Bangladesh and Pakistan where secondary school enrolment ratios for boys are nearly double those for girls (Table 2).

The majority of older South Asian adolescents are not in school, except in Sri Lanka (Table 2). Some are unemployed, while others work for pay, or work without remuneration in households, family farms and businesses. Surveys suggest that labour force participation rates are relatively high—both among older adolescents aged 15–19 and among younger adolescents aged 10–14 (Table 3). In Bangladesh, for example, a 1995–1996 survey found that over one-quarter and one-third of younger adolescent females and males were economically active, as were about half and two-thirds of older adolescents, respectively. Labour force participation of younger adolescents is also high in other countries—among males in Nepal and Pakistan, for example. By ages 15–19, large proportions of South Asian males (36–66%) and females (21–49%, excluding Pakistan) are engaged in economic activity. Rural adolescents are more likely to work and less likely to study than their urban counterparts. Caution in interpreting sex specific figures is advised since surveys can underestimate girls' contributions to household labour and consequently their economic activity rates (see, for example, Jejeebhoy, 1993).

Health status of adolescents in South Asia

As noted in the global overview by Paul Van Look, adolescence is generally a period of life free from both childhood diseases and the ravages of ageing. Consequently, as in other settings, mortality rates

Figure 1. Per cent of women with 7+ years of education, by generation

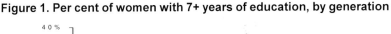

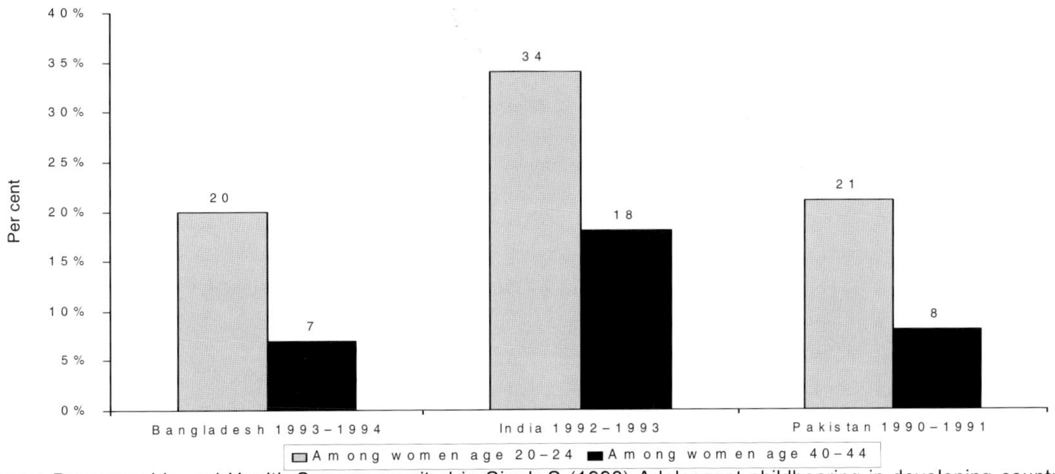

Source: Demographic and Health Surveys as cited in Singh S (1998) Adolescent childbearing in developing countries: a global review. *Studies in Family Planning*. 29(2):117–163.

among adolescents and young people in this region are generally lower than those observed at younger and older ages. However, unlike in other countries, adolescent and young women in the countries of South Asia, with the exception of Sri Lanka, experience somewhat higher mortality rates than males at the same ages (Table 4). Disparities are particularly evident among young people aged

Table 2. Secondary school enrolment and illiteracy rates among adolescents in South Asia and other selected Asian countries, 1995–1997

	Secondary school enrolment ratios (% of # enrolled to # in applicable age groups		Per cent of teens aged 15–19 who are illiterate	
Country	***Boys***	***Girls***	***Boys***	***Girls***
South Asia				
Bangladesh	25	13	58	71
India	59	39	20	44
Nepal	51	33	26	51
Pakistan	33	17	56	74
Sri Lanka	72	78	9	10
Other Asian Countries				
China	74	67	3	8
Indonesia	55	48	2	3
Philippines	77	78	4	1
Thailand	38	37	1	2
Viet Nam	48	46	7	7

Source: Population Reference Bureau (2000) *The World's Youth 2000.* Washington, DC, Population Reference Bureau, Measure Communication.

Table 3. Labour force participation rates of adolescents and youth by sex and age group

	Females (%)			Males (%)		
Country and year	**Aged 10–14**	**Aged 15–19**	**Aged 20–24**	**Aged 10–14**	**Aged 15–19**	**Aged 20–24**
South Asia						
Bangladesh (1995–96)*	28.1	47.8	58.7	37.8	65.5	82.0
India (1991)*	5.1+	26.2	33.5	5.7+	43.8	74.7
Nepal (1991)*	28.0	49.0	54.0	18.1	49.2	80.0
Pakistan (1999)**	5.8	9.6	11.7	16.5	51.1	85.5
Sri Lanka (1999)***	3.1	21.2	50.6	3.3	35.8	87.1
Other Asian countries						
China (1990)*	na	68.3	89.6	na	61.5	92.6
Indonesia (1999)***	na	90.6	53.8	na	45.5	33.6
Philippines (1999)***	na	25.8	52.7	na	45.1	81.0
Thailand (1999)***	8.3++	29.1	67.9	9.0++	37.7	77.9
Viet Nam (1989)*	37.4++	73.3	88.8	29.5++	67.4	94.4

* International Labour Organisation (1998) *Yearbook of Labour Statistics 1998.* Geneva, ILO.

** International Labour Organisation (1999) *Yearbook of Labour Statistics 1999.* Geneva, ILO.

***International Labour Organisation (2000) *Yearbook of Labour Statistics 2000.* Geneva, ILO.

+ Aged 5–14; ++ aged 13–14.

na: not available.

15–19 and 20–24, and this may well be explained by the poorer reproductive health of females in these countries.

Gender disparities in health are particularly significant in South Asia. In terms of food intake, access to health care and growth patterns, girls are worse off than their brothers. Disparities become evident soon after birth, and, by adolescence, many girls are grossly underweight (Jejeebhoy, 2000). Adolescent girls contribute long hours to the household economy, but their activities are largely invisible and undervalued since they draw no income. Gender roles and expectations have such a profound impact on the lives of adolescents that nearly every author in this collection explores some dimension of the ways in which gender roles affect adolescents' lives.

Adolescent sexual and reproductive health in South Asia

Two papers in this collection provide comprehensive overviews of South Asian adolescents' sexual and reproductive health, namely, a regional overview by Ena Singh and a national overview of the Indian situation by A.R. Nanda. Together, these papers outline the many factors that undermine adolescents' ability to make informed sexual and reproductive choices in South Asia. For example, South Asian societies have traditionally placed high priority on preserving young women's chastity before marriage—a concern that has important implications for their education, age at marriage, autonomy and mobility. Seclusion norms are widespread in the region from puberty onwards. As a result, adolescent girls in many South Asian settings are unlikely to have much exposure or physical access to the outside world. Few services cater to their needs for health care, nutrition, vocational skills, economic opportunities or information. A sizeable proportion of women in South Asia marry well before age 18, and early pregnancy further exacerbates their poor reproductive health and the poor survival chances of the infants they bear. These papers also highlight the factors that prevent boys from making informed decisions, including lack of knowledge about sex and reproduction, and social pressure to have sex

Table 4. Age-specific death rates of adolescents and youth by sex and age group

Country and year	Females (%) Aged 10–14	Females (%) Aged 15–19	Females (%) Aged 20–24	Males (%) Aged 10–14	Males (%) Aged 15–19	Males (%) Aged 20–24
South Asia						
Bangladesh (1986)	1.1	2.3	3.1	1.7	2.0	2.2
India (1997–98)	1.4	2.5	3.8	1.0	1.8	2.7
Nepal (1986–87)	6.6+	4.1++	3.3+	4.3++		
Pakistan (1996–97)	2.5	1.9	3.9	2.6	1.9	2.9
Sri Lanka (1995)	0.4	0.9	1.0	0.5	1.7	3.6
Other Asian countries						
Philippines (1991)	0.6	0.7	0.9	0.7	1.2	2.3
Thailand (1997)	0.3	0.6	1.1	0.5	2.1	3.3

+ Aged 5–14; ++ aged 15–24, further breakdown not available.

Sources: ***Bangladesh:*** United Nations (1997) *Demographic Yearbook 1995*. New York, United Nations (ST/ESA/STAT/SER. R/26); ***Philippines, Sri Lanka, Thailand:*** United Nations (2000) *Demographic Yearbook 1998*. New York, United Nations (ST/ESA/STAT/SER. R/29); ***India:*** International Institute for Population Sciences & Macro (2000) *National Family Health Survey (NFHS-2) 1998–99: India*. Mumbai, International Institute for Population Sciences; ***Nepal:*** Central Bureau of Statistics, Nepal (1995) *Population Monograph of Nepal*. Kathmandu, Government of Nepal, Table 1.4, p. 33; ***Pakistan:*** Hakim et al. (1998) *Pakistan Fertility and Family Planning Survey 1996–97 (PFFPS)*. Islamabad, Pakistan, National Institute of Population Studies (December).

under unsafe conditions, placing them at risk of sexually transmitted infections.

The other papers in this collection explore all these dimensions in more depth, including papers from Bangladesh, China, India, Pakistan, Nepal, Sri Lanka and Thailand. The first half of the collection presents empirical evidence about adolescents' situation and needs that form the basis for programmes and policies discussed in the second half.

Married adolescents: the health consequences of early marriage and childbearing

International attention on adolescent sexual activity tends to focus on *premarital* sex. However, in South Asia, sexual debut among adolescent girls occurs largely within marriage. Despite rising age at marriage and laws prohibiting marriage before age 18 for women and before age 21 for men in most South Asian countries, the majority of women marry as adolescents in Bangladesh, India and Nepal (Figure 2 and Table 5). Correspondingly, most South Asian women experience sexual debut as married adolescents. Moreover, large surveys have found that almost half of all women aged 20–24 are married by age 15 in Bangladesh, as are nearly one-fourth (24%) in India and one-fifth (19%) in Nepal. In contrast, South Asian boys rarely marry as adolescents. For example, the recent National Family Health Survey (NFHS-2) in India found that only 6% of adolescent boys were married (Kulkarni, this volume).

Over the past decade, adolescent fertility has dropped in nearly all South Asian countries. However, due to the persistence of early marriage, pregnancy during adolescence is still common (Figure 3 and Table 7). The 1996–1997 Bangladesh Demographic and Health Survey found that 14% of 15 year-old girls were either already mothers or pregnant with their first child (Mitra et al., 1997). Many girls become pregnant before they reach physically maturity, which has adverse health consequences, both for young women and their children.

Several papers in this collection explore the social context and health consequences of early marriage

Figure 2. Per cent of women aged 20–24 married by age 18 in South Asia and other selected Asian countries

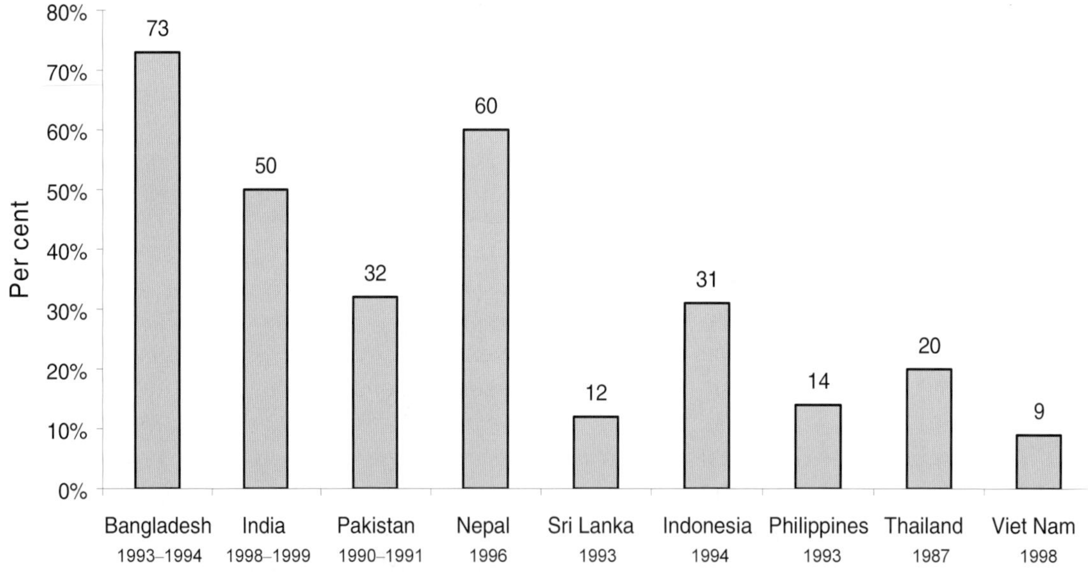

Sources: National Demographic and Health Surveys from various years as noted. Figures cited in the following sources: ***India:*** International Institute for Population Sciences & Macro (2000); ***Pakistan:*** Blanc & Way (1998); ***All other countries***: De Silva W (1998).

Table 5. Per cent of women aged 20–24 married by age 15, 18 and 20 in South Asia and other selected Asian countries

Country and year	By age 15 (%)	By age 18 (%)	By age 20 (%)
South Asia			
Bangladesh (1993–1994)	47	73	82
India (1998–1999)	24	50	na
Nepal (1996)	19	60	76
Pakistan (1990–1991)	na	32	na
Sri Lanka (1993)	1	12	24
Other Asian countries			
Indonesia (1994)	9	31	48
Philippines (1993)	2	14	29
Thailand (1987)	2	20	37
Viet Nam (1998)	1	9	31

na: not available.

Sources: National Demographic and Health Surveys from various years as noted. Figures cited in the following sources: ***India:*** International Institute for Population Sciences & Macro (2000); ***Pakistan:*** Blanc & Way (1998); ***All other countries***: De Silva W (1998).

Table 6. Median age at first marriage and per cent of teenage girls ever married

Country and year	Median age at first marriage among women aged 20–24	Per cent of girls aged 15–19 ever married
South Asia		
Bangladesh (1996–1997)	15	50
India (1998–1999)	18	34
Nepal (1996)	17	44
Pakistan (1990–1991)	20	25
Sri Lanka (1993)	24*	7
Other Asian countries		
Indonesia (1997)	20	18
Philippines (1998)	na	8
Thailand, na	na	17
Viet Nam (1998)	22.5	8

* Among women aged 25–29; na: not available.

Sources: National Demographic and Health Surveys various years as noted. Data cited in following sources: ***Sri Lanka:*** De Silva W (1997); ***Thailand:*** Population Reference Bureau (2000); ***All other countries:*** www.measuredhs.com.

and childbearing. Kulkarni and Adhikari each present a national profile of married adolescents' reproductive health in papers from India and Nepal, respectively. Kulkarni analyses data from the 1998–1999 National Family Health Survey, India (NFHS-2), that focus on young women aged 15–19, while Adhikari draws from published and unpublished research on women aged 15–24, including the 1996 Nepal Family Health Survey.

These papers describe a situation applicable to many South Asian settings (with the possible exception of Sri Lanka). Surveys from the late 1990s suggest that over two-fifths of adolescent girls in Nepal and nearly one-third of those in India have ever been married. Both Adhikari and Kulkarni present evidence that a substantial proportion of young girls enter marriage already malnourished. For example, a study from three rural areas of Nepal found that 72% and 45% of girls aged 10–14 and 15–18 were stunted and undernourished. In India, the NFHS-2 found that nearly 15% of ever-married adolescent women were stunted, and about one-fifth had moderate to severe anaemia.

Figure 3. Per cent of married women aged 20–24 who gave birth by age 20, from national surveys in the 1990s.

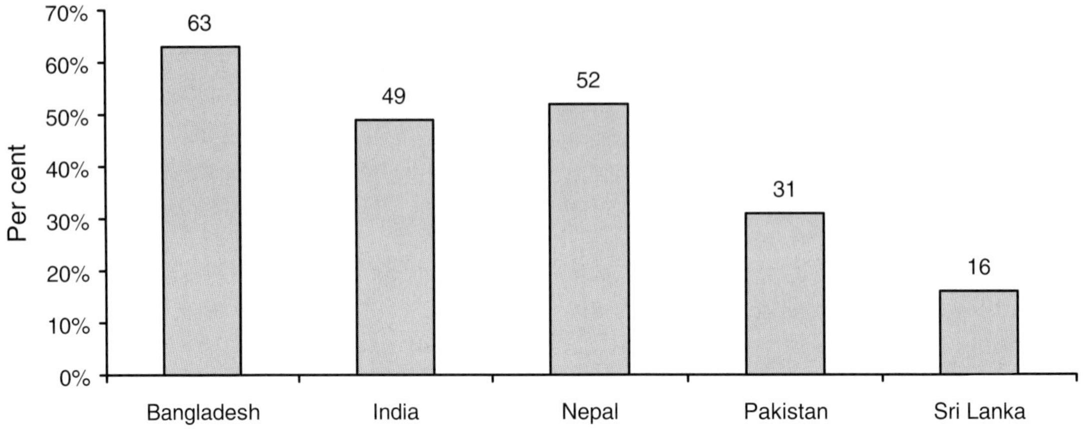

Source: Population Reference Bureau (2000) *The World's Youth 2000.* Washington, DC, Population Reference Bureau, Measure Communication.

The combination of poor nutrition and early childbearing expose young women to serious health risks during pregnancy and childbirth, including damage to the reproductive tract, maternal mortality, pregnancy complications, perinatal and neonatal mortality and low birth weight. International analyses suggest that, at the global level, girls aged 15–19 are twice as likely to die from childbirth as are women in their twenties, while girls younger than age 15 face a risk that is five times as great (United Nations Children's Fund, 2001). These sources report that more adolescent girls die from pregnancy-related causes than from any other cause (Population Reference Bureau, 2000). Kulkarni and Adhikari support such findings with data from India and Nepal. For example, studies from Nepal found higher rates of obstetric morbidity among adolescents than among adult women, as

Table 7. Childbearing among adolescents in South Asia and other selected Asian countries

Country	Per cent of women aged 20–24 who gave birth by aged 20*	Per cent of TFR attributed to births by mothers aged 15–19*	Teenage fertility rate (births per 1000 girls aged 15–19) circa 1999**	Per cent of births to women aged 15–19 attended by trained personnel*
South Asia				
Bangladesh	63	18	140	14
India	49	18	107	34
Nepal	52	13	117	14
Pakistan	31	9	100	17
Sri Lanka	16	5	21	82
Other Asian countries				
China	8	1	15	na
Indonesia	31	11	57	32
Philippines	21	6	43	51
Thailand	24	20	76	61
Viet Nam	19	5	na	76

na: not available; TFR: total fertility rate

Sources: *Population Reference Bureau (2000) *The World's Youth 2000.* Washington, DC, Population Reference Bureau, Measure Communication. **World Bank (2001) *World Development Indicators.* Washington, DC, World Bank.

well as a 25–66% higher incidence of low birth weight among children of adolescent mothers. Both authors report considerably higher rates of neonatal and infant mortality among children of adolescent mothers. Despite greater risks, both authors cite evidence that adolescents do not receive more antenatal or intrapartum care than older women. Adhikari argues that adolescent girls in Nepal actually receive less prenatal care than older women.

The social context of early marriage

Within the age- and gender-stratified family structure that characterizes much of South Asia, young, newly married women are particularly powerless. The average adolescent bride is unlikely to have had a say in the decision about whom or when to marry, whether or not to have sexual relations, and when to bear children. On the contrary, society often places strong pressures on young women to prove their fertility, and, in many settings, bearing sons is the only means by which young women can establish social acceptance and economic security in their marital homes. Lack of autonomy within their marital homes often means that married girls have limited access to health care or participation in decisions about their own health. For example, Kulkarni notes that in some Indian states, such as Maharashtra and Madhya Pradesh, fewer than one-third of adolescent women surveyed reported any involvement in decision-making about their own health.

Two papers in this collection focus on the social context of married adolescents. Both Chowdhury (Bangladesh) and George (India) present qualitative findings from small-scale, in-depth studies with select groups. Findings from these studies are not necessarily representative of larger populations, but they provide an important complement to the quantitative evidence, by describing experiences of new wives and mothers in their own words.

George highlights young wives' lack of sexual autonomy in a review of two qualitative studies among poor urban women in India. Those studies gathered retrospective data from women who married as adolescents. Most women in these studies reported that they were unprepared for, and ignorant about, sexual intercourse until the first night with their husbands. Many experienced some form of sexual coercion, and many described their first sexual experience as traumatic, distasteful, painful and involving the use of physical force.

Chowdhury presents preliminary findings from a study on first-time parents in Bangladesh. Women reported that they did not have a choice as to whom or when to marry, or when to begin childbearing. As echoed by many papers in this collection (for example, see Rashid), many male and female respondents told researchers that they would have liked to have waited longer before getting married. Lack of decision-making authority permeated all aspects of young women's lives—including food intake during pregnancy, workload, mobility, and access to health care. Young women reported heavy workloads during pregnancy, which only increased after the birth of their child, and some expressed great unhappiness about their situation.

Other papers in this collection explore the context of early marriage as one among many issues that concern adolescents. Though it was not the central focus of their research, Waszak, Thapa and Davey describe similar experiences involving young married women in Nepal, based on 71 focus group discussions. Young women suggested that young pregnant girls often have low priority when food is distributed in their husbands' family. Heavy workloads are common and supported by local beliefs such as: "the more you work, the lighter your body becomes and easier it is at delivery". Newly married girls are expected to tolerate sexual coercion from their husbands, to prove their fertility as soon as possible after marriage, and to allow family elders to limit their food intake and health care during pregnancy.

Many authors in this collection argue that girls who postpone marriage and stay in school longer are better off than those who marry early. This is not only because they will reach physical maturity before childbearing, but also because they may be better able to negotiate with their in-laws and voice their own needs.

Social and economic factors behind early marriage

Many papers in this collection examine why early marriage persists in South Asia. Again, such research findings tend to emerge from qualitative studies that cannot be generalized to the tremendously diverse population of South Asia as a whole. Furthermore, it is important to note that marriage trends are in flux, and average age at which girls marry in South Asia is rising. Nevertheless, this collection of studies offers important insights into the factors that contribute to early marriage among girls—in the words of both adolescents and their parents.

Rashid presents findings that emerged from focus group discussions in the Nilphamari district of Bangladesh. In this district, girls still marry as young as age 11. Mothers explained that the main reason for early marriage was parents' fear that daughters would be raped, become pregnant or elope. The knowledge that a girl has had premarital sex (even resulting from rape) can ruin the status and reputation of the entire family. Respondents suggest that attitudes towards early marriage may be changing, as parents increasingly appreciate the value of education and the negative health consequences of early childbearing. Nevertheless, they noted that parents who wait too long to marry their daughters often face community pressure, including derogatory comments from community elders. Chowdhury also cites evidence that early marriage of girls in Bangladesh may stem from financial pressures, a father's death or a large of number of daughters.

Waszak, Thapa and Davey analysed focus group discussions (FGDs) held in 11 districts in Nepal. During FGDs stratified by age, sex, marital status and residence, researchers explored gender norms that affect work, education, marriage and childbearing among young people aged 14–22. On the one hand, respondents suggested that families have increasingly recognized the benefits of education for girls (though parents still generally invest more resources in sons). On the other hand, families face social pressure to marry their daughters early as a way to protect their "character". The longer a girl stays at home, the longer she is at risk of running away or having a love marriage—all of which could bring dishonour on the family. Adolescents described norms that condone premarital sexual activity among boys, but ruin girls who do the same. Parents' fear about their daughters' sexual chastity often pressures them to end their schooling and arrange early marriages. Marriage usually ends a girls' education, because her increased household responsibilities are generally incompatible with attending school. The respondents also described how gender norms pose different challenges for young men. Pressure to achieve financial stability before marriage often forces them to delay marriage, increasing pressures and opportunities for young men to engage in unsafe sexual activity.

Attitudes and risk behaviours of unmarried adolescents

Given highly conservative attitudes about sex in South Asia, few studies have successfully elicited information on sexual behaviour. Most explore premarital rather than marital sex, men's behaviour rather than women's, and young people's current experiences or retrospective experiences of adults. Samples tend to be small and drawn from urban areas rather than rural communities or slums. Results, therefore, tend to be unrepresentative of the general population. While generalization is difficult, findings of the few available studies (see for example, Jejeebhoy, 2000, for India; or Abraham, this volume) generally suggest that between 20% and 30% of young men and between 0% and 10% of young women report premarital sexual experience. Sexual initiation occurs earlier than many assume, and is often unplanned and unprotected. Moreover, as noted in many papers in this volume, substantial proportions of young men report having sex with sex workers—usually without condoms.

Several papers in this collection present findings on the sexual behaviour and attitudes of South Asian adolescents before marriage, including studies from Bangladesh, India, Nepal, Pakistan and Sri Lanka. Understandably, these studies are quite diverse, having used different methodologies among diverse populations. Study populations included low-income urban college students in India, young people from provincial settings in Pakistan and a nationwide sample in Nepal. Methodologies ranged from a combination of qualitative and quantitative in India and Sri Lanka, to a pilot survey in Pakistan, and focus group discussions in Nepal and Bangladesh.

Studies suggest that most South Asian adolescents have conservative attitudes towards marriage and sex. For example, in studies from Bangladesh, Nepal and Sri Lanka, young people told researchers that they generally disapprove of love marriages, premarital sex (particularly by girls), and often for that matter, social interaction between unrelated women and men. In some cases even the hint of a friendship with a boy can ruin a girl's reputation, her marriage prospects and the social status of her entire family. While few studies have considered social constraints on adolescent boys, it is clear that their behaviour is less closely supervised than that of girls. Many young people feel that society condones premarital sexual activity among boys and even puts social pressure on boys to become sexually active at an early age.

Rashid presents findings from discussions with adolescents in Bangladesh about love and romance. Most adolescents did not approve of "love" (*prem*) and instead felt that young people should marry whomever their parents chose for them. They described heavy sanctions and punishments that befall girls discovered to be involved in sexual relationships. Nevertheless, some respondents expressed attitudes that—in the author's view—were "considered unthinkable for previous generations". For example, some had secretly fallen "in love". Many distinguished between "pure" love as a relationship that leads to marriage, and "impure" love as a relationship that does not lead to marriage or involves sex.

Abraham presents focus group discussion and survey data gathered among low-income, urban college students aged 16–18 and 20–22 in Mumbai. Young respondents reported friendships with members of the opposite sex, despite strong parental disapproval of such behaviour. The author describes different categories of friendship, including platonic (*bhai-behen)*, romantic with the intention of marriage ("true love"*)* and transitory sexual relationships ("time pass"). The boundaries of these categories are fuzzy, as is the extent of physical intimacy. Authors note that many researchers have not adequately explored different kinds of sexual activity. While only 26% of young men and 3% of young women reported penetrative sex, as many as 49% and 13%, respectively, reported other forms of physical intimacy. Young women almost unanimously reported monogamous and committed relationships. By contrast, young men reported a range of partners, including sex workers and "aunties" (older married women in the neighbourhood).

Silva and Schensul report considerable premarital relationships between young men and women in Sri Lanka, according to survey data gathered among low-income youth and university students aged 17–28. Contrary to what the authors expected, this study found that university students were somewhat more likely than less educated young people to oppose premarital sex among women. Similar to the study among Indian college students, young men were considerably more likely than young women to approve of premarital sexual activity. Unlike the Indian case, however, differences between women and men reporting a "love partner" (not necessarily a sexual partner) were marginal. Over 50% of both young women and young men reported having such a partner. This study found that young people generally preferred behaviours perceived to protect female virginity, such as inter-femoral and other forms of non-penetrative sex. Even so, as in India, a large number of young boys and men reported sexual relations with commercial sex workers.

Bhuiya and colleagues present findings from a community-based survey in two rural sites in Bangladesh, which found relatively lower rates of premarital sexual activity among 2626 unmarried adolescents aged 13–19. In this study, 9% of 1462 boys and three of 1164 girls had ever engaged in premarital sexual relations. (Two of the three girls reported forced sex.) Once again, evidence suggests that sexual relations are often unsafe and sometimes non-consensual. Two-fifths of the sexually experienced males reported sex with commercial sex workers. Less than one-quarter of sexually experienced males reported condom use at first sex. Twelve per cent reported a sexually transmitted infection (STI) symptom in the previous six months, and 6% (7 adolescents) reported having experienced coerced sex.

Non-consensual sexual activity among adolescents

As a taboo subject, sexual violence is rarely reported or studied. Hence it is difficult to estimate how many young people suffer from sexual abuse, violence, coercion, incest, rape or sexual trafficking. Nevertheless, evidence suggests that a disturbingly large number of adolescent girls and boys are subjected to coercion in South Asia. Several small studies suggest that sexual coercion and rape often occur within marriage, and adolescents may be more likely to experience such violence than older women. Sexual coercion can have considerable health consequences, including sequelae related to unsafe abortion.

Many papers in this collection cite evidence of sexual coercion against young people, including Waszak, Thapa and Davey (Nepal), George (India), Bhuiya et al. (Bangladesh), and Qazi (Pakistan). Three papers from India explore sexual coercion in more depth, including papers by Ramakrishna et al. among street boys in Bangalore, by Sodhi and Verma among young people in a low-income area of Delhi, and by Patel et al. among school-going adolescents in Goa. None of these studies was designed to explore sexual coercion exclusively; instead they focused on coercion as one of several risk behaviours. Given the sensitive nature of the topic, researchers typically learned the most about these experiences from in-depth interviews rather than surveys.

As one might expect, evidence suggests that street children are highly vulnerable to coercion. Ramakrishna and colleagues offer insight into the context of coercion among street boys in Bangalore, a city with an estimated 85 000–100 000 street children. Using a variety of qualitative methods and sample recruitment strategies, their study found that some 74 of 121 street boys aged 9–21 were sexually experienced. Forty had their first sexual experience by age 12. A large proportion of boys reported coercive experiences, both as victims and perpetrators, often involving exchange of money, gifts or other favours, as well as physical force. Sexual coercion is so pervasive on the streets that street boys rated rape and forced sex as among the most pleasurable ways of seeking sexual gratification. Authors argue that social conditions, poverty and drug use shape concepts of sexuality and coercion among street boys.

Sodhi and Verma's study among low-income adolescents in Delhi, India, supplements this profile of coercion. During 71 in-depth interviews with youth, respondents described widespread verbal harassment of women as well as 32 instances of sexual coercion, including forced sex. Both girls and boys reported experiences of coercion, including cases in which girls were forced to engage in sex against their will, sometimes with multiple partners. Double standards are pervasive, and young women who experience forced sex often face severe reprisals should their experience be disclosed. Some are even forced to continue coercive relationships under threat of disclosure from the perpetrator. Echoing other studies in this collection, young married women also reported widespread marital rape, which they tended to view as "normal" male behaviour.

Patel and colleagues present the findings of a survey that explored the prevalence and consequences of abuse and violence among 811 students in the first year of higher secondary school (average age 16). Researchers asked adolescents about forced or unwanted verbal or physical sexual coercion in the last 12 months. As many as one-third of students—both male and female—reported a coercive experience in the past year, and 6% reported forced sexual intercourse. Nearly half of all adolescents who experienced coercion reported more than one such experience. Students and friends were the most commonly reported perpetrators, followed by strangers, neighbours and others; abuse by parents and teachers was also reported. Most suffered the abuse in silence. The authors found strong associations between forced sex and and a number of variables, including poor school performance, self-reported mental and physical health and subsequent consensual sexual relations.

Together these studies suggest that for many young people, homes, schools and neighbourhoods do not provide a safe and supportive environment. Societal norms and double standards often perpetuate violence by condoning harassment and abuse perpetrated by young men, while blaming victims. Their findings suggests that researchers and service providers need to pay more attention to factors such as violence and sexual abuse that impact young people's mental and emotional health.

Adolescents' use of condoms and contraceptives

In light of evidence that substantial proportions of South Asian adolescents are sexually active, many papers in this collection explored the extent to which adolescents take measures to protect themselves from unwanted pregnancy and STIs. At the global level, adolescents are far less likely than adults to use contraception, either in or out of marriage. Not all contraceptive methods are suitable for adolescents, and those that are appropriate may be inaccessible or simply unavailable. Not surprisingly therefore, a substantial proportion of sexually active adolescents—both married and unmarried—have an unmet need for contraception and are at risk of STIs, including HIV/AIDS.

While an array of contraceptive methods exists, evidence of their suitability, safety and efficacy among adolescents is incomplete. Questions remain about their clinical performance and their effects on adolescents who have not reached physical maturity. Meirik reviews the existing literature on these issues, which suggests that certain methods, such as Depot-medroxyprogestrone acetate (DMPA) and the intrauterine device (IUD), are not advisable for adolescents. While evidence is still inconclusive, some data suggest that DMPA may reduce adolescents' bone mass, thereby increasing the risk of fracture later in life. Concerns about the IUD arise from its possible link with increased risk of pelvic inflammatory disease (PID), to which young women are at higher risk than adult women. In contrast, recent evidence demonstrates that combined oral contraceptives do not adversely affect either the maturation of the hypothalamic-pituitary-ovarian system or the risk of breast cancer later in life, as was previously feared. The author argues that combined oral contraceptives and male condoms are clearly safe for adolescents. However, he notes that only condoms offer dual protection against unwanted pregnancy and STIs, including HIV.

Pachauri and Santhya's review of available data on married adolescents' contraceptive use in South Asia confirms that the proportion of married adolescents who use contraception in these countries remains low, even though significant minorities of young women say they want to delay or space births. In large surveys, 41% of sexually active married adolescents aged 15–19 in Nepal reported an unmet need, as did 16% in Bangladesh, 14% in India and 8% in Pakistan (Table 8). In India, Nepal and Pakistan, fewer than 10% of married adolescent women or their partners practise contraception, compared to about one-quarter in Bangladesh and one-fifth in Sri Lanka

(Alan Guttmacher Institute, 1998). In addition, discontinuation and failure rates for contraceptive use are more pronounced among adolescents than among older couples. The authors argue that the unmet need for reversible methods is particularly great. They cite the example of India where the leading method used by married adolescents is sterilization, a method that, by definition, cannot be used to delay or space births.

Few studies have looked at the extent to which adolescents protect themselves from pregnancy or STIs during pre- or extra-marital sexual activity. The few studies that have done so generally focus on young men's use of condoms, including papers in this collection by Tamang and Nepal (Nepal) and Abraham (India). Tamang and Nepal offer a rare look at factors that inhibit condom use among young, unmarried men aged 18–24 in border towns of Nepal. That study found that nearly one-third of respondents initiated sexual activity before age 18, and more than one-fourth reported "casual" sexual relations in the previous 12 months, including with commercial sex workers. Less than half of the respondents who engaged in casual sex reported condom use in their last sexual contact. Alcohol consumption was strongly associated with unprotected sex. When researchers asked young men why they did not use condoms, however, the most common responses were that they did not feel at risk; they expressed fatalistic attitudes or they thought that condoms would reduce pleasure.

Abraham's study also found that male college students in Mumbai used condoms rarely and irregularly. Despite the fact that most sexually experienced young men reported multiple partnerships, fewer than one in six young men who engaged in sexual relations with a casual partner said that they "always" used a condom. All those who admitted to having sex with commercial sex workers reported having used a condom at least once. The majority, however, used them rarely, and not a single student reported regular use of condoms during sex with sex workers. Meanwhile, few young people perceived themselves to be at risk of contracting an infection. The author notes that young women seem oblivious to the possibility that the unprotected sexual behaviour of their future husbands may eventually expose them to infection, even if they themselves practise strict abstinence before marriage.

Numerous factors contribute to low contraceptive use rates among adolescents, ranging from lack of knowledge to gender imbalances that prevent communication between partners and exclude young women from decisions about when to have children. Pachauri and Santhya note that while adolescents' awareness of at least one method of

Table 8. Current contraceptive use among adolescents (aged 15–19) in South Asia and other selected Asian countries

Country, year of survey	Per cent of married women aged 15–19 currently using any method of contraception	Estimated per cent of women aged 15–19 with an unmet need for contraception
South Asia		
Bangladesh 1997	33	19
India 1998–1999	8	27
Nepal 1996	7	41
Pakistan 1996–1997	6	23
Sri Lanka 1987	20	na
Other Asian countries		
Indonesia 1997	36	9
Philippines 1998	18	32
Thailand 1997	43	na

Sources: All figures from Demographic Health Surveys cited in Pachauri & Santhya (2002).

contraception is nearly universal in South Asian countries (with the exception of Pakistan), adolescents are not necessarily aware of reversible methods that might be most appropriate for their situation, such as oral contraceptives or condoms. Furthermore, many young couples do not know how to obtain such methods or understand how to use them correctly. As many papers in this volume illustrate, adolescents who want to protect themselves from pregnancy and STIs/HIV face a host of obstacles including lack of access to services, poor quality of care, and provider attitudes that adolescents find threatening, disrespectful or indiscrete.

Few studies have explored the ways that provider attitudes may inhibit contraceptive use among unmarried adolescents. Two papers in this collection shed light on this issue, including Gao et al. (China) and Naravage (Thailand). Gao and colleagues provide a rare look at provider attitudes in China. They report that as many as 40% of providers disapproved of supplying contraceptives to unmarried young people. Their findings suggest that even in settings such as China, where family planning is so well accepted, provider attitudes may discourage sexually active unmarried youth from using methods to protect themselves against unwanted pregnancy or STIs.

Emergency contraception (EC) has increasingly been recognized as a useful backup method for adolescents who have unprotected sex, but few studies have explored the acceptability or use of EC among youth in South Asia. The paper by Naravage suggests that misinformation and barriers to access may undermine the potential benefits of EC. The study found that both distributors and purchasers had a poor understanding of how to use EC correctly. Furthermore, young women told researchers that they were reluctant to purchase EC for fear of disclosing the fact that they were sexually active. Many purchasers reported using EC incorrectly or using it on a regular basis, which is contrary to its intended purpose. These findings suggest that the introduction of EC must be accompanied by clear and accurate instructions, as well as efforts to raise awareness among both potential users and distributors about how to use EC correctly and how to choose a contraceptive method that is appropriate for regular or long-term use.

Unplanned births and induced abortion among adolescents

Because so many adolescents have sex without protection (both in and out of marriage), the proportion of adolescent births that are unplanned, unwanted or mistimed is relatively high, as illustrated by Figure 4, reprinted from Pachauri and Santhya (this volume).

Worldwide, many unplanned births end in induced abortion, often under unsafe conditions. Data on the numbers of adolescent abortions are scarce, but estimates for developing countries range from 1 to 4.4 million (McCauley & Salter, 1995). Some evidence suggests that adolescents—particularly unmarried adolescents—are more likely than older women to seek abortions from untrained providers, to undergo second trimester abortions and to suffer complications. Fear, shame and lack of access to both services and resources inhibit adolescents from seeking safe and early abortions on the one hand, and from seeking care in case of complications on the other (Bott, 2000).

The abortion scenario varies considerably within South Asia. In India, abortion has been legal since 1972, but limited availability and poor service quality keep safe abortion beyond the reach of most poor women. In Bangladesh, abortion has been available since 1999 for up to 12 weeks of gestational age in the form of "menstrual regulation", and large proportions of women use these services. In Sri Lanka, abortion is legally restricted, but available, and women have access to relatively safe services. In Nepal and Pakistan, it remains severely restricted and women who undergo an abortion are liable to prosecution.

Few studies have explored the context of abortion among young women in South Asia. The majority

Figure 4. Per cent of births to married adolescent girls that are unplanned in selected countries of South Asia and South-East Asia

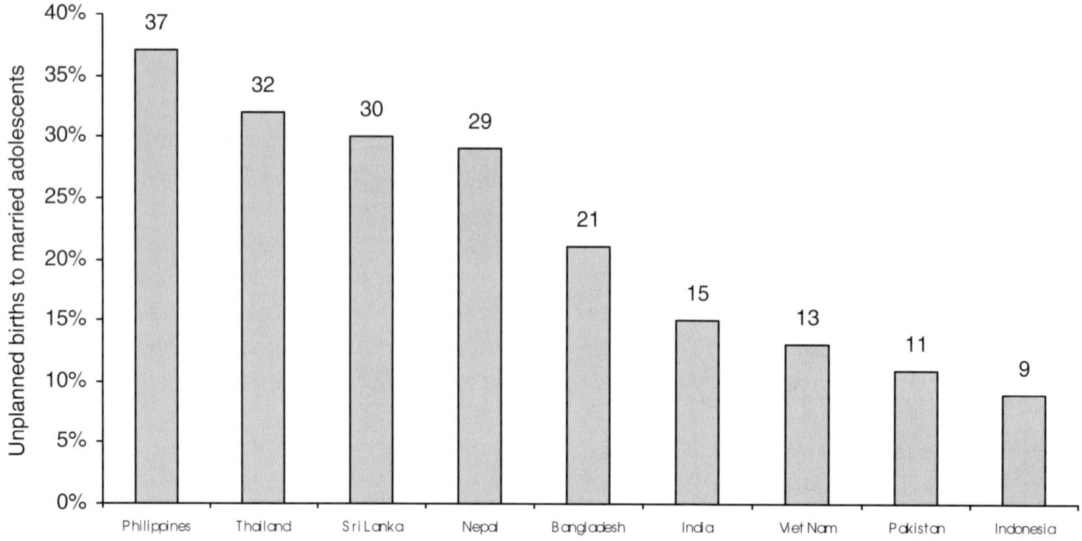

Sources: Figure reprinted with permission from Pachauri & Santhya, this volume, Figure 3, p. 111. Data for: ***Bangladesh:*** National Institute of Population Research and Training et al. (1997); ***India***: International Institute for Population Sciences (IIPS), Macro International (2000); ***Indonesia:*** Central Bureau of Statistics (CBS), Indonesia et al. (1998); ***Nepal:*** Pradhan A et al. (1997); ***Pakistan and Thailand:*** Alan Guttmacher Institute (1998); ***Philippines:*** National Statistics Office (NSO), Philippines et al. (1999); ***Sri Lanka:*** Department of Census and Statistics, Sri Lanka et al. (1998); ***Viet Nam***: National Committee for Population and Family Planning (NCPFP), Viet Nam et al. (1999).

of these studies have been hospital-based rather than community-based, urban rather than rural, and conducted among married women rather than all women. Two papers in this collection, Akhter (Bangladesh) and Ganatra & Hirve (India) present rare data on adolescent abortion. Their evidence paints a disturbing picture.

Akhter reviews various studies from Bangladesh. Because abortion services are available only up to the 12th week of pregnancy, women who want such services must recognize their pregnancy as early as possible. This poses a major obstacle for adolescent girls who may not recognize their pregnancy or find the resources to access services in time. Akhter reports that while adolescents constituted 9% of women who received services from "menstrual regulation" clinics, they constituted 15% of those rejected by the clinics, presumably because their pregnancies were too far along. As a result, many adolescent girls are hospitalized for complications of induced abortion after undergoing an abortion by traditional birth attendants or after attempting to self-induce. About half of these girls resorted to unsafe methods such as inserting a solid stick or rubber catheter, or ingesting medicines. Researchers observed life-threatening complications such as severe infection, mechanical injury to the cervix or vagina, and evidence of a foreign body having been inserted into the vagina, cervix or uterus. Awareness and prior practice of contraception were found to be limited among young women in the study.

Ganatra and Hirve describe a rare community-based study of abortion in a rural Indian setting. The study found that young women age 15–24 constituted over half of all abortion-seekers in the area. About 14% of married women who had recently experienced an induced abortion were younger than age 20, and another 40% were aged 21–24. Although abortion among unmarried women in India is a highly sensitive topic, researchers were able to identify 43 unmarried adolescents who admitted to having had an induced abortion. Their results suggest a number of important differences between married adolescent and adult abortion-seekers. First, adolescents reported considerably less decision-making authority than older abortion-seekers. They were less likely to have been allowed a major role in the decision, more likely to have been coerced into an abortion, and conversely, more likely to have faced opposition from their families. As in Bangladesh, young women's knowledge about and use of contraception were limited, yet their need to space births was a leading reason for seeking abortion. Finally, providers were more likely to insist on spousal consent from younger abortion-seekers than from adult women, even though such consent is not legally required.

The study found several important differences between married and unmarried adolescent abortion-seekers. While no evidence indicated that ***married*** adolescents delayed seeking services compared to older married women, it was clear that ***unmarried*** adolescents sought abortions further along in their pregnancy than their married counterparts. While married adolescents preferred the private sector, unmarried adolescent abortion-seekers reported higher use of traditional providers as a result of less family support, less money, and concerns about confidentiality and provider attitudes. Adolescents tended to believe that abortion services were not legally available to unmarried women. Researchers also found that some providers charged unmarried women a higher price for their services. Regardless of marital status, however, almost three-quarters of adolescent abortion-seekers reported post-abortion morbidity. Drawing on findings from other studies, the authors suggest that deaths related to abortions and unwanted pregnancies account for a significantly larger proportion of pregnancy-related deaths among adolescents than among older women. They also noted that suicides related to unwanted pregnancy constitute a substantial portion of maternal deaths in the area.

Reproductive tract and sexually transmitted infections among adolescents

In his address to the 6th International Congress on AIDS in Asia and the Pacific, Peter Piot, the Executive Director of the Joint United Nations Programme on HIV/AIDS (UNAIDS), stated his conviction that, "Asia and the Pacific hold the key to the global future of the epidemic". Compared to the African region, many Asian countries have seen only limited spread of HIV. Nonetheless, several worrisome indicators suggest that South Asia is at risk of sharp future increases in the numbers of HIV/AIDS cases. Estimates suggest that nearly four million people were living with HIV/AIDS in India by the end of 2000, and some surveillance sites in Southern India have found that more than 2% of pregnant women are infected with HIV (Monitoring the AIDS Pandemic & Joint United Nations Programme on HIV/AIDS, 2001). Sex workers throughout the region are at higher risk, as are men who purchase sex, and their wives. As several studies in this collection suggest, this situation poses a serious concern for male adolescents, young men and their future wives.

In their global overview, Mane and McCauley discuss the physiological, behavioural and social risk factors surrounding STIs/HIV among adolescents. They point out that physiologically, adolescents are more vulnerable to STIs than adults, and girls are more vulnerable than boys. Gender power imbalances, societal norms, poverty and economic dependence all contribute to young people's risk of STIs. Many young people lack control over the choice of their marital and sexual partners, how many partners they have, the circumstances and nature of sexual activity and the extent to which sex is consensual or protected. Many lack information about condoms or are unaware of the risk. It is not surprising, therefore, that global estimates suggest that more than half of all new HIV infections occur among young people age 15–24. Mane and McCauley note that the pandemic also has an impact on young people who live with an HIV-infected parent. For these young people, adolescence ends prematurely. They often face early withdrawal from school and entry into economic activity, stigma, poverty and psychological suffering from losing a parent.

Few researchers have studied reproductive tract

infections (RTIs) or STIs among South Asian adolescents. Nonetheless, evidence suggests that young people constitute a neglected but high-risk group. The typical STI patient is a young man barely out of adolescence (modal ages are 20–25), of relatively low socioeconomic status. Likewise, the proportion of young women attending STI clinics has been increasing (see, for example, Ramasubban, 2000).

Girls who marry early begin sexual activity when they are physiologically more vulnerable to infection. Boys who have unprotected sex expose not only themselves but also their future wives to infection. Since discussion of sex is taboo, young people often lack reliable information and misconceptions abound. Gender imbalances ensure that girls are particularly uninformed about their bodies and STIs. With limited power to negotiate safer sex, young women in South Asia are at risk of STIs/HIV no less than young men. Young people who experience an STI suffer not only health consequences, but also shame and social stigma. Fear of reprisal often prevents young people from getting timely treatment for an STI, thus worsening the situation and facilitating HIV infection.

Several studies in this collection highlight the prevalence of reproductive tract infections, including STIs among adolescents, particularly among girls. Kulkarni and Adhikari cite evidence from India and Nepal that adolescent women report relatively high rates of gynaecological morbidities—of particular concern in settings where girls have limited access to adequate health care. The 1998-1999 NFHS-2 in India found that nearly two in five ever-married adolescent women reported some reproductive health problem.

Joseph and colleagues present a rare community-based study of RTI prevalence among 451 married women aged 16–22 in rural Tamil Nadu, India. This study found alarming levels of morbidity. As many as 49% of women in the study suffered from one or more RTI, not counting cases of infertility, urinary tract infections and prolapse. Clinical and laboratory examination diagnosed 18% with an STI, including chlamydia, trichomoniasis and syphilis. Researchers found that wives of truck drivers and army personnel seemed more likely than other women to experience sexually transmitted morbidity, although the multivariate analysis found that length of marriage was the only statistically significant variable. These data clearly suggest that husbands' unsafe sexual behaviours transmit infections to their young wives—an alarming finding, given that many infected women are asymptomatic and are unlikely to seek medical care even when symptoms do appear. In fact, the authors report that two-thirds of women with symptoms did not seek care, and among those who did, over three in four sought treatment from unqualified sources, such as home treatment or untrained private practitioners.

Even when adolescents seek care, a host of barriers may prevent them from receiving appropriate care. Ranjha and Hussain carried out research on the *Hakims* who provide services at "Sex Clinics" throughout Pakistan and much of South Asia. These clinics are more accessible and perceived to be less judgmental than public sector facilities. They are often the first place that adolescents seek care. A nongovernmental organization (SAHIL) in the area found that more than half of the adolescents seeking counselling services at their centres had previously sought care from *Hakims* at local sex clinics. Researchers found that *Hakims* were poorly informed about sexual and reproductive health matters and lacked even the vocabulary to address sexual and reproductive health issues. They knew little about STIs, their diagnosis or treatments. Their services reinforced myths and misinformation and bordered on outright quackery. The medicine they prescribed contained potentially dangerous substances such as appetite stimulants, steroids, male and female hormones, and narcotics. Additionally, researchers posing as mystery clients reported incidents of sexual harassment by the *Hakims.*

Awasthi, Nichter and Pande report findings from an innovative, interactive programme designed to raise awareness of risk behaviours and sexually transmitted infection among some 377 boys residing in a slum in Kanpur in north India. As other studies have shown, a sizeable proportion of boys had engaged in sexual activity, some with casual partners and some with sex workers. Misperceptions concerning disease transmission were widespread, and condom use minimal. The intervention included three educational sessions using a host of communication strategies, such as "teaching by analogy" and responding to questions dropped anonymously in a sealed letter box. Messages drew upon previously conducted qualitative research with young males and used analogies drawn from events that were familiar to these urban slum residents. Exposure to the intervention succeeded in significantly reducing misconceptions about STI transmission among participants—for example, that one can only be infected by having sex with a prostitute. The intervention also raised awareness of basic facts such as the asymptomatic nature of STIs and the days during a woman's cycle when she is least likely to become pregnant. The intervention made some headway in changing the misconception that taking medicines before or after sex, using a vaginal birth control tablet or washing the penis after sex with disinfectant would reduce chances of acquiring sexually transmitted infections. In short, the study demonstrated that to be effective and acceptable to young men, STI education requires innovative and confidential approaches that address both medical and cultural concerns.

Communication between adolescents and adults about sexual and reproductive health

Adolescents in South Asia tend to be poorly informed about their own bodies and matters related to sexuality and health. The information they have is often incomplete and confused. Low rates of schooling, limited access to sex education and attitudes that prohibit discussion of sex exacerbate their ignorance. As gatekeepers who should play a central role in enabling adolescents to protect their health, parents often obstruct rather than facilitate informed choice. Adolescents commonly report that discussions with parents about sex or reproduction are taboo. In both rural areas and urban slums, parents often want and expect their adolescent children, particularly daughters, to remain uninformed about sex. Educational systems also tend to be ambivalent about sex education, though this has begun to change in the wake of the HIV/AIDS pandemic. In many cases, sex education continues to stress biological and scientific information over broader issues of sexuality. Teachers often find the topic embarrassing or shameful, and may avoid such issues, even in schools that supposedly teach a family life/sex education curriculum. As a result of adults' reticence to address these issues, young people tend to rely on peers and mass media for information about sex, reproduction and STIs including HIV/AIDS.

Qazi presents data from a pilot survey in Pakistan that explored knowledge about sex and reproduction among adolescents aged 13–21 . The survey found that adolescents' knowledge tended to be limited, with many misconceptions regarding pregnancy, contraception and STIs (including HIV/AIDS). The study also found that although sex and pregnancy were considered taboo topics of discussion, many young people do indeed discuss them, often with peers. Qazi points out that in the conservative setting of Pakistan, parents are often reluctant to discuss matters of sex and reproductive health with their adolescent children, and many young people do not turn to their parents for such information.

Bhuiya and colleagues cite similar survey data suggesting that communication between parents and children on topics of sexuality and reproduction in Bangladesh is limited—particularly between parents and boys. The study found that although a majority of girls had discussed reproductive health issues with their mothers, very few boys had discussed such matters with their parents or other family members, (2% with fathers, 3% with mothers and 6% with other family members).

Three papers, namely those by Rashid

(Bangladesh), ul Haque and Faizunnisa (Pakistan) and Masilamani (India), explore communication between adolescents and adults based on focus group discussions in Bangladesh and Pakistan, and more informal discussions and programme experience in India. In all three settings, parents reported embarrassment about discussing issues with adolescent children—including menstruation. They generally preferred to leave this responsibility to textbooks, teachers and others. In all three settings, parents argued that they themselves lacked the knowledge and even the vocabulary to discuss such sensitive issues. As a result, Rashid reports that many young girls knew nothing about menstruation before it began. Unable to ask for help from their parents, many believed that they were sick or dying. Concern for the sexual security and chastity of daughters dominates parental relationships with adolescent girls. This concern leads to close supervision of daughters and strict limits on their mobility. In contrast, sexual activity among adolescent sons tends to be condoned. In many cases, as Masilamani notes, parents believe that talking to adolescents about these matters will imply approval of premarital sexual activity. Adolescents perceive discussions with parents about sexual and reproductive topics to be taboo and express embarrassment at the prospect. As a result, adolescents tend to get their information from peers and the media, despite the fact that adolescents often express a desire to be able to turn to parents for information and counsel. These papers clearly suggest a need for educators and parents to improve their ability to communicate with young people.

A fourth paper describes family relationships and the extent to which these can be dominated by fear and violence. Bella Patel Uttekar and colleagues present findings from a study of domestic violence in the homes of 382 adolescents aged 10–19 living in a slum area of Allahabad, India. The authors describe a situation in which adolescents' home environments are frequently characterized by high levels of physical and verbal violence perpetrated by fathers against mothers and children. As many as 49% of boys and 16% of girls reported that they themselves had been beaten by their fathers, and a quarter reported that their mothers were verbally abused or beaten. Clearly, intra-family dynamics of this nature can severely impede the ability and willingness of adolescents to communicate with parents on any threatening topic, let alone sexual issues.

Programmes that address the sexual and reproductive health of adolescents

Equipping adolescents to make informed sexual and reproductive choices requires multi-pronged activities, including efforts to enhance knowledge and awareness, change attitudes and strengthen skills, such as the ability to negotiate with peers, partners and family members. At the facility level, programmes have tried to design "youth-friendly" services. At the household and community level, programmes have tried to enhance parents' ability and willingness to communicate with adolescents. Through a multitude of ways, programmes have tried to educate young people, build life skills and address the myriad of concerns that young people express that go beyond sexual and reproductive health.

Authors in this collection highlight several broad, but important lessons learned from adolescent programmes. First, evidence suggests that youth are reluctant to patronize clinics. Hence, the programmes that do not reach out beyond the clinic facility are unlikely to reach many young people. Second, in the process of preparing for adulthood, young people face a plethora of challenges and concerns, and projects intended to enhance the exercise of informed sexual and reproductive choices among them need to be delivered within the context of other issues that adolescents consider to be relevant to their immediate needs. Finally, effective programmes need to use multiple strategies. Most effective programmes have not limited themselves to family planning, clinical services or education alone. They combined multiple strategies, including education, counselling, and building links with services, to name but a few. The rest of this chapter reviews the papers in this collection that focus on programme experiences and recommendations.

Family life and sex education programmes

A variety of educational programmes are under way in the region, implemented by both the public and nongovernmental sectors. According to a recent UNAIDS report, in the wake of new epidemiological evidence about the spread of HIV/AIDS, as many as 25% of schools in India will have launched AIDS education programmes by 2001 (Monitoring the AIDS Pandemic-MAP & the Joint United Nations Programme on HIV/AIDS, 2001). Chakrabarti reviews population and sex education programmes within the formal and informal educational sectors in India. With UNFPA funding and government collaboration, the National Population Education Project reached about 154 million students in 2000. She argues that such programmes must complement sex education with strategies such as telephone counselling, peer counselling, life skills education, health camps, and efforts to change attitudes and awareness among teachers and parents.

In addition to governmental efforts to educate youth, the nongovernmental sector has designed many innovative sexuality education programmes throughout South Asia, many of which use the strategies that Chakrabarti recommends. Case studies in this collection illustrate such efforts, including programmes run by Indian nongovernmental organizations (NGOs), such as the Family Planning Association of India (Brahmbhatt) and Parivar Seva Sanstha (Tewari & Taneja), that work in schools, colleges, non-formal education sectors and community-based centres. Activities include counselling centres that offer services individually, in groups, by correspondence, telephone hotlines and a variety of peer-led activities. In addition, they direct their programmes at gatekeepers, such as parents, teachers and service providers. Both programmes underscore the importance of flexibility to youth-friendly services. Aside from convenient locations, affordable fees, and specially trained staff, central elements of programmes aiming to communicate with youth are anonymity and drop-in hours.

Rashid describes the efforts of BRAC, an NGO in Bangladesh that provides reproductive health education in conjunction with a three-year non-formal education programme conducted for adolescents who have never attended school. Introduced in the last year of the three-year programme (and corresponding to the government secondary school programme), the curriculum informs adolescents about puberty, reproduction and contraception and sensitizes them about gender equity and responsible relationships. Tiedemann and DasGupta describe similar efforts among youth organizations (namely the Scouts and Guides Associations) in West Bengal, India. This programme is designed to use the "learning-by-doing" approach of the Associations. The programme involves providing education, building links with local health providers and training Scouts and Guides to become peer leaders. Since large numbers of youth sign up to become Scouts and Guides in West Bengal, the programme hopes to reach thousands of young people.

In short, all these programmes include a range of activities intended to enhance young people's knowledge and communication skills, change attitudes, dispel misconceptions, prevent risky behaviour and address traditional gender norms. A typical curriculum addresses physiological changes during puberty, menstrual hygiene, reproduction, contraception, gender equity, and skills needed to manage relationships. In communities where early marriage for girls is common, programmes often provide premarital counselling and sensitization on responsible parenthood. Nearly all organize peer education, along with strategies to reach parents, teachers and service providers. Many emphasize counselling services, including face-to-face counselling, written correspondence and telephone counselling. They all aim to communicate with young people in direct, non-judgmental yet culturally sensitive ways.

A number of papers in this collection describe evaluations of programmes that inform adolescents about sexual and reproductive health issues. Tiedemann and DasGupta describe the evaluation plans—including a study/control design—that will be used to evaluate the programme among Scouts and Guides in West Bengal. Papers by Teiwari & Taneja and by Rashid report tentative observations of changes in awareness among adolescents exposed to education programmes. Both report a considerable increase in awareness of issues relating to sex, contraception and infection. In addition, Rashid describes how adolescents exposed to the programme reported improved menstrual hygiene as well as attempts to break down communication barriers between themselves and their parents—in particular about their request to delaying early marriage. Nevertheless, several conference participants noted that programme evaluation remains a weakness of many NGOs. They argued that policy-makers and donors need rigorous evidence about which strategies have produced results and are therefore worth scaling up.

Building self-efficacy among adolescents

Many programmes include "life skills" either as one component or as the central focus of their work. In the early 1990s, the World Health Organization defined life skills (World Health Organization, 1993; 1994) as the "abilities for adaptive and positive behaviour that enable individuals to deal effectively with the demands and challenges of everyday life". WHO identified a group of core life skills that include problem-solving, decision-making, goal setting, critical and creative thinking, values clarification, communication skills, inter-personal and negotiation skills, as well as self-awareness, self-esteem and understanding how to cope with stress.

Papers by Seth, and Levitt-Dayal and colleagues describe life skills programmes in India. Seth describes a programme that trains teachers to conduct life skills programmes among youth in rural Rajasthan. Anecdotal feedback from participating teachers suggested that such training empowered trainers to communicate sexual and reproductive health information more effectively and with fewer inhibitions. Preliminary observations also suggest that such training may benefit teachers themselves, as well as young people. Levitt-Dayal et al. describe programmes in rural Gujarat, rural Madhya Pradesh and periurban areas of Delhi that aim to enhance life skills among young women. These programmes use a combination of nonformal, family life and vocational education, combined with the provision of services. They give young women the opportunity to learn to use banks and public transport, to participate in recreational activities and to receive leadership training. These programmes are among the few that have evaluated the impact of their efforts by gathering follow-up data among their alumnae and among a control group of girls who did not participate in their programmes. Compared to controls, alumnae were more likely to remain in school and to have greater decision-making authority within their families, particularly with respect to decisions about when to marry and whether to continue their education. The alumnae demonstrated higher levels of self-esteem, assertiveness, mobility and exposure to media and new ideas. Married alumnae were also more likely to have married at age 18 years or older, and were more likely to obtain appropriate care during pregnancy, compared to those who had not participated in the programmes.

Making health services accessible and friendly

While the need to provide accessible and friendly services to youth is generally acknowledged, there is less clarity about what is meant by "youth-friendly" services. What is evident is that in most settings, adolescents face obstacles in accessing health services. Reviewing the global situation, Epstein, and Chandra Mouli highlight the many obstacles that may discourage young people from seeking health care. These include an inability to access services independently from their families, fear of discovery by family or community members, inconvenient locations and hours, long waits at clinics, high costs, and providers whom adolescents perceive to be threatening, judgmental or unwilling to respect their confidentiality. Using survey data from Bangladesh, Bhuiya and colleagues underline adolescents' reluctance to use health services. They hold the perceived unfriendliness of providers responsible for much of this reluctance. Only 1% of adolescents surveyed had visited a facility in the prior six months, and concerns about how they would be treated were clearly an issue. Only 15% of boys and 1% of girls believed that providers would treat them with respect if they sought contraceptive services, and 26% and 7%, respectively, believed that providers would treat them respectfully if they sought care for STI symptoms. The adolescents' perceptions of pharmacies were similar, if not worse.

The literature often mentions the need for services to be "youth-friendly", but this term is not always clearly defined. However many authors (such as Epstein, Mehta, Poonkhum, Brahmbhatt, Tewari & Taneja and Chandra Mouli) note that, when asked, adolescents generally cite a number of fundamental characteristics that make services "youth-friendly". These include special hours or settings for adolescents, convenient access, a place that does not look like a clinic, a place used by their peers, affordable fees, drop-in hours, staff who are empathetic, knowledgeable and trustworthy, staff that are non-judgmental and non-punitive, and services geared towards young people's needs and interests. Epstein points to adolescents' need for related services such as counselling in managing friendships, partner and family relationships, and life skills development activities that help young people develop practical and applied skills in many areas of life.

Few organizations in South Asia have implemented, let alone evaluated, models for delivering such "youth-friendly" services—although such efforts seem to be on the rise. Chandra Mouli describes a number of models of youth-friendly services: integrated comprehensive services that offer a range of services including sexual and reproductive; community-based health facilities that provide stand-alone sexual and reproductive health services (such as those offered by Marie Stopes International or Profamilia) or those that are offered through a district or municipal health system; community-based centres that offer an array of personal development activities and a limited health focus; and outreach activities designed to enhance access to services. Chandra Mouli stresses that priorities in adolescent-friendly health services need to vary according to the nature of the health services provided and to the specific adolescent group to be reached. For example, approaches that make services friendly to sexually active males may not be wholly adaptable to girls in their early adolescent years. In short, programmes must be tailored to meet the special needs of the adolescents who are being addressed, keeping in mind such issues as social and cultural sensitivities, feasibility and sustainability. Clearly, strategies should be adapted to different sociocultural and programme settings, but what is needed are supportive policies, involvement of the community and adolescents in the design of services, and competent and committed providers.

This volume includes several case studies of youth-friendly services. Bhuiya and colleagues describe efforts to establish "youth-friendly" services in existing NGO clinics, complemented with other outreach efforts in north-west Bangladesh. That project introduced designated hours for adolescent clients, strengthened privacy and confidentiality, expanded the range of services offered, and made an effort to ensure that physicians have the skills to provided counselling. They supplemented these services with efforts to educate community members, provide telephone counselling and establish community-based reproductive health programmes for young people.

Two case studies from Thailand (Poonkhum) and India (Mehta) describe efforts to set up "youth-friendly" services in specially designated areas within government hospitals. These programmes involved remarkably similar preparatory steps, activities and experiences. Both designed the projects based on discussions with adolescents.

Counselling on a variety of topics was the cornerstone of the projects. To avoid using the term "clinic", the project in Thailand delivered services in "adolescent-friendly rooms". Services were free and offered during extended hours. Both maintained confidentiality through anonymous record-keeping. The projects developed training materials and fact sheets (India) or manuals containing frequently asked questions (Thailand). In addition, they trained peers, teachers and parents on reproductive health knowledge and life skills. In Thailand, the project promoted its services with the help of radio DJs who had a wide following among adolescents.

Preliminary findings from both interventions suggest that establishing adolescent-friendly services at government hospitals is feasible and sustainable. However, both found it difficult to attract adolescents to the hospital setting, despite efforts to promote the services widely. Both found that adolescents preferred telephone counselling rather than face-to-face services, probably because it provided greater privacy and anonymity. In Thailand, the Department of Health has considered setting up services in sites outside hospitals that would be more acceptable to adolescents.

Reflecting on lessons learned from experiences around the world, Epstein suggests that the public sector may not be the best entity to deliver such services. In many settings, adolescents perceive NGO services to be less threatening and more acceptable than public services. Furthermore, the public sector tends to take the clinic-based approach, the limitations of which are illustrated by examples in this collection. Several innovative programmes have explored alternatives in the private and NGO sectors, such as training pharmacists or doctors in the private, for-profit sector to serve adolescents, providing counselling and contraceptive services at workplaces and military sites, setting up emergency drop-in centres, offering special hours or facilities for boys, developing long-term adult/adolescent mentoring programmes, and providing discussion opportunities for young couples on marriage and parenthood. Given the limited success of public sector programmes, Epstein argues for a model in which governments support NGOs to scale up successful adolescent reproductive health services.

Regardless of the approach used, Epstein argues that cross-referrals are crucial, because adolescents' needs go beyond the capacity of any one sector. For example, hotline services need to establish formal agreements with other services, such as pharmacies, private physicians, neighbourhood depot holders, abuse/violence crisis centres, mental health counsellors, lawyers and legal services centres, micro-credit facilities, or job training programmes in order to best serve the needs of adolescents. Such cross-referrals require considerable cooperation across public and private sectors and between organizations that provide different services to youth.

Finally, Epstein points out that existing programmes are rarely designed in ways that facilitate rigorous evaluation. Evaluations of adolescent programmes tend to rely on pre- and post-intervention assessments of reproductive health awareness. Because most programmes focus on small populations and evaluations do not include comparisons or controls, it remains difficult to determine whether an outcome is directly attributable to the programme alone, and therefore, whether a finding has programme or policy implications. Furthermore, while many programmes measure changes in knowledge, few are able to measure behaviour change, which would be a more important indicator of success. Epstein argues for building rigorous evaluations into all stages of programmes—a recommendation that has major implications for those who fund programmes, because it would require investing substantial resources in evaluation.

Conclusions

This overview has sought to provide a profile of the sociodemographic and sexual and reproductive health situation of adolescents in South Asia. More significantly, it has attempted to record the evidence and insights that emerged at the conference and to synthesize from these a summary of what is currently known about the sexual and reproductive health risks and challenges faced by adolescents and young people in the region. The findings generally emphasize the considerable risks that adolescents continue to face, extending from unsafe or unwanted sexual activity to such consequences as unwanted pregnancy, abortion and infection, and from misperceptions to a lack of life skills and wide gender power imbalances. They also underscore the vast obstacles that must be overcome in order to access contraceptive and other reproductive health information and services.

At the same time, however, several encouraging signs are evident. The sexual and reproductive health needs of adolescents and young people are firmly on national agendas in the South Asian region. There is growing recognition that adolescents themselves must be given a role in articulating and designing such programmes. Finally, a growing number of programme experiences already exist that appear to respond successfully to young people's sexual and reproductive health needs in innovative and acceptable ways.

Nonetheless, throughout this volume, authors suggest ways in which policy-makers, programme managers, researchers and service providers could do more to improve the lives of South Asian adolescents. The final chapter of this collection summarizes their recommendations—both for research and programmes. These recommendations should be seen as a call to action by all those who care about the well-being of the next generation.

References

Alan Guttmacher Institute (1998) *Into a New World: Young Women's Sexual and Reproductive Lives.* New York, Alan Guttmacher Institute.

Blanc A, Way A (1998) Sexual behavior and contraceptive knowledge and use among adolescents in developing countries. *Studies in Family Planning*, 29(2):106-116.

Bott S (2000) Unwanted pregnancy and induced abortion among adolescents in developing countries: Findings from WHO case studies. In: Puri CP and Van Look PFA, eds. *Sexual and Reproductive Health: Recent Advances, Future Directions.* Mumbai, New Age International (P) Limited, Publishers.

Brown A, Jejeebhoy SJ, Shah I, Yount KM (2001) *Sexual Relations Among Young People in Developing Countries: Evidence from WHO Case Studies.* Geneva, World Health Organization, Department of Reproductive Health and Research (WHO/RHR/01.8).

Central Bureau of Statistics (CBS), Indonesia et al. (1998) *Indonesia Demograhic and Health Survey 1997.* Calverton MD, USA, Macro International.

De Silva W (1997) The Ireland of Asia: Trends in marriage timing in Sri Lanka. *Asia-Pacific Population Journal,* 12(2):3–24.

De Silva W (1998) *Socio-economic change and adolescent issues in the Asian and Pacific region, Report and Recommendations of the Expert Group Meeting on Adolescents: Implications of Population Trends, Environment, and Development.* Bangkok, ESCAP (Asian Population Studies Series, No. 149).

Department of Census and Statistics, Sri Lanka (1988) *Sri Lanka Demographic and Health Survey 1987.* Columbia MD, USA, Institute for Resource Development/Westinghouse.

Department of Census and Statistics, Sri Lanka (1995) *Demographic and Health Survey 1993 Sri Lanka.* Colombo, Department of Census and Statistics, Sri Lanka.

Hakim A, Cleland J, Bhatti MH (1998) *Pakistan Fertility and Family Planning Survey 1996–1997. Preliminary Report.* Islamabad, Pakistan, National Institute of Population Studies and London School of Hygiene and Tropical Medicine.

International Institute for Population Sciences, Macro (2000) *National Family Health Survey (NFHS-2) 1998–1999: India.* Mumbai, International Institute for Population Sciences.

International Labour Organisation (1998) *Yearbook of Labour Statistics 1998*. Geneva, International Labour Organisation.

International Labour Organisation (1999) *Yearbook of Labour Statistics 1999*. Geneva, International Labour Organisation.

International Labour Organisation (2000) *Yearbook of Labour Statistics 2000*. Geneva, International Labour Organisation.

Jejeebhoy S (1993) Family size, outcomes for children and gender disparities: A case of rural Maharashtra. *Economic and Political Weekly*, 28(35):1811–1822.

Jejeebhoy S (2000) Adolescent sexual and reproductive behaviour: A review of the evidence from India. In: Ramasubban R, Jejeebhoy S, eds. *Women's Reproductive Health in India*. Jaipur, Rawat Publications.

Macro International (2002) Demographic Health Surveys, Stat Compiler [Online data base available at http://www.measuredhs.com].

McCauley AP, Salter C (1995) Meeting the needs of young adults. *Population Reports*, Series J, No. 41, Vol. XXIII, 3 (October).

Mitra SN, Al-Sabir A, Cross AR, Jamil K (1997) *Bangladesh Demographic and Health Survey 1996-1997*. Dhaka, Bangladesh, National Institute of Population Research and Training (NIPORT).

Monitoring the AIDS Pandemic (MAP), Joint United Nations Programme on HIV/AIDS (2001) *The Status and Trends of HIV/AIDS/STI Epidemics in Asia and the Pacific, Provisional Report.* Melbourne, Australia, MAP, UNAIDS. [Available at: www.unaids.org/hivaidsinfo/statistics/MAP/index.html]

National Statistics Office (NSO), Republic of the Philippines (1999) *Philippines National Demographic and Health Survey 1998,* Manila, NSO and Macro International.

National Committee for Population and Family Planning (NCPFP), Viet Nam (1999) *Viet Nam Demographic and Health Survey 1997.* Hanoi, NCPFP.

Nepal Central Bureau of Statistics (1995) *Population Monograph of Nepal.* Kathmandu, Central Bureau of Statistics.

Pachauri S, Santhya KG (2002) Reproductive choices for Asian adolescents: a focus on contraceptive behaviour. *International Family Planning Perspectives,* 28(4):186–195.

Population Reference Bureau (2000) *The World's Youth 2000.* Washington, DC, Population Reference Bureau, Measure Communication.

Pradhan A et al. (1997) *Nepal Family Health Survey 1996.* Kathmandu and Calverton, MD, Nepal Ministry of Health, New ERA and Macro International, Inc.

Ramasubban R (2000) Women's vulnerability: The recent evidence on sexually transmitted infections. In: Ramasubban R, Jejeebhoy S, eds. *Women's Reproductive Health in India*. Jaipur, Rawat Publications:280–330.

Singh S (1998) Adolescent childbearing in developing countries: a global review. *Studies in Family Planning,* 29(2):117–163.

United Nations (1997) *Demographic Yearbook 1995*. New York, United Nations (ST/ESA/STAT/SER. R/26).

United Nations (1999) *World Population Prospects: the 1998 Revision. Volume II: The Sex and Age Distribution of the World Population.* New York, United Nations.

United Nations (2000) *Demographic Yearbook 1998*. New York, United Nations (ST/ESA/STAT/SER. R/29).

United Nations Children's Fund (2001) *The Progress of Nations 2001.* New York, UNICEF.

World Health Organization (1993) *Increasing the Relevance of Education for Health Professionals.* Geneva, World Health Organization (WHO Technical Report Series, No. 838).

World Health Organization (1994) *The Development and Dissemination of Life Skills Education: an Overview.* Geneva, World Health Organization (MNH/PSF/94.7).

II

Inaugural presentations

On being an adolescent in the 21st century

Paul F.A. Van Look

Background

The World Health Organization defines "adolescence" as 10–19 years old, "youth" as 15–24 years old, and "young people" as 10–24 years old. Nevertheless, adolescence should be considered a phase rather than a fixed age group, with physical, psychological, social and cultural dimensions, perceived differently by different cultures. As a group, adolescents include nearly 1.2 billion people, about 85% of whom live in developing countries (United Nations, 1999) (Figure 1). Behaviours formed in adolescence have lasting implications for individual and public health and, in many ways, a nation's fate lies in the strength and aspirations of its youth—important reasons to invest in adolescent health and development. This presentation describes the general situation of adolescent health (exploring adolescent sexual and reproductive health in particular) and highlights some key elements of successful programmes.

Figure 1. World population of adolescents, 1950–2050, medium fertility scenario

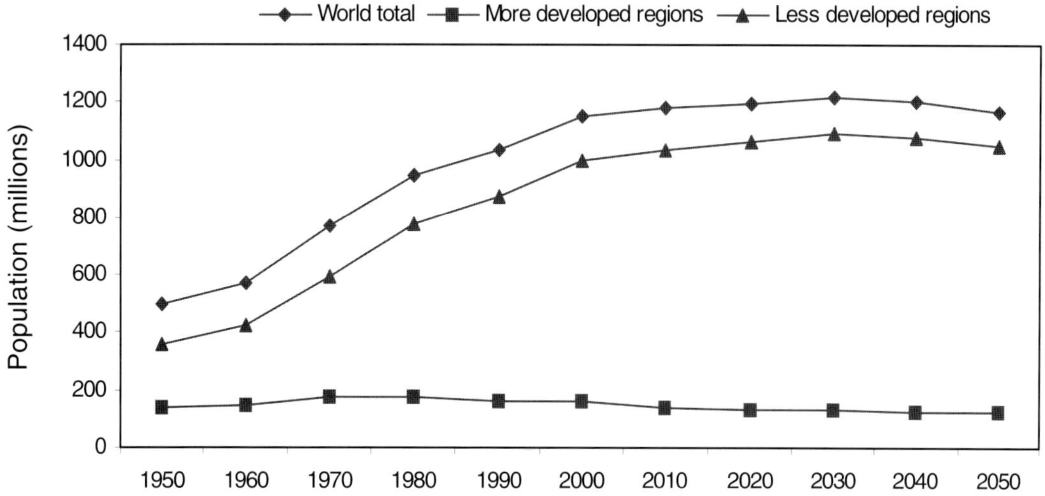

Source: United Nations (Department of Economic and Social Affairs, Population Division) (1999) *World Population Prospects. The 1998 Revision. Volume 1. Comprehensive Tables.* New York, United Nations (document ST/ESA/SER.A/177).

The health status of adolescents

In the absence of a single measure that can express the health status of a population in a general sense, it is difficult to assess the health of a population group. About ten years ago, researchers attempted to create such a measurement unit, called the DALY (Disability-Adjusted Life Years), in order to quantify the global burden of disease throughout the world (Murray & Lopez, 1996). This measure tries to capture two elements at once—years of life lost due to premature mortality and years of healthy life lost from disability, adjusted for severity of the disability. For example, DALYs lost due to heart attack may include years lost as a result of premature death, as well as healthy years lost due to disability such as becoming bedridden.

Researchers have used DALYs to quantify the burden of each disease in the world in specific regions and in different population groups. For example, Chris Murray and Catherine Michaud attempted to quantify the degree of ill-health in adolescents in terms of DALYs in both developing and developed regions of the world. At the global level, they found that adolescents bore nearly 10% (6.6% in developed regions) of the ill-health present in the world in 1990. We typically think of adolescence as being the prime of life—relatively free from infectious diseases of childhood and from conditions associated with ageing. Thus, one would expect that the proportion of ill-health attributable to adolescents would be small. But clearly it is not the case. In 1990, most DALYs (92.0%) among adolescents were lost in developing regions, which is not surprising, since that is where most adolescents live. Adolescents in developed regions were slightly healthier in terms of DALYs than their counterparts in developing regions.

Table 1 presents the 10 most common factors that led to death and disability among adolescents globally in 1990, as measured in terms of DALYs. The worldwide list mirrors the conditions that affect developing countries, including infectious diseases, diarrhoeal diseases, iron-deficiency anaemia, accidents, injuries, war and suicide attempts. Perhaps surprisingly, the top ranked condition is a mental health problem—unipolar major depression. Altogether the top ten conditions represent more than one-third of DALYs lost among adolescents worldwide (Table 1).

Looking at developed and developing regions separately, factors leading to death or disability in developing regions are the same as for the world as a whole, but the pattern is quite different in developed regions. Only three factors appear on both lists. Instead of infectious diseases and anaemia that are prominent in developing regions, the list for developed regions includes several other mental health problems, such bipolar disorders, obsessive-compulsive disorders (which include, for instance, anorexia and bulimia) and schizophrenia. Drug and alcohol use, which are often associated with mental health disorders, are also high on the list. Altogether, the top ten factors represent more than 50% of the total amount of DALYs lost among adolescents in developed regions (Table 2).

One major limitation of using DALYs to measure ill-health among adolescents is that DALYs only capture those problems that are manifest at that moment in time. However, many events and behaviours that begin during adolescence lead to serious problems later in life. Substance abuse patterns, such as smoking and drinking, often

Table 1. Causes of DALYs (per cent of total) in descending order among adolescents globally, 1990 (Total DALYs in thousands = 132 562)

Rank	Disease or injury	Per cent of total
1	Unipolar major depression	6.9
2	Road traffic accidents	4.9
3	Falls	4.0
4	Iron-deficiency anaemia	3.7
5	War	3.5
6	Lower respiratory infections	3.3
7	Drowning	2.8
8	Self-inflicted injuries	2.7
9	Alcohol use	2.3
10	Diarrhoeal diseases	2.3
	Total:	36.3

Source: Murray & Michaud (1996, unpublished data).

Table 2. Causes of DALYs (per cent of total) in descending order among adolescents in developing and developed regions, 1990

Developing regions			Developed regions		
Rank	**Disease or injury**	**Per cent of total**	**Rank**	**Disease or injury**	**Per cent of total**
1	Unipolar major depression	6.5	1	Road traffic accidents	12.3
2	Road traffic accidents	4.2	2	Unipolar major depression	11.3
3	Falls	4.2	3	Alcohol use	8.3
4	Iron-deficiency anaemia	3.9	4	Schizophrenia	4.4
5	War	3.6	5	Drug use	3.5
6	Lower respiratory infections	3.5	6	Bipolar disorder	3.4
7	Drowning	2.9	7	Obsessive-compulsive disorders	3.3
8	Self-inflicted injuries	2.7	8	Asthma	2.6
9	Diarrhoeal diseases	2.4	9	Osteoarthritis	2.5
10	Malaria	2.2	10	Self-inflicted injuries	2.3
TOTAL		**36.3**	**TOTAL**		**54.0**
(Total DALYs in thousands:121 927)			(Total DALYs in thousands: 10 635)		

Source: Murray & Michaud (1996, unpublished data).

develop in adolescence but do not cause ill-health until adulthood. For example, young people who start drinking before age 15 are four times more likely to become alcoholics than those who start at age 21 or later, and most adults who smoke began during adolescence (World Health Organization, 2001).

The Bulletin of the World Health Organization recently published the results of the Global Youth Tobacco Survey[1] (Warren et al., 2000). Researchers concluded that in spite of efforts to counter it, tobacco use among children and adolescents is increasing, and the average age of initiating smoking is declining. In many countries, between one-third and three-fourths of 13–15 year-olds have smoked cigarettes, and around 20–35% of these young people are current users (Figure 2). Once children and adolescents start smoking cigarettes, it becomes extremely difficult for them to stop, even when they have a strong desire to do so. The survey found that a large majority (between 60% and 80%) of 13–15 year-olds who smoke expressed a desire to quit the habit. The per cent who have been unsuccessful was nearly equally high (50–70%). If these trends continue, tobacco will kill 250 million people who are children or adolescents today.

Adolescent sexual and reproductive health

Though early marriage continues to be the norm in some areas, age at marriage among both sexes is rising in virtually every country of the world.

Age at first sexual activity has not followed this trend, however, and in many areas tends to begin at a younger age than in the past. As a result, there is a growing window of opportunity for premarital sexual activity. A recent report by the Population Reference Bureau (2000) compares the median age at marriage (both formal marriage and cohabitation) and the median age at first intercourse. As Table 3 illustrates, a large proportion of adolescents experience first intercourse before marriage in all countries listed. In other words, the evidence clearly indicates that a large proportion of adolescents—if not the majority—are engaging in premarital sexual activity.

Aggregate data often hide important differences between subgroups, including differences between the sexes. Over the past decade, WHO has supported a series of studies involving young people, which have shed light on these differences. Data extracted from 29 of these studies (Brown et al., 2001) indicate that a higher proportion of boys

1 As an aside, it is noteworthy that even WHO has difficulty using consistent terminology. By WHO's own definition, youth begins at 15 years old, yet the Global Youth Tobacco Survey included 13–15 year-olds.

Table 3. Age at marriage and age at first sexual intercourse among young women*— selected countries

Country	Median age At marriage**	Median age at first intercourse
Cameroon	18.0	15.9
Kenya	20.2	16.8
Niger	15.3	15.3
Bolivia	20.9	19.0
Brazil	21.0	18.8
Guatemala	19.2	18.6
Haiti	20.5	18.7
Indonesia	19.9	19.8
Philippines	22.7	22.8

*Among women interviewed when 25–29 years old.
**Includes formal marriage and cohabitation.

Source: *Population Reference Bureau (2000) The World's Youth 2000.* Washington, DC, Population Reference Bureau.

than girls report having engaged in premarital sex in nearly all countries. In some countries, that proportion is as high as 70% among boys, whereas among girls it tends to be below 40% (Figure 3). While part of this difference may be due to the tendency of males to over-report and females to under-report premarital sexual activity, much of this difference seems to be genuine, reflecting gender-related double standards.

These studies suggest other important differences between the sexes in terms of numbers and types of partners. For example, boys tend to report more sexual partners than girls in all countries (Figure 4).

In the majority of cases, girls reported having first sexual intercourse with a boyfriend or fiancé, and only rarely with casual partners. Boys, on the other hand, reported a greater diversity of types of first partners. Around 60% of boys reported that fiancées were their first partner, but a large proportion of boys had sexual partners who were commercial sex workers (Figure 5).

Figure 2. Percentage of students aged 13–15 years smoking cigarettes (Global Youth Tobacco Survey, 1999)

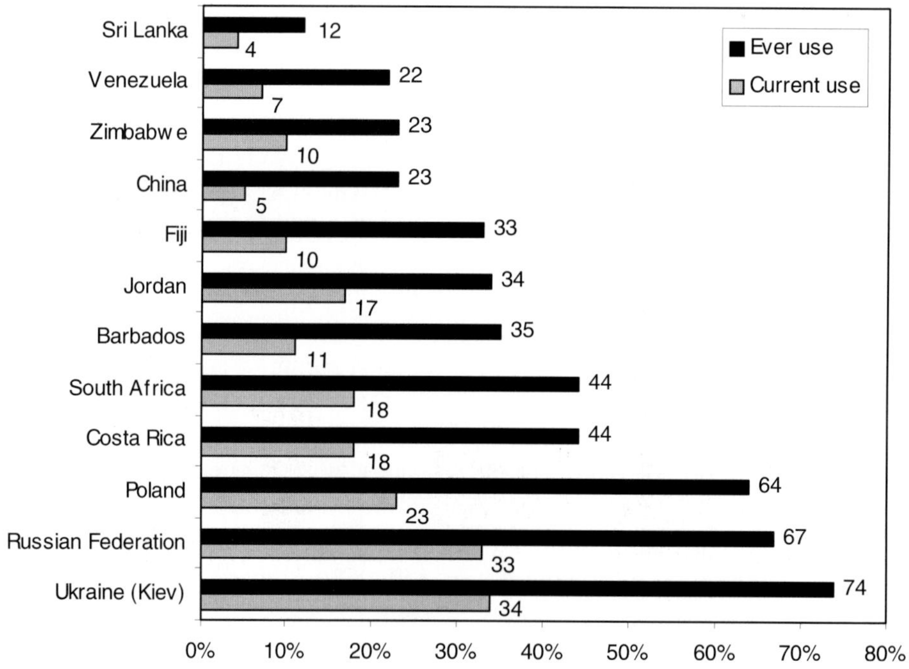

Source: Warren CW et al. (2000) Tobacco use by youth: a surveillance report from the Global Youth Tobacco Survey project. *Bulletin of the World Health Organization*, 78(7):868–876.

Figure 3. Proportion of young people reporting premarital sexual activity during the 1990s — selected studies*

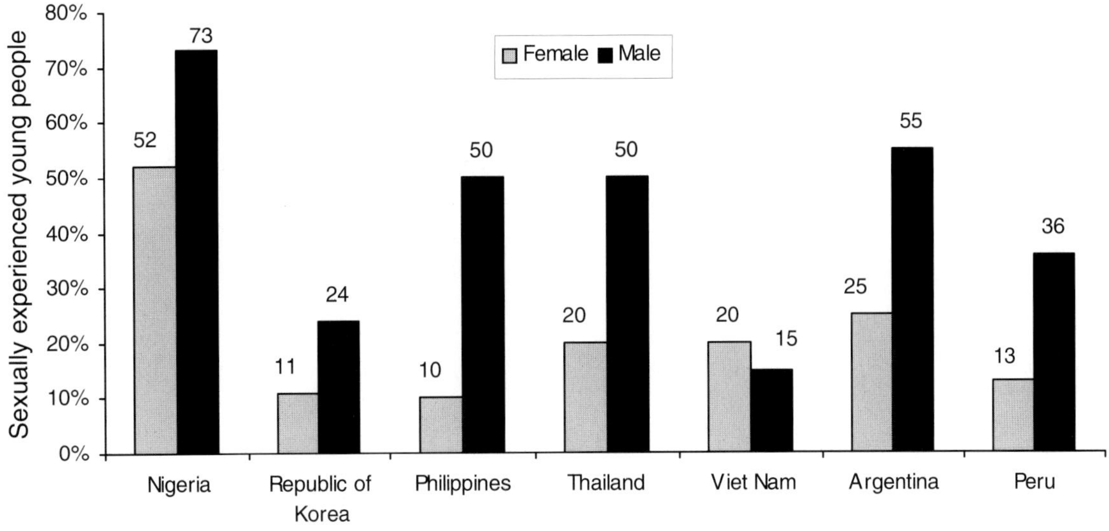

*Note: The studies were not designed to be similar. Hence the samples, methodologies and age ranges varied.

Source: Brown A et al. (2001) *Sexual relations among young people in developing countries. Evidence from WHO case studies.* Geneva, World Health Organization (WHO/RHR/01.8).

Figure 4. Proportion of young people reporting two or more sexual partners—selected studies

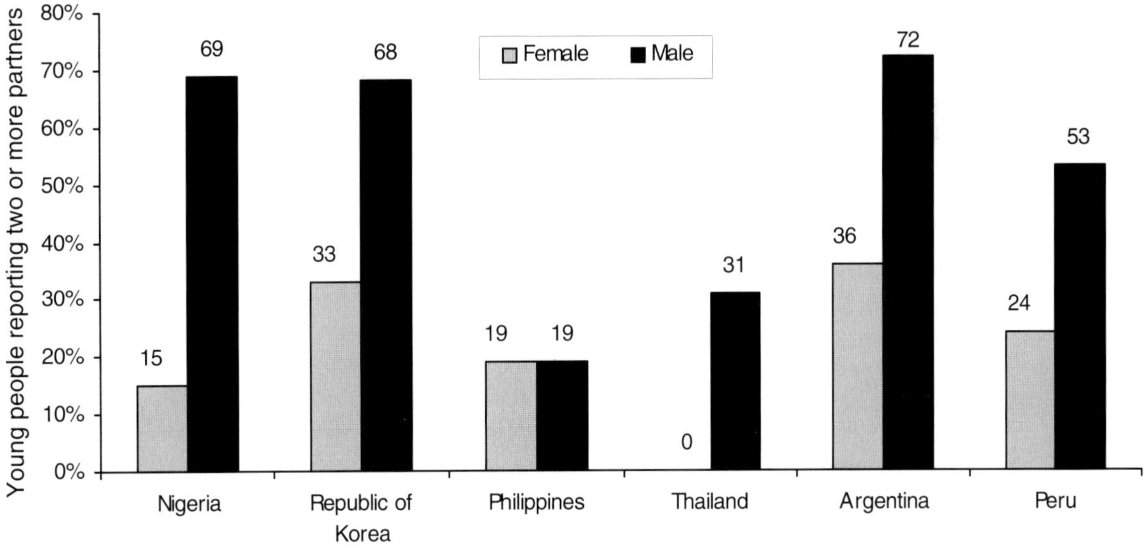

Source: Brown A et al. (2001) *Sexual relations among young people in developing countries. Evidence from WHO case studies.* Geneva, World Health Organization (WHO/RHR/01.8).

Figure 5. Type of sexual partner at debut, or currently, by sex—selected studies

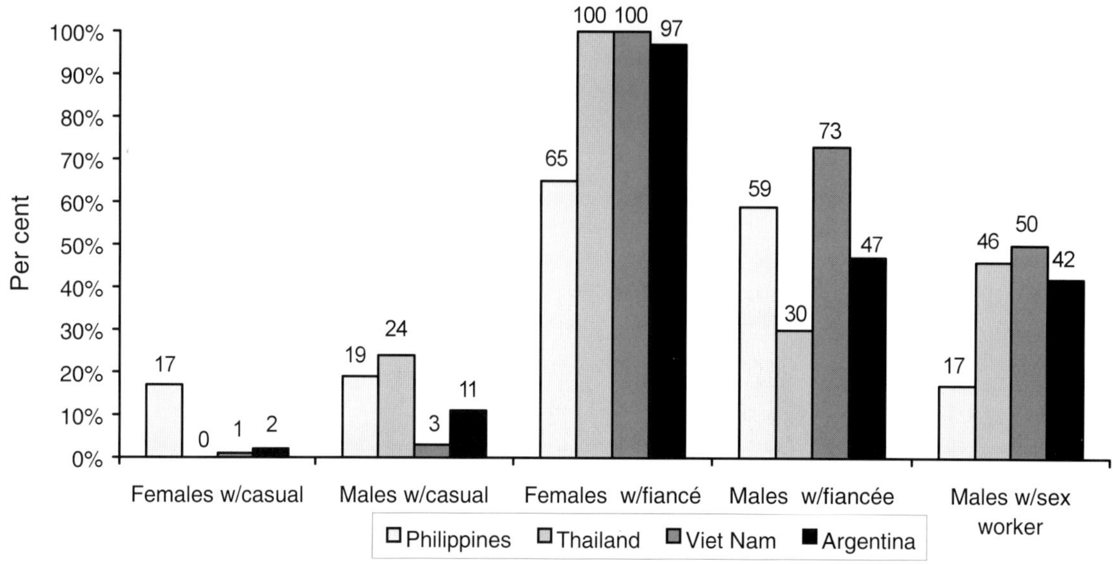

Source: Brown A et al. (2001) *Sexual relations among young people in developing countries: Evidence from WHO case studies.* Geneva, World Health Organization (WHO/RHR/01.8).

These studies also found that a high proportion of girls reported coercive sexual experiences, in some cases as many as 40%. Boys also reported coercive experiences, but did so much less frequently (Figure 6).

This collection of studies suggests that premarital sexual intercourse is often not premeditated and happens at the spur of the moment. Contraception is rarely and irregularly used at sexual debut. After sexual initiation, the pattern of adolescent sexual

Figure 6. Proportion of young people reporting a coercive sexual experience—selected studies

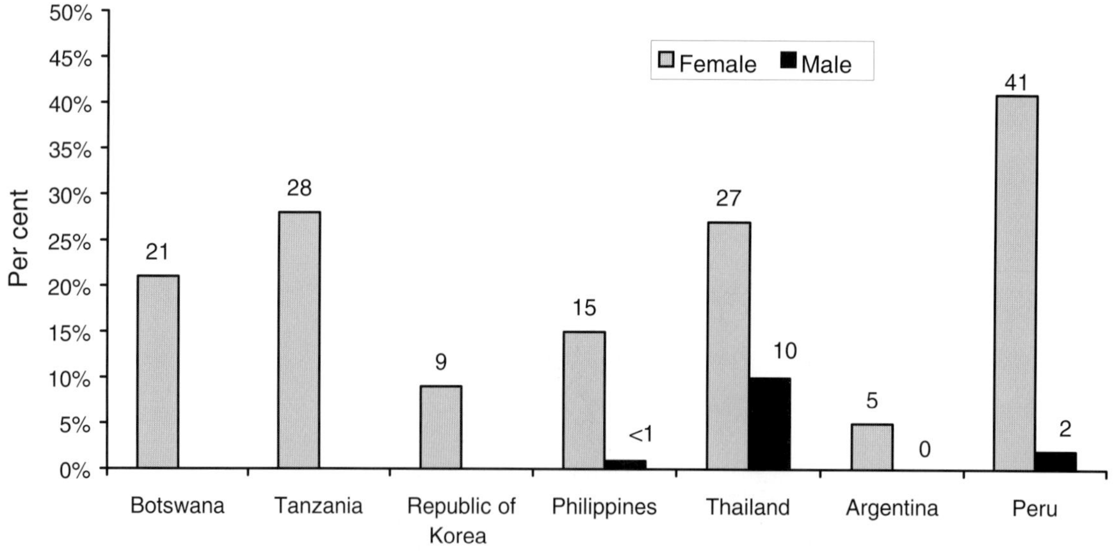

NB: Data not available for males in three countries. Studies measured coercion in different ways. For example, data from Argentina refer only to "rape".

Source: Brown A et al. (2001) *Sexual relations among young people in developing countries: Evidence from WHO case studies.* Geneva, World Health Organization (WHO/RHR/01.8).

Figure 7. Contraceptive use among single, sexually active 15–19 year-old women—selected studies

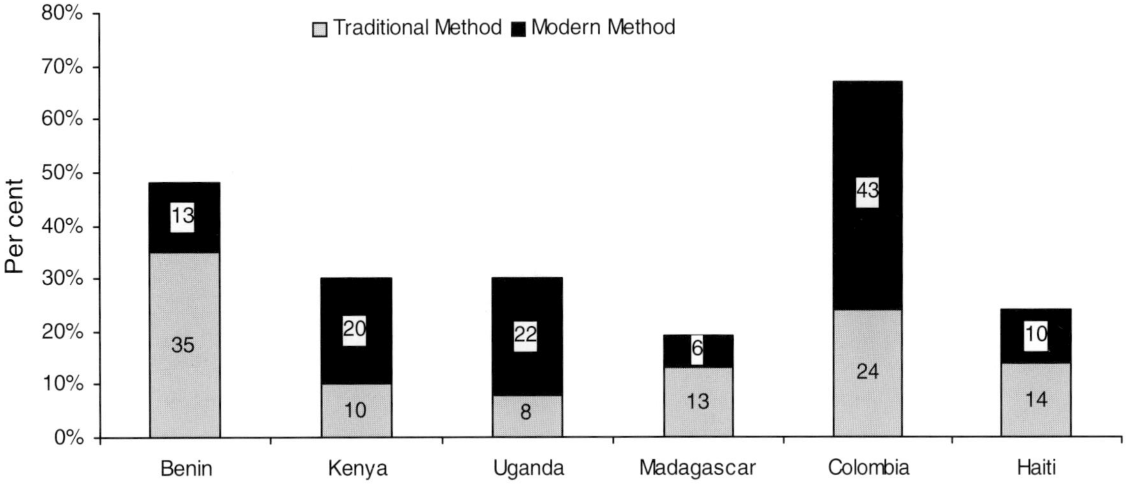

Source: Population Reference Bureau (2000) *The World's Youth 2000*. Washington, DC, Population Reference Bureau.

behaviour is often erratic, and few young people report consistent and correct use of contraception.

Using data from Demographic and Health Surveys, the Population Reference Bureau recently analysed contraceptive use among single, sexually active 16–19 year-old women in a number of countries (Population Reference Bureau, 2000). Their analysis found that many single, young, sexually active women do not use contraception, and a high proportion of those who do, use less effective, traditional methods (Figure 7).

Over 14 million adolescents give birth each year, and about 85% of those births occur in developing countries (Alan Guttmacher Institute, 1998) (Figure 8). Adolescent pregnancies and births carry higher risks— for both the mother and the newborn—than births and pregnancies among older women. The maternal mortality rate among this age group is twice as high as for women in their 20s, and more adolescent girls aged 15–19 die from pregnancy-related causes than from any other cause (United Nations Children's Fund, 1998). In addition, the risk of death during the first year of life is 1.5 times

Figure 8. Births to adolescent women each year, by region (total 14 million)

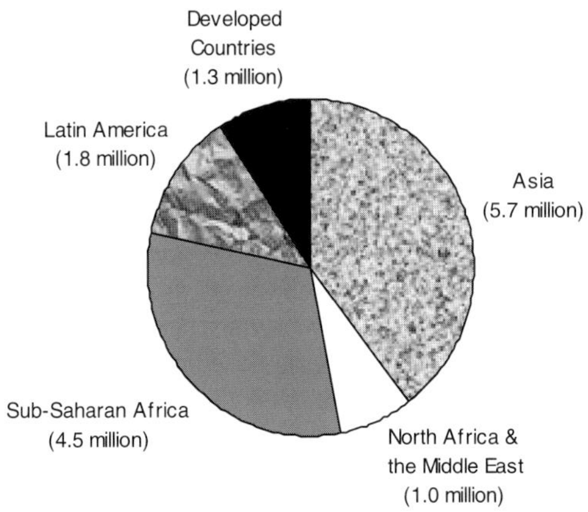

Source: Alan Guttmacher Institute (1998) *Into a New World: Young Women's Sexual and Reproductive Lives*. New York, Alan Guttmacher Institute.

higher for infants born to mothers before the age of 20 than for infants born to women in the third decade of their life (Population Reference Bureau, 2000).

Data compiled by the Alan Guttmacher Institute suggest that between 33% and 66% of births among teenagers are unplanned in most countries (Figure 9).

Many adolescents who experience an unplanned pregnancy resort to abortion—often under unsafe conditions, or late in pregnancy when abortions carry higher risk. Evidence suggests that adolescents have abortions in high numbers, irrespective of the type of abortion laws that exist in a country (Alan Guttmacher Institute, 1998). For example, high numbers of abortions occur in countries with very restrictive abortion laws, such as the Dominican Republic, as well as in countries with less restrictive laws such as the United States of America (Figure 10).

Other important consequences of unprotected intercourse include sexually transmitted infections (STIs). Here again, for biological and social reasons, adolescents are at a high risk. Out of an estimated 340 million cases of curable STIs in the world, at least one-third occur in young people under age 25. This means that more than one out of 20 adolescents contract a curable STI each year. In addition to curable STIs, many cases of STIs occur for which no cure exists—foremost among them HIV infection. According to estimates, half of all new HIV infections currently occur among 15–24 year-olds, the equivalent of 2.5 million new infections each year (Joint United Nations Programme on HIV/AIDS, 2001).

To demonstrate what might have happened in sub-Saharan Africa if HIV/AIDS did not exist, Figure 11 illustrates the HIV/AIDS pandemic's impact on projected life expectancy in 29 African countries. Without HIV/AIDS, life expectancy should have increased over time. Instead, since the emergence of HIV/AIDS, life expectancy has decreased in these countries. According to some estimates there will be a difference of nine years between what it would have been with and without HIV/AIDS by 2010–2015 (United Nations, 2000). In terms of life expectancy, HIV/AIDS has wiped out decades of work of eradicating infectious diseases and

Figure 9. Per cent of adolescent births that are unplanned

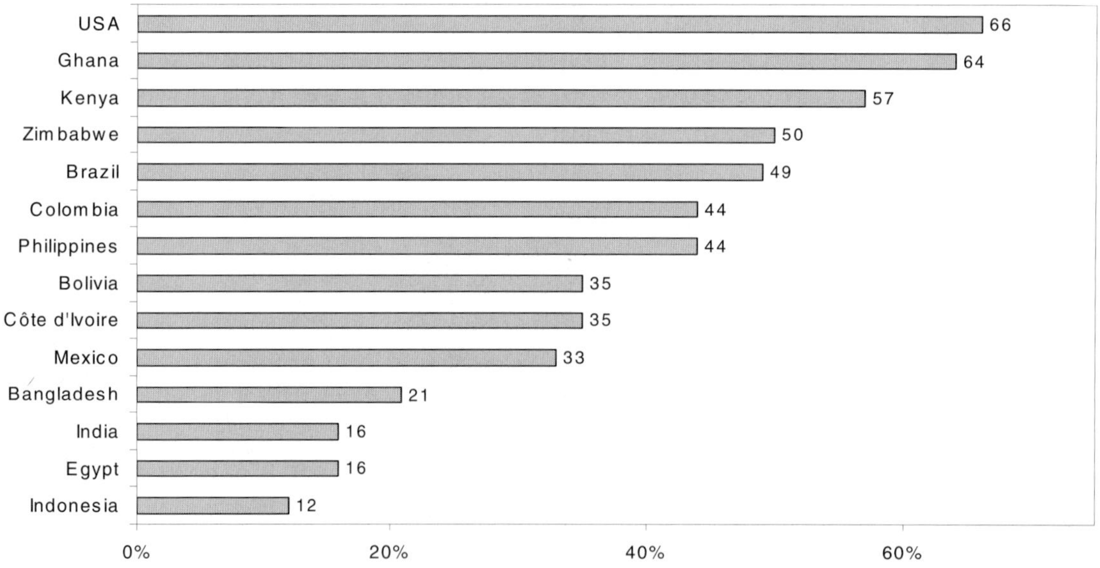

Source: Alan Guttmacher Institute (1998) *Into a New World: Young Women's Sexual and Reproductive Lives.* New York, Alan Guttmacher Institute.

Figure 10. Number of abortions per 100 adolescent women aged 15–19, selected countries

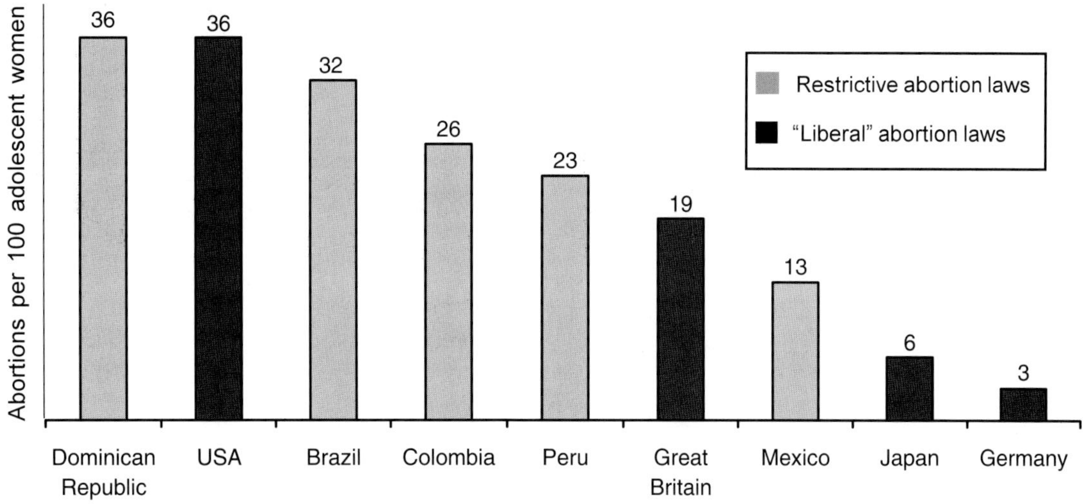

Source: Alan Guttmacher Institute (1998) *Into a New World: Young Women's Sexual and Reproductive Lives.* New York, Alan Guttmacher Institute.

improving health systems in the space of ten years (Figure 11).

Despite the burden of sexual and reproductive ill-health among adolescents in the world today, there are many reasons to be optimistic about adolescents' health and well-being. First, more people are gaining access to information as a result of increased exposure to mass media. Levels of education are rising among girls and boys in virtually every country, and evidence suggests that educated people are better able to look after their own health (The World Bank, 1993). In addition, declining levels of early marriage in nearly all countries should positively influence maternal and newborn health, provided that young unmarried people have access to appropriate reproductive health services, particularly contraceptive services. Use of contraceptives by adolescents is increasing (Population Reference Bureau, 2001), and this may lead to fewer unplanned pregnancies; increased condom use should also lower rates of STI

Figure 11. Life expectancy at birth in 29 African countries with and without AIDS

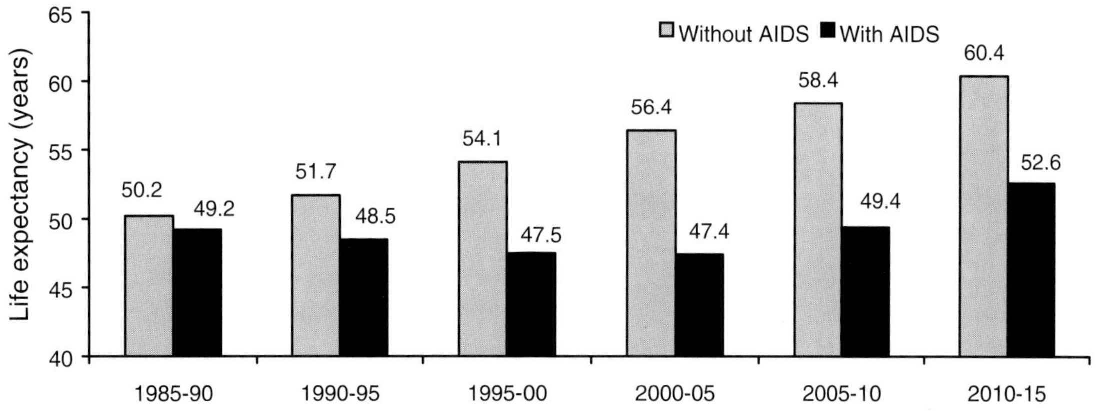

Source: United Nations (Department of Economic and Social Affairs, Population Division) (2000) *World Population Prospects. The 1998 Revision. Volume 3, Analytical Report.* New York, United Nations (document ST/ESA/SER.A/186).

Figure 12. HIV prevalence rate among 13–19 year-olds, Masaka, Uganda, 1989–1997

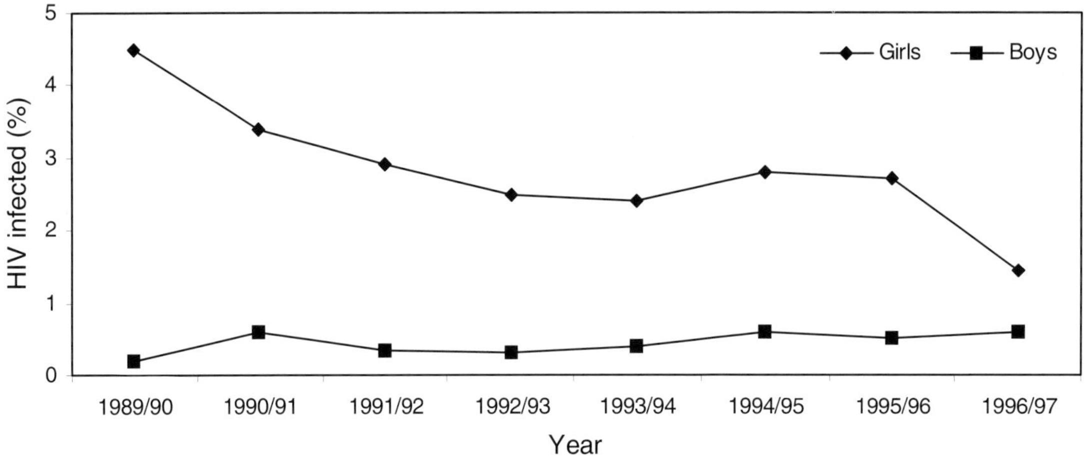

Source: Joint United Nations Programme on HIV/AIDS (2000) *Report on the Global HIV/AIDS Epidemic, June 2000.* Geneva, UNAIDS.

infection. Finally, there have even been positive results in the area of HIV/AIDS. For example, as a result of prevention efforts, HIV prevalence in Uganda has gradually declined among 13–19 year-old girls from about 4.5% to 1.5% since the beginning of the 1990s (Joint United Nations Programme on HIV/AIDS, 2000) (Figure 12).

Similarly, in Zambia, intensive prevention efforts have helped bring down HIV levels among young women attending antenatal clinics. Various clinics in Lusaka reported levels of HIV infection higher than 25% in 1993. These levels have since dropped below 17%, demonstrating that it is possible to influence trends in HIV prevalence (Joint United Nations Programme on HIV/AIDS, 2000) (Figure 13).

Figure 13. HIV prevalence rate among pregnant 15–19 year-olds, Lusaka, Zambia, 1993–1998

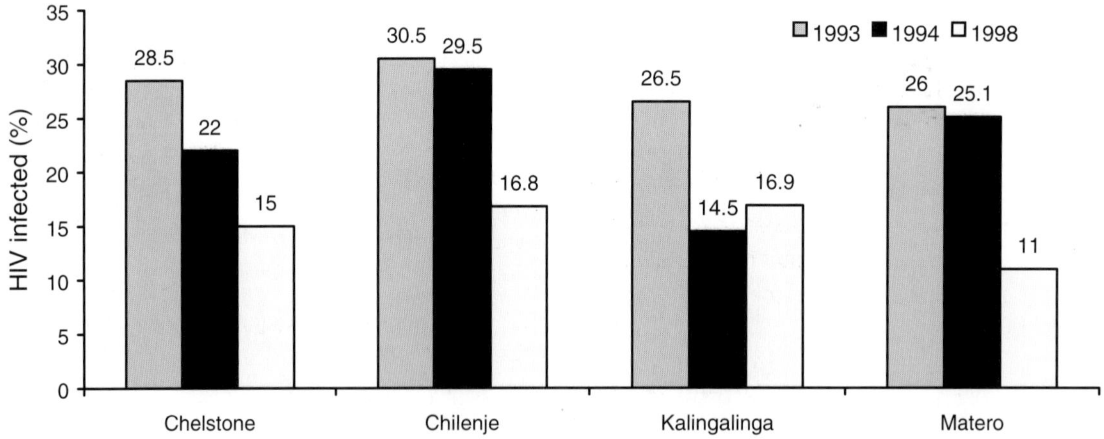

Source: Joint United Nations Programme on HIV/AIDS (2000) *Report on the Global HIV/AIDS Epidemic, June 2000.* Geneva, UNAIDS.

Conclusions: key elements of successful programmes

In 1999, Dr Gro Harlem Brundtland, Director General of WHO, addressed the ICPD + 5 in The Hague. During her address, she argued that, "there is a deep-seated discomfort when dealing with adolescent sexuality. We need to change this." As researchers, policy-makers and programme managers address adolescent sexuality and search for ways to improve young people's lives, they should consider a number of elements that seem to be key to successful programmes. First, adolescents themselves need to participate in programme planning and design. Second, programmes need to address health problems in a comprehensive manner. Many problems that adolescents experience have common roots and common determinants. It makes little sense to address one particular health problem while ignoring others.

In addition, programmes should combine interventions from different areas, such as health, education and life skills development, micro-credit, small business development and safe environments for entertainment. Whenever possible, programmes should build links with existing services in order to achieve cost-effectiveness and avoid duplication. To reinforce services, ways need to be found to provide young people with more supportive environments within their families, schools and communities.

All these recommendations require strong programme management. It is not easy to develop comprehensive programmes for adolescents that are able to deal with many facets of adolescent life. To meet the needs of different categories of adolescents in ways that respect cultural diversity requires great skill from service providers and programme managers.

The above recommendations have emerged from lessons learned or current thinking about programming for young people, but more work is needed to define the elements of successful programmes on the basis of empirical evidence. We hope that this Conference contributes to that effort.

References

Alan Guttmacher Institute (1998) *Into a New World: Young Women's Sexual and Reproductive Lives.* New York, Alan Guttmacher Institute.

Brown A, Jejeebhoy SJ, Shah I, Yount KM (2001) *Sexual Relations Among Young People in Developing Countries: Evidence from WHO Case Studies.* Geneva, World Health Organization (WHO/RHR/01.8).

Joint United Nations Programme on HIV/AIDS (2000) *Report on the Global HIV/AIDS Epidemic, June 2000.* Geneva, UNAIDS.

Joint United Nations Programme on HIV/AIDS (2001) *Children and Young People in the World of AIDS.* Geneva, UNAIDS.

Murray CJL, Lopez AD, eds. (1996) *The Global Burden of Disease: A Comprehensive Assessment of Mortality and Disability from Diseases, Injuries and Risk Factors in 1990 and Projected to 2020.* Global Burden of Disease and Injury Series, Vol. 1. Cambridge, MA, Harvard School of Public Health on behalf of the World Health Organization and the World Bank.

Murray CJL, Michaud C (1996) *Recalculation of DALYs according to age groups pertaining to adolescents, youth, and young people—Description of methodology and data used for calculation* (unpublished paper).

Population Reference Bureau (2000) *The World's Youth 2000.* Washington, DC, Population Reference Bureau.

Population Reference Bureau (2001) *Youth in Sub-Saharan Africa: A Chartbook on Sexual Experience and Reproductive Health.* Washington, DC, Population Reference Bureau.

United Nations (Department of Economic and Social Affairs, Population Division) (1999) *World Population Prospects. The 1998 Revision. Volume 1: Comprehensive Tables.* New York, United Nations (ST/ESA/SER.A/177).

United Nations (Department of Economic and Social

Affairs, Population Division) (2000) *World Population Prospects. The 1998 Revision. Volume 3: Analytical Report*. New York, United Nations (ST/ESA/SER.A/186).

United Nations Children's Fund (1998) *Progress of Nations 1998*. New York, UNICEF.

Warren CW et al. (2000) Tobacco use by youth: a surveillance report from the Global Youth Tobacco Survey project. *Bulletin of the World Health Organization*, 78(7):868–876.

The World Bank (1993) *World Development Report 1993—Investing in Health*. Oxford, Oxford University Press on behalf of the World Bank.

World Health Organization (2001) Briefing note 3 on adolescent health—Provision of health services. *Briefing Notes on Selected Adolescent Health Issues*. Geneva, World Health Organization, Department of Child and Adolescent Health and Development.

Paul F.A. Van Look, MD, PhD, FRCOG
Director
Department of Reproductive Health and Research
World Health Organization
1211 Geneva 27
Switzerland

Addressing the reproductive health needs of adolescents in India: directions for programmes

A.R. Nanda

Background

The World Health Organization defines "young people" as those between the ages of 10 and 24. This age group is composed of two overlapping subgroups, namely "adolescents" (aged 10–19) and "youth" (aged 15–24). The Planning Commission of India estimates that as of March 2000, adolescents aged 10–19 comprised 23% of the Indian population, i.e. almost 230 million. Such a large group represents a major human resource that can and must contribute to the overall development of the country. Addressing their needs will contribute not only to social and economic development, but also to social harmony, gender parity, population stabilization and improved quality of life for all Indians.

Health programmes generally make provisions for adults and young children, but adolescents have largely been overlooked. Adolescence is a period of tremendous opportunity as well as of risk, characterized by physical, psychological and social change. While adolescents are not yet adults, neither are they completely out of childhood. The 1994 International Conference on Population and Development held in Cairo recommended that governments focus more attention on adolescents through an integrated approach to their health, education and social needs.

Official statistics in India do not completely correspond with emerging international definitions. Much information about the age group 15–19 needs to be estimated or disaggregated from information about the age group 15–24. Better quality data are available for older adolescents (age 15–19) than for younger adolescents (age 10–14). Gender-disaggregated data for adolescents are limited and are generally available only for recent years. More qualitative data are also needed, especially to explore issues of gender discrimination and reproductive behaviour. Nevertheless, this paper reviews the data that are available on adolescents' situation in India in terms of employment, literacy and health. The paper goes on to make recommendations for programming and reviews ongoing government policies and programmes aimed at young people.

Employment, education and literacy

Data from the Ministry of Human Resource Development indicate that nearly 90% of children aged 6–11 are enrolled in school, but enrolment falls to 59% among 11–14 year-olds. An obvious gender bias operates in the education sector; two-thirds of boys aged 11–14 are enrolled in school compared with less than half of girls in that age group. The dropout rate for girls in high school is as high as 72% (Government of India, Ministry of Human Resource Development, Department of Education, 1999).

There is a close association between educational attainment and age at marriage, fertility regulation and health-seeking behaviour. Studies from India reveal that while age at marriage among illiterate women is 15 years, age at marriage among girls who have completed high school is significantly higher, at 22 years (United Nations Population Fund, 1998). Globally, women with seven or more years of education tend to marry four years later and have 2.2 fewer children than women with no schooling (United Nations Population Fund, 1996).

A large proportion of adolescents are employed. The 1994–95 National Sample Survey Organisation found that the work participation rate among rural adolescents aged 15–20 years was 77% for young men and 31% for young women. Many adolescents, including those younger than age 14, work in occupations such as bidi-making, gem-polishing, coir-making, paper bag manufacturing, embroidery, zari embroidery, and the lock, glass and carpet industries. Many adolescents work in the agricultural sector or for local village industries as a part of a family labour force. In urban areas, girls form a large part of the unorganized sector working as domestic help. Besides receiving unequal wages, working girls are more vulnerable to sexual abuse and violence than older women.

Adolescent marriage and childbearing

In many parts of India, early marriage for girls is a religious and social imperative. Despite laws that specify the legal age of marriage for girls as 18 years, cultural pressures often force parents to marry off their daughters at a younger age. In 1996, an average of 38% of girls aged 15–19 were married (Jejeebhoy, 1998). This rate was significantly higher in rural areas where 46% of girls in this age group were married, compared with 22% of girls aged 15–19 in urban areas. Age at marriage varies from state to state, however. Early marriages are common in Madhya Pradesh, Andhra Pradesh, Rajasthan and Bihar, where more than 50% of young women aged 15–19 are married. In Haryana and Uttar Pradesh, 40–44% of young women aged 15–19 are married. Women in Kerala, Punjab, Goa, Manipur, Mizoram and Nagaland tend to marry later, and in those states fewer than 15% of girls aged 15–19 are married.

Because of early marriage, adolescent fertility in India is relatively high. This should be a cause for concern since many younger adolescents are physiologically immature for reproduction. Compared to adult women, childbearing during adolescence poses greater health risks to both the mother and the newborn. Fertility during this period contributes to maternal morbidity and mortality, high incidence of low birth weight babies and neonatal morbidity and mortality (Jejeebhoy, 1998). Not surprisingly, 1997 age-specific fertility rates (ASFR) among 15–19 year-olds reveal a major urban–rural differential. At 20.3 per thousand, the rural ASFR was more than double the urban ASFR of 9.8 per thousand (International Institute for Population Sciences, 1995).

Sexual behaviour and knowledge among adolescents

Studies suggest that adolescents have limited knowledge about sexual and reproductive health, and know little about the natural processes of puberty, sexual health, pregnancy or reproduction. This lack of knowledge about reproductive health —including the emerging threat of HIV/AIDS—may have grave consequences for the country.

Countrywide information on adolescents' sexual behaviour is not available. However, contrary to general expectations, small-scale studies suggest that sexual activity begins at a relatively early age. As reported in a review of adolescent sexual and reproductive behaviour in India, a 1993–94 study conducted by the Family Planning Association of India among educated urban youth revealed that the average age of first sexual experience among

15–19 year-olds was age 14.8 for males and age 16.1 for females; another 1995 study found that only 38% of young men and 63% of young women disapproved of premarital sexual relationships (Jejeebhoy, 1998). While these studies are not representative of the entire country, they do suggest that a substantial proportion of adolescents are sexually active. The need of the hour is to obtain more culturally and context specific data for formulating interventions that address sexual decision-making, gender roles and power relations between the sexes.

Knowledge and use of contraception

Large-scale studies such as the National Family Health Survey suggest that at least half of all young women in India are sexually active by age 18—mostly within marriage—and almost one in five are pregnant by age 15. Well over half of all married women aged 15–19 have experienced a pregnancy or given birth (United Nations Population Fund, 1998). Nevertheless, the 1995 National Survey on Fertility and Family Planning Practices (International Institute of Population Sciences, 1995) found that adolescents had relatively low levels of knowledge about reversible contraceptive methods. The study revealed that while 89% of adolescents were aware of sterilization, less than 50% were aware of oral contraception and only 39% knew about IUDs. In view of the previous discussion about sexual activity among younger age groups, it is disheartening to note that such a small percentage of adolescents are aware of spacing methods that would be most suitable for their contraceptive needs.

Evidence suggests that contraceptive use rises with age. The 1992–93 National Family and Health Survey (International Institute for Population Sciences, 1995) indicated that no more than 5% of married women aged 13–14 and no more than 7% of married women aged 15–19 were practicing contraception. These low levels contrast with 21% of women aged 20–24 and 61% of women aged 35–39 using contraceptives.

Programme recommendations

Many health programmes view the needs of adolescents with a narrow focus on reproductive health. While reproductive health is undoubtedly important, programmes need a wider perspective that considers adolescents' broader emotional and physical needs as well. For example, risk-taking behaviour and employment in hazardous industries place young people at risk of physical injury. Adolescent health programmes also need to consider relatively high rates of substance abuse, violence—especially sexual violence—and trafficking of children and adolescents for commercial sex work.

A programme's willingness to address issues that may not relate directly to health can have a profound effect on both the acceptability and cost-effectiveness of those interventions. Programmes should focus not only on counselling services, contraception, nutrition, and rehabilitation of the abused or exploited, but also on factors such as life skills, protection from abuse and vocational guidance.

Programmes for adolescents also need to recognize the vast diversity among this segment of the population. Adolescents include a wide spectrum of categories: in-school and out-of-school; married and unmarried; tribal, rural and urban; the employed and the unemployed; those who have been sexually exploited; those in institutions; those who are disabled and those in conflict with the law.

Finally, programmes need to involve adolescents themselves and other stakeholders at every stage —from conceptualization to programme design and evaluation. Because adolescent sexual and reproductive health is such a sensitive issue, programmes must consult community leaders, religious groups, parents and teachers in order to ensure the acceptability and effectiveness of their interventions.

Institutional versus outreach models

Services for adolescents can be delivered through institutions or through outreach schemes. At present, hospital services do not cater to adolescents. To become more acceptable to adolescents, hospital services need to give adequate attention to their particular concerns, such as privacy. Although this may not require many additional resources, it does require sensitivity and reorganization of clinical services in some health facilities. The Safdarjung Hospital in New Delhi, which is one of the largest public hospitals in the country, has begun a two-year pilot project to test the feasibility of such an approach.

Because a vast majority of the Indian population lives in rural areas, outreach efforts are also needed to reach many adolescents. For example, health camps held at regular intervals in remote and far-flung areas can provide basic reproductive health services, as well as services such as counselling, nutritional advice, rehabilitative services, life skills, and vocational guidance. Ideally, governmental and nongovernmental organizations (NGOs) would collaborate in this endeavour.

Government programmes for adolescents

While the Government of India has not yet formulated specific programmes for adolescents, several ongoing programmes have components that address their needs. For example, the National Population Policy has recognized adolescents as an underserved category that will have a central role in determining the size of the population in coming decades. The policy aims to provide for adolescents' nutritional, contraceptive and information needs. Other policy documents have also addressed adolescents' diverse needs: for example, the National Nutrition Policy (1983) identified adolescent girls as a vulnerable group; the National Education Policy (1986) reaffirmed the commitment of the government to eradicating illiteracy in the age group 13–35; and the National Plan of Action for Children devoted a separate section to adolescent girls. The draft National Youth Policy 2000 calls for a multi-dimensional integrated approach to youth development. This policy focuses on youth empowerment, gender justice, youth participation in decision-making, establishment of a strong intersectoral approach and building a robust information and research network to address needs of the young population.

Several government schemes provide vocational training, education, social development and empowerment of girls, including Training of Rural Youth for Self Employment (TRYSEM), Vocational Guidance and Employment Scheme, Balika and Sarv Sksha Ahiyan, adolescent girls' scheme under the Integrated Child Development Scheme (ICDS), Nehru Yuvak Kendra Sangthan and the National Service Scheme, among others. In addition, NGO programmes in several parts of the country address adolescents' needs, including reproductive health, rehabilitation of sexually abused children, street children, gender equity, employment and other issues.

Conclusions

This Conference on reproductive health is taking place at an opportune moment for the Ministry of Health and Family Welfare. The Ministry is in the early stages of formulating future strategies that will succeed the current Reproductive and Child Health Programme. The deliberations and recommenda-tions of this Conference will undoubtedly help in this task.

References

Government of India, Ministry of Human Resource Development, Department of Education (1999) *Selected Educational Statistics*. New Delhi, Government of India.

International Institute for Population Sciences (1995) *National Family Health Survey (MCH and Family Planning), India 1992–93*. Mumbai, International Institute for Population Sciences.

Jejeebhoy S (1998) Adolescent sexual and reproductive behaviour: a review of the evidence from India. *Social Science and Medicine*, 10:1275–1290.

United Nations Population Fund (1996) *The State of the World's Population*. New York, UNFPA.

United Nations Population Fund (1998) India Country Paper. Paper presented at the *South Asia Conference on the Adolescent, New Delhi*.

A.R. Nanda
Secretary, Family Welfare
Ministry of Health and Family Welfare
Government of India
Nirman Bhavan
New Delhi 110011
India

Adolescent reproductive health in South Asia: key issues and priorities for action

Ena Singh

Background

Adolescents make up one-fifth of the world's population—over a billion people. In South Asia that proportion is even greater. Programmes aimed at adolescents affect not only their lives and the lives of their future offspring, but also the lives of their younger siblings, mothers and fathers—in fact, all of society. No matter which "sector" we come from—whether reproductive health, education, gender, violence, drug abuse or indeed any area of serious concern to society today—we must realize the importance of working with adolescents. That is why so many national policies include references to adolescents, including policies related to youth, women, children, population, education, health, nutrition and HIV/AIDS. This paper reviews the situation of adolescents in South Asia in terms of education, labour participation, sexual and reproductive health and violence. The paper then explores recommendations for designing successful programmes to address the wide range of issues that adolescents face.

Education and employment of adolescents

Despite improved educational opportunities in recent decades, a sizeable proportion of adolescents remain illiterate in South Asian countries; Sri Lanka and the Maldives are the exceptions. In much of the rest of the region, between one-third and two-thirds of younger adolescent girls are illiterate, as are one-fifth to one-half of younger adolescent boys. Moreover, in many countries in the region, secondary school enrolments are low, and a large proportion of older adolescents aged 15–19 engage in economically productive activities. For example, older adolescents' labour participation rates range from 18% in Sri Lanka, to 49% in Nepal, to 67% in Bangladesh, while they average 33% for the rest of the region (United Nations Population Fund, 1998). Adolescents, especially girls, are subject to many types of exploitation—including sexual exploitation and trafficking as well as economic exploitation such as organized begging (see, for example, Mundigo & Indriso, 1999).

Sexual and reproductive health

Adolescents in South Asia often lack reproductive choice, such as whether, when and whom to marry; whether and when to have children and how many to have; whether to abort a female fetus; whether to use contraceptives and where to get them. More broadly, adolescents often lack choice about whether they can study and learn, work and earn, keep their own earnings or have to give them to their elders or spouses, and whether they can send their children to school. In many cases, adolescents have dreams and aspirations, but little freedom to shape their own lives.

The age at which young girls marry is distressingly low in most of South Asia. Early marriage for girls is the norm in most countries of the region, despite laws prohibiting marriage before age 18 for girls, and before age 21–24 for boys. Nearly two-thirds of girls in most South Asian countries marry by age 18, while one-fourth marry by age 15. Again, Sri Lanka is an exception (United Nations Population Fund, 1998).

Nevertheless, age at marriage is rising throughout the region (see, for example, United Nations Population Fund, 2000). This trend raises its own set of issues and concerns. South Asia societies generally consider sex outside marriage immoral and condemn adolescents—girls in particular—who engage in it. However, rising age at marriage and more schooling, combined with increased migration and urbanization have led to more opportunities for premarital sex. In Bangladesh, for example, one survey found that 60% of unmarried urban adolescent boys and 10% of unmarried urban girls reported sexual experiences (United Nations Population Fund, 1998). In India, one study found that 20–25% of unmarried adolescent boys reported engaging in sexual relations (United Nations Population Fund, 1998).

More opportunities for premarital sex combined with a lack of knowledge about the body and contraception may be responsible for increasing the number of unwanted pregnancies and abortions among adolescent girls. Studies suggest that not only do many unmarried girls lack knowledge of contraceptives, but many hesitate to use them, because this would conflict with their self-image as moral beings (United Nations Population Fund, 1998). Sadly, "Had I known..." is a phrase often heard from young women who did not have basic knowledge of contraception and did not fully understand the consequences of unprotected sex, the risks of pregnancy, or the dangers of unsafe abortion.

Because of delays in making a decision or reaching a service provider, adolescent abortions are often second trimester, illegal and unsafe. Unfortunately, service providers are known to take advantage of adolescents' vulnerability, often asking for money or favours that they would not ask from older, married women. Abortion thus remains an urgent issue for young people. Options such as increasing adolescents' access to emergency contraception must be seriously explored.

Young people are not only at high risk for pregnancy, but also for sexually transmitted infections (STIs). The available data show high prevalence levels of reproductive tract infections (RTIs) and STIs among married and unmarried adolescent girls and boys. For example, a study in Bangladesh found that 40% of adolescent girls (including both married and unmarried) and 20% of unmarried adolescent boys reported symptoms of RTIs and STIs (United Nations Population Fund, 1998). A study in Sri Lanka found that 7% of adolescent boys had an STI (United Nations Population Fund, 1998).

Many adolescents, particularly girls, experience violence, such as sexual abuse, trafficking, rape and "honour killings". In Bangladesh, one thousand rapes were reported in 1995, 20% of which were committed against minors (United Nations Population Fund, 1998). This is only the tip of the iceberg. Most often, the perpetrators are boys or men whom adolescents know and trust. In addition to the trauma of violence, young girls often suffer additional shame and guilt inflicted by society upon the victim.

Programmes

Because education, work, sex and violence are all part of adolescents' lives, those who work with adolescents must let the boundaries of their specializations blur. Effective programmes for adolescents quickly become trans-sectoral, meaning that they integrate different sectors into a single programme, rather than being multisectoral, which implies the mere inclusion of many separate interventions. Because adolescents will not accept programmes that do not relate to their lives, most successful programmes address life skills such as self-esteem, self-awareness, communication and negotiation. Indeed, in programmatic jargon, adolescents and life skills seem to have become synonymous.

This conference has provided an opportunity to discuss how to design, initiate and sustain life skills programmes. In this context, the most important question is what we teach young people in these programmes. In a book entitled *Conversations with God, Book I,* Neale Donald Walsch (1995) states:

> *Most people have misunderstood the meaning, the purpose, and the function of education, to say nothing of the process by which it is best undertaken. People think that the purpose of education is to pass on knowledge; that to educate someone is to give them knowledge. Yet, education has very little to do with knowledge. It has to do with Wisdom. Wisdom is knowledge applied… we mustn't ignore wisdom in favour of knowledge… It would kill education. It* ***is*** *killing it. We are teaching our children what to think instead of how to think. Lessons in critical thinking, problem solving, and logic are considered by many parents to be threatening. And well they might. Because children who are allowed to develop their own critical thinking process are very much likely to* ***abandon*** *their parent's morals, standards and entire way of life.*

This quote addresses the perpetual question of how to balance parents' responsibilities with adolescents' rights, a question that generated much heated debate at ICPD + 5 (5-Year Review and Appraisal of Implementation of the ICPD Programme of Action) and other fora. No other topic in these debates evokes more intense discussion than the topic of sexuality and sex education. We have a great deal of evidence that when sexuality is openly discussed and when young people learn about their bodies and their emotions, they are better able to cope with sexual maturation. Sexual crimes, RTIs and unwanted births would not pose problems of such magnitude if such issues were more openly discussed. If each birth is to be considered a blessing and each sexual encounter an expression of love, not an irresponsible experiment or an act of aggression, then we must talk openly about sex.

Because most reproductive health programmes originated from concern about population growth, they viewed adolescent fertility with concern. From a demographic perspective, one-fifth of births occur in adolescence, and adolescent girls have shorter birth intervals than older women. As a society, however, we have had to ask whether it is acceptable to tell unmarried adolescents about contraception. Even if we can agree that it is acceptable to ***tell*** them about contraception, what about ***giving*** them contraception? Many argue that we might let unmarried boys have access to condoms, but are more ambivalent about giving pills to unmarried girls. Health workers are often left to sort out these dilemmas according to their own value systems or the administrators' preferences.

There ***is*** a solution, however. First, each country or state must make clear choices and must act on those choices. Second, we must not propose solutions that do not match the problem. Denying contraception will not mandate morality. Morality depends on the way that men and women treat each other, the way that the media creates aspirations, and the way that society defines success—issues that should be tackled at their own levels. Responsible sex education and contraceptives should not be denied to people who are at risk of disease or unwanted pregnancies.

Many countries have begun to provide sexual and reproductive information in a responsible and sensitive way, though often in response to concerns about HIV/AIDS rather than unwanted pregnancy or unsafe abortion. Those who design education, services and counselling programmes for adolescents must consider that young people have their own language about the body, sex and pregnancy. It is crucial to understand who influences girls' decisions to have sex or to abort a pregnancy, and what role their partners play. Can they turn to a mother, sister, aunt or friend when in trouble? Who will pay? Lack of money is a common theme in young girls' stories, including lack of money to raise the child they carry, or lack of money to pay for a safe abortion.

Programmes for adolescents confront issues as complex as life itself—education, nutrition, contraception, disease control, reproductive choices and rights, reproductive safety, employment, skills and mental health. They all merit priority. Although this conference focuses on reproductive health, we must remember that programmes cannot improve adolescents' reproductive health if they ignore the rest of adolescents' often turbulent lives.

A few broad principles should guide those of us who work with adolescents from a reproductive health perspective. First, help adolescents to know their potential to become knowledgeable, confident, responsible, and caring adults, whether this is achieved through camps, life skills programmes or regular education. Healthy reproductive health choices will follow. Such programmes may be expensive, but failure to help adolescents achieve their potential will be even more costly.

Second, we need to think beyond the scope of our particular sectors for a while. Programmes for adolescents can begin with focus on a single issue, but they need to grow into broader programmes covering the issues that are the wants and needs of young people. If individual reproductive health issues are important, their turn will come. Most adolescents want information about love, sex, marriage and children. With time, reproductive health issues emerge as a priority—though not necessarily the highest priority.

Third, we should collaborate with all those who work with adolescents. Reproductive health programmes do not have to start from scratch or work in isolation. We can help professionals from other sectors to address reproductive health issues effectively. Often they ignore reproductive issues not because they discount their importance, but because they may not know how to talk about reproductive and sexual health concerns in sensitive and engaging ways.

Fourth, we need to work with young people, not "work at" them. The conference session on youth-friendly services sheds light on how this can be done. One lesson is that young people's comfort with their own sexuality is a prerequisite to responsible and caring reproductive behaviour. But as counsellors, service providers or managers, we need to be comfortable with our own sexuality before trying to teach young people to be comfortable with theirs.

Finally, do not forget boys. Many initiatives have been preoccupied with girls, perhaps because they emerged from efforts devoted to girls' education, reproductive health or women's empowerment. It is good for programmes to concentrate on girls. However, I recall several occasions when organizations denied funding for boys simply because they had defined girls as a priority. Interventions for boys and girls do not need to be mutually exclusive.

In this regard, we need to remember that educating and sensitizing boys are not shortcuts or substitutes for empowering girls, though such efforts may support that objective. We must preserve the spaces that have been carved out for girls and women at great cost. Involving men and boys can be a double-edged sword; it can cut through centuries of bias and patriarchy, but such involvement can also threaten the tender ropes that women have so recently woven to pull themselves out of prison. We need to exercise the utmost care not to allow this to happen.

Before closing, I would like to recall the collective words of the young people who attended a South Asia Conference on Adolescents held in New Delhi in 1998 (United Nations Population Fund, 1998):

We adolescents are not only conscious of our rights but we also feel responsible for moving away from the "me" decade in which we are living, to a decade where adolescents will prove to be an important human resource for the betterment of the region. We pledge to make this a reality.

Our perspective is that we feel neglected, and so we need more attention, care and support from all. We feel we do not have the right to make our own choices, even after learning about all the alternatives and choices related to our careers, friends, movements and life partners. We greatly lack proper and correct information and guidance, especially related to our bodies' physiological and psychological changes. We are not allowed to express our emotions and our thoughts. We feel increasingly 'self abused' through frequent exposure to pornography, blue films, sex shops and obscene advertisements.

To our parents, we say that we need you to listen to us, to our dreams, our experiences, our explanations. Give us your time—you gave us life, now we want your time. Don't hide things from us, especially when they are related to us. Give us the privacy and the space to grow. Guide us; don't drive us.

To our Governments, we say that our biggest dilemma is why girls are discriminated against. Do something. Review the education system, especially the way you evaluate us. Don't experiment with us and change curricula frequently. Make education more relevant and interesting. Provide non-formal education programmes for adolescents who can't go to school. Include lessons on life skills and sex education in formal and non-formal education programmes. Provide adolescents with professional and confidential counselling services on sexual and reproductive health issues. Eliminate child labour, child abuse and all types of violence against adolescents, including trafficking. Take legal action against immoral acts such as pornography, blue films, sex shops, and obscene advertisements. Don't just make laws; enforce them. Require law enforcement agencies to be more sensitive towards physical abuse cases. Let us support you and join hands to fight the menace of drugs.

Our declaration ends here, but not our desire to do something for millions of adolescents we represent.

With such a force on our side, is change not inevitable? Often I have heard people say that they love working with adolescents because their efforts are met with enthusiasm, and because the transformation of young people is fast and dramatic. It is a very rewarding experience. How fortunate that it is so. Under such circumstances, surely we will succeed.

References

Mundigo I, Indriso C, eds. (1999) *Abortion in the Developing World*. Delhi, World Health Organization and Vistaar Publications.

United Nations Population Fund (1998) *Report of the South Asia Conference on Adolescents. New Delhi, July 1998*. Kathmandu, UNFPA Country Support Team for Central and South Asia.

United Nations Population Fund (2000) *Adolescents in India: A Profile*. New Delhi, UNFPA for the United Nations System in India.

Walsch ND (1995) *Conversations with God, Book I*. London, Hodder and Stoughton.

Ena Singh
UNFPA
55 Lodi Estate
New Delhi 110013
India

III

Sexual and reproductive health of married adolescents

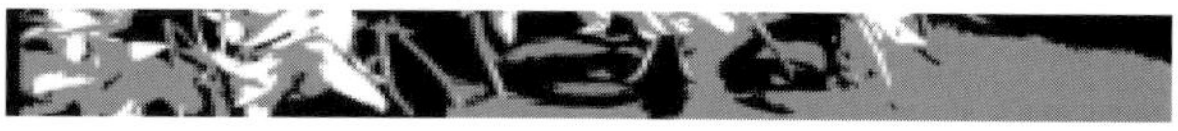

The reproductive health status of married adolescents as assessed by NFHS-2, India

Sumati Kulkarni

Background

Adolescence is the transition period between childhood and adulthood. However, in many Asian countries, early marriage and childbearing deprive girls of this transitional phase and push them to shoulder responsibilities for which they are not fully equipped. As a result, married adolescents form one of the most vulnerable sections of the population in a country like India. In order to formulate policies and programmes for this group, it is essential to know about the risks that they face and the extent to which the present health system meets their needs. This paper presents findings of the second National Family Health Survey (NFHS-2) that pertain to ever-married women in the age group 15–19, defined as adolescents in this paper.

Methods

The International Institute for Population Sciences (IIPS) undertook the NFHS-2 in 1998–1999, in collaboration with ORC Macro, USA. The study covered a representative sample of 89 199 eligible women aged 15–49, from 91 196 households in 26 states. The survey included 8182 married adolescent women (aged 15–19), who formed nearly 9.2% of the women interviewed in the survey. During two phases of data collection in November 1998 and March 1999, the survey gathered data on fertility, family planning, maternal and child health, utilization of health services, women's autonomy, reproductive health and nutritional status. One unique feature of the survey was blood testing for haemoglobin levels, which made it possible to measure levels of anaemia among the respondents.

Key findings

The survey revealed that nearly one-third of female adolescents were ever married compared to only 6% of male adolescents. In addition, one-third of ever-married women aged 25–49 were married by age 15, while two-thirds were married by age 18. This situation remained unchanged since the NFHS-1 was conducted in 1991–1992. For the majority of women in the age group 25–49, the age at first cohabitation with their husbands was 17 years, but it varied from 15 years in Andhra Pradesh to 23 years in Goa.

During the last 15 years, there has been a 33% decline in adolescent fertility. Nevertheless, currently married adolescent women (aged 15–19 at the time of the survey) reported 4209 births during the three years preceding the survey, one-fourth of which were second or higher order births. This indicates the extent of physical strain on these women at a tender age. The NFHS-2 found wide regional variations in adolescents' contribution to total fertility rates, however. In states such as Maharashtra, Madhya Pradesh and Andhra Pradesh, the share of total fertility contributed by adolescents was between 21% and 29%. In contrast, the corresponding share in Goa, Kerala and Punjab was 10% or less.

Since the NFHS-1, the ideal reported family size among adolescents declined from 2.7 to 2.5 in the NFHS-2. Among currently married adolescent women, about 13% had ever used contraception and 8% were current users at the time of survey. About 7% of all sterilized women and wives of sterilized men were adolescents. About one-fourth of currently married adolescents had an unmet need for family planning, mostly for spacing. In light of these findings, intensive efforts to reach this group need to be given high priority.

The infant mortality rate (IMR) was much higher among children born to adolescent mothers compared to those born to mothers aged 15–49 (93 versus 73 dying before age 1 among 1000 live births). The neonatal mortality rate (risk of dying within the first month of life) was also higher for children of adolescent mothers, compared to children of mothers aged 15–49 (63 compared to 48 per 1000 live births). However, both the IMR and the neonatal mortality rate declined since the NFHS-1, which found an IMR of 107 and a neonatal mortality rate of 71 for children born to mothers below age 20.

In NFHS-2, adolescent mothers (those under age 20 at the time of delivery) reported a total of 7589 births during the three years preceding the survey. About two-thirds of these mothers reported receiving a check-up from a health professional and the recommended tetanus toxoid vaccination during their pregnancy; the corresponding figure for such health care in NFHS-1 was only 55%. In NFHS-2, 59% of adolescent mothers received an adequate supply of iron and folic acid (tablets or syrup), and nearly one-third of all births took place in institutional facilities, compared with one-fourth in NFHS-1. As for postpartum check-ups, 80% of all births outside institutional facilities to adolescent mothers were followed by a check-up within two months ofr delivery (Table 1).

Each of the two postpartum complications, massive vaginal bleeding and very high fever, were reported in about 13% of births by adolescent mothers during the three years preceding the survey (Table 2).

Two out of every five currently married adolescent women reported some reproductive health problem.

Table 1. Antenatal, natal and postnatal care received by mothers: comparison of adolescent mothers and mothers in other age groups (as a per cent of births* during three years preceding the survey, NFHS-2, India, 1998–1999)

Indicator	Woman's age (years)		
	< 20	20–34	35–49
All births to adolescent mothers*	*N = 7589*	*N = 23 469*	*N = 1335*
Per cent with no antenatal check-up (%)	31.7	33.6	54.9
Per cent that received two or more tetanus toxoid injections (%)	67.6	67.6	47.0
Per cent given iron and folic acid tablets or syrup (%)	58.8	58.4	36.6
Per cent that gave birth in institutional facility (%)	31.8	35.0	19.9
Per cent with delivery assisted by a health professional (%)	41.6	43.4	27.4
Non-institutional births to adolescent mothers	*N = 5148*	*N = 15 184*	*N = 1059*
Per cent of non-institutional births in which the mother had a postpartum check-up within two months after delivery (%)	18.1	16.4	10.5

*Refers to per cent of two most recent births during three years preceding the survey.

Source: *National Family Health Survey (NFHS-2), All India, 1998–1999.* India, Mumbai, International Institute for Population Sciences, USA, ORC MACRO.

Table 2. Postpartum complications among ever-married women, by age group (as a per cent of births* during 2–35 months preceding the survey, NFHS-2, India, 1998–1999)

	Woman's age		
Per cent* having postpartum complications within two months after delivery	**< 20 years old (*N* = 7311)**	**20–34 years old (*N* = 22 329)**	**35–49 years old (*N* = 1262)**
Massive vaginal bleeding (%)	12.2	10.5	11.2
Very high fever (%)	13.3	12.3	15.9

*Refers to two most recent births during 2–35 months preceding the survey.

Source: *National Family Health Survey-2, All India, 1998–1999*. India, Mumbai, International Institute for Population Sciences, USA, ORC MACRO.

Among ever-married women of age 15–19, one out of every four had abnormal vaginal discharge, and one out of every six reported symptoms of urinary tract infections. Among currently married women almost the same proportion (16%) reported experience of painful intercourse, but only 4% reported bleeding after intercourse. The percentage of currently married adolescent women reporting any reproductive health problem was somewhat lower (37.9%) than for ever-married women aged 15–49 (39.2%), but younger women may be less likely to report such problems. These figures need to be interpreted with caution; they represent only women's reports of symptoms experienced and were not corroborated by laboratory tests or clinical examination (Table 3).

Being stunted (height below 145 cm) and having a body mass index (BMI) below 18.5 kg/m^2 (weight in kilograms divided by height in metres squared) indicate poor nutritional status. The survey found that about 15% of ever-married adolescent women were stunted. Nearly two of every five adolescent ever-married women had a BMI below 18.5 kg/m^2. Based on measures of haemoglobin levels, the survey found that one of every five ever-married adolescent women had moderate or severe anaemia, which is a matter of serious concern.

Table 3. Health status and symptoms of reproductive health problems among married women*, by age group, NFHS-2, India, 1998–1999

Age group (years)	**Any abnormal discharge (%)**	**Symptoms of urinary tract infections (%)**	**Any reproductive health problem* (among currently married women) (%)**	**Stunted (with height below 145 cm) among ever-married women (%)**	**Chronic energy deficiency (BMI below 18.5 kg/m^2 among ever-married women (%)**	**Any anaemia** (%)**	**Moderate anaemia** (%)**	**Severe anaemia** (%)**
15–19	26.2	16.1	37.9	14.7	38.8	56.0	17.9	1.9
20–24	29.3	17.1	39.7	13.0	41.8	53.8	17.0	2.0
25–29	32.5	18.3	41.6	12.4	39.1	51.4	14.7	1.9
30–34	33.2	18.6	41.9	12.3	35.0	50.5	13.7	1.9
35–39	32.2	18.1	40.5					
40–44	27.3	18.0	35.7	3.7	31.1	50.5	13.6	1.9
45–49	20.7	15.5	30.3					
15–19	*N= 8182*	*N=8182*	*N=8014*	*N=6707*	*N=6707*	*N=7117*	*N=7117*	*N=7117*
15–49	*N=81149*	*N =89 199*	*N=83 649*	*N=77 119*	*N=77 119*	*N=79 663*	*N=79 663*	*N=79 663*

* "Any reproductive health problem" refers to currently married women. All other columns refer to ever-married women; **Any anaemia: haemoglobin level below 10.9 g/dl for pregnant women and below 11.9 g/dl for non-pregnant women. Moderate anaemia: haemoglobin level 7.0–9.9 g/dl. Severe anaemia: haemoglobin level less than 7.0 g/dl.

Source: *National Family Health Survey-2, All India, 1998–1999*. India, Mumbai, International Institute for Population Sciences, USA, ORC MACRO.

Fewer than two out of every five adolescent ever-married women had heard about AIDS. Among those who had heard of it, 80% had heard about it from television; however, 45% of ever-married adolescent women had not been exposed to any media. One-third of those who had heard of AIDS could not state how to avoid the infection. This suggests that intensive information, education and communication (IEC) activities for this vulnerable group should be given high priority.

Nearly one out of every three female adolescents was illiterate, while one out of five had completed at least a high school education. Nearly one-fourth were not involved in any decision-making in the household, and only two out of five were involved in decision-making about their own health care, which reflects the low level of autonomy that married adolescent women have in the Indian setting.

Conclusion

The NFHS-2 revealed many ways in which the reproductive health of married adolescent women needs to be improved. However, a single uniform strategy across India would not be successful, owing to extreme inter-state variations in reproductive health, average age at marriage, contraceptive use and decision-making. For example, among all ever-married women aged 15–49, only 2–3% were in the age group 15–19 years in Kerala and Himachal Pradesh. In contrast, the corresponding percentage in Madhya Pradesh and Bihar was as high as 12–13%.The proportion of adolescent women using contraception ranged from 2–4% in Bihar and Rajasthan to 33% in West Bengal. In Maharashtra and Madhya Pradesh, fewer than one-third (31%) of married adolescents were involved in decision-making about their own health care, but in Himachal Pradesh and Punjab as many as 74–84% were involved. State-specific strategies targeted at married adolescent women are urgently required to ensure that young women receive antenatal, natal and postnatal services, as well as clinical testing for reproductive tract infections. Apart from these direct measures, what would really bring about change would be an effective strategy to empower married adolescents. Ideally, no adolescent girl would marry. Strict implementation of the law regarding legal minimum age at marriage as well as IEC activities to create awareness about reproductive health issues and to change attitudes are long-term solutions.

References

International Institute for Population Sciences (1995) *National Family Health Survey (NFHS), 1992–1993.* India, Mumbai, IIPS.

International Institute for Population Sciences, ORC MACRO (2000) *National Family Health Survey (NFHS-2), All India 1998–1999.* India, Mumbai, IIPS, USA, ORC MACRO.

Professor Sumati Kulkarni
Consultant to ORC-MACRO & PRB
Retd. Professor, IIPS. Mumbai,
E-2, Himachal Housing Society,
Sector 17, Plot 22, Vashi,
Navi Mumbai - 400 703

Pregnancy and postpartum experience among first time young parents in Bangladesh: preliminary observations

Syeda Nahid M. Chowdhury

Background

The majority of adolescents in South Asia who bear children do so within marriage, and young couples generally face social pressure to have a child soon after marriage. As relatively new family members, young mothers are isolated and vulnerable. They have limited control over their lives and lack social support. However, the first birth may offer a unique opportunity to improve the prospects of young mothers. Because the young women are about to give birth to the next generation, husbands and husbands' families may be open to new information and behaviour change.

This paper presents preliminary findings from the first phase of a study that was designed to increase understanding of the sociology of the first birth. The second phase will use these findings to develop and test interventions to make services more responsive to young mothers' needs. During the qualitative phase of this research, we focused on the roles and influence of spouses, mothers-in-law, and other family members, in an attempt to understand why young women do not access health services, breastfeed, or have safe sex. The study also focused on the vulnerability that comes with girls' young age and position in the family and how the young women's social status affects the first birth and vice versa.

Methods

The study is being carried out in 24 villages in southeast Bangladesh. The area is predominantly Muslim and has a population of over 28 000 people. Researchers randomly selected eight of the 24 villages and identified all 40 households in those villages that had young, first-time pregnant or postpartum women. In-depth interviews were then conducted with the young women, their husbands, senior women in the household including sisters-in-law and mothers-in-law, peers, and service providers. In addition, researchers conducted focus group discussions with husbands and peers. The study gathered information on issues such as marriage patterns; knowledge, attitude, and practices related to family planning, pregnancy and workload; food intake; mobility; social support; and health-seeking behaviours during pregnancy, delivery and post-partum.

Key findings

The young women interviewed included girls between the ages of 13 and 19. All had a few years of school education, but not all were married to literate men. Nearly all respondents, both men and women, mentioned that they would have liked to have married later, and some women had even pursued this issue with their parents or guardians.

In most cases, however, their requests were ignored. A father's death, a large number of daughters, and poor financial conditions influenced families' decision to marry their daughters early. Parents arranged the marriages, and girls did not get an opportunity to meet their prospective husband before marriage. Some men had had a chance to see their prospective bride, but again the decision depended on the parents. Dowries are common in this area and can involve cash or in-kind payments, as well as promises to help obtain jobs within or outside the country. To marry their daughters, families often agreed to the demands of the husband's family, which they then often failed to meet. Their inability to meet such demands affected the girls' relationships and position within the marital family.

In general, the young women in the study did not plan their pregnancies. All young women knew the name of some family planning methods, but none had actually used them. Their perception was that once they were married, they would have a baby. Many believed that getting pregnant soon after marriage was god's will. Mothers-in-law were aware that their daughters-in-law were not using family planning, but we found that they did not actively try to influence the young couples' decision-making. As one mother-in-law said, the "*husband and wife must decide, but they must take into consideration the opinion of the elders*". Nevertheless, in-laws had a general expectation that couples should have a baby soon after marriage. Even when young women expressed a desire to postpone childbearing, they did not necessarily delay pregnancy. One respondent said, "*I wanted a child after two or three years, but after one year when I did not conceive, my sister-in-law and neighbour started taunting me, saying that I was barren. That is why I wanted to have a baby.*"

The study gathered information on what changes occurred once girls conceived, especially in terms of food intake, workload and mobility. We found many food taboos in the community, but no evidence that young women were given extra food or particularly nutritious food during pregnancy. The young women tended to be in charge of cooking, but other family members were responsible for dishing out the food. As a result, pregnant girls had little control over their own food intake. Apart from work that required heavy lifting, young mothers continued to have a heavy workload during pregnancy. After delivery, their workload actually increased because they had to take care of the new child as well as do all the household work. The young women in the study expressed great unhappiness about this situation.

In general the young women had limited mobility, as these villages are fairly conservative. There are many taboos surrounding mobility during pregnancy. For example, pregnant women are not supposed to go out during the afternoon or evenings; nor are they supposed to go into the backyard of the house for fear that they might become possessed by evil spirits.

The study found that young women went to spiritual healers to protect them against possession by evil spirits, but none of the young women had gone for antenatal check-ups during their pregnancy, despite the presence of NGOs and government facilities in the area. In comparison, the 1996–1997 Demographic and Health Survey found that nationally, 71% of pregnancy women below age 20 received no prenatal care (Mitra et al., 1997). Young women in this study were not aware of the need for medical care during pregnancy or delivery. They had little idea about what to expect during pregnancy and delivery, and only vague ideas about possible complications.

Objections of in-laws and financial concerns were major barriers to seeking health care. The negative attitude of one mother-in-law towards prenatal care was captured in the following quote:

> *To go to a doctor you need money, after taking money they do not provide medicine... Everywhere there is a doctor. They only take money, but they know nothing.*

Most women expected to deliver at the marital home aided by a traditional birth attendant, as is the norm in these communities. Mothers-in-law make this decision, however, and young women do not have any say in the matter.

Conclusions

Researchers hope that this study will shed light on the sociology of first birth in rural Bangladesh. Preliminary findings reinforce the need for interventions to take into consideration young women's social networks. Once researchers finish analysing the qualitative data, they will design an intervention to investigate whether they can a) increase the level of agency through social support and health programmes, and b) adapt health services to reflect the realities and needs of first time mothers.

Reference

Mitra SN, Al-Sabir A, Cross AR, Jamil K (1997) *Bangladesh Demographic and Health Survey 1996–1997*. Dhaka, Bangladesh, National Institute of Population Research and Training [NIPORT].

Dr Syeda Nahid M.Chowdhury
Programme Manager
Operations Research
Reproductive Health Alliance Europe
443 Highgate Studios
53–79 Highgate Road
London NW5 1TL
United Kingdom

Early marriage and childbearing: risks and consequences

Ramesh K. Adhikari

Background

In South Asia, early marriage is a social norm, and marriages are expected to result in childbirth within a few years of couples living together. It is important to review how this influences the physical and social well-being of young women in order to develop relevant policies and programmes. This paper reviews several studies from Nepal, including the 1996 Nepal Family Health Survey (NFHS) (Nepal Ministry of Health et al., 1996), a 1994 longitudinal study of factors influencing the nutritional status of adolescents, several hospital-based studies on outcomes of adolescent pregnancy, as well as information from the international literature. The paper highlights the physical and social consequences of early marriage and childbearing among women aged 15–24 and puts forward some recommendations for policy consideration. For the purpose of this paper, adolescents are defined as the age group 15–19 years, young adults as the age group 20–24 years and youth as the age group 15–24 years.

Adolescents and the youth population in Nepal: some characteristics

Historically, child marriages were common in Nepal, and the 1971 census noted that 2.4% of children aged 6–9 were married. After 1962, the legal minimum age for marriage was raised to 16 and 18 years for women and men, respectively, with parental consent, and 18 and 21 years without consent. Mean age at marriage has increased from 15.4 years in 1961 to 18.1 years in 1991, though there is great geographic variation among districts in Nepal, ranging from 15.1 to 23 years (Thapa et al., 1997). According to the 1996 NFHS, nearly half (44%) of all female adolescents were married in 1996. Early marriage almost always leads to early childbearing. Over half (54.3%) of the married adolescent girls in the 1996 NFHS were already mothers or were pregnant, as were 90% of married young adult women aged 20–24.

Nationwide information about the nutritional status of adolescents is not available; however, one study conducted in three remote rural areas found that the majority of adolescent girls were stunted and undernourished, including 72% of girls aged 10–14 and 45% of girls aged 15–18. The majority (70%) of younger girls had a body mass index (BMI) less than 5%, as did 15% of girls aged 15–18. The same study found that adolescent girls achieved menarche later and continued to grow beyond the period when girls in the reference population stopped gaining height, and the final height attained by the majority of girls remained below the third percentile (Regmi & Adhikari, 1994). Similar observations have been reported from other developing countries, including Colombia, Guatemala and India (Kurz, 1996).

Health consequences of early marriage and childbearing

It is generally accepted that childbearing among women aged 15–19 doubles the risk of death due to pregnancy-related causes compared to women in their twenties (Population Reference Bureau, 2000). Hospital-based studies from Nepal have shown an association between teenage pregnancy, pregnancy-induced hypertension and anaemia. The same studies found that fetal loss and abnormal deliveries were higher among teen mothers (Malla & Shrestha, 1996). The percentage of pregnant women attending antenatal care (ANC) is low in Nepal, probably due to a lack of adequate services. Even in urban areas, where health facilities are within easy reach, pregnant adolescents attend antenatal facilities at lower rates than adult women (Adhikari & Amatya, 1996).

Several studies from Nepal have documented poorer outcomes for children born to adolescent mothers compared to older mothers. The NFHS found that neonatal mortality among children of adolescent mothers was 73% higher than children of older mothers, and 25% higher than children of mothers aged 30–39. Studies have also found a 25%–66% higher incidence of low birth weight among children of adolescent mothers (Dali et al., 1989; Adhikari & Amatya, 1996). One hospital-based study found a perinatal mortality rate that was twice as high among children of adolescent mothers compared to children whose mothers were older than age 19 (40.5 versus 18 per 1000 births) (Adhikari & Amatya, 1996). In addition, evidence suggests that children of older adolescents (aged 17–19) fare better than those born to younger adolescents (aged 16 or younger), when outcomes such as low birth weight and pre-term birth are compared (Dali & Pradhan, 1992).

Social consequences of early marriage and childbearing

In addition to health consequences, early marriage and childbearing have consequences for women's education. Although literacy among youth has gradually increased over the years, only 55% of adolescents and 44% of young adults were literate as of 1991, according to the National Census (Central Bureau of Statistics, Nepal, 1995). The 1996 NFHS found a gender difference in schooling levels. Only 15% of male adolescents had never attended school compared to 53% of female adolescents. Women who marry "early" in their teens tend to have even fewer educational opportunities and a higher dropout rate. In the 1996 NFHS, 32% of women who had dropped out of school cited marriage as the reason for discontinuing school. The 1996 NFHS also revealed a close relation between education and childbearing among adolescents. Thirty-two per cent of illiterate adolescents had already begun childbearing, compared to only 10% of those who had secondary education.

Finally, women who marry early and begin childbearing in adolescence are expected to have a higher total fertility rate (TFR), though contraceptive use may offset this. For example, although the teenage contribution to TFR is high in Bangladesh (18%) relative to Nepal (13%) and Pakistan (9%), the overall TFR in Bangladesh is relatively low (3.3) compared to Nepal (4.6) and Pakistan (5.6). The lower TFR among young Bangladeshi women is apparently due to the higher prevalence of contraceptive use among adolescents in that country (33%) compared to Nepal, India (both 7%) and Pakistan (3%) (Population Reference Bureau, 2000). Thus, until adolescent marriages can be delayed, adolescent-friendly contraceptive services may help keep down fertility rates.

International comparisons

Studies from Nepal seem to confirm that adolescent pregnancy confers higher risk for mothers and infants. Most studies from developing countries—including Dali & Pradhan (1992), Malla & Shrestha (1996) and Adhikari & Amatya (1996) from Nepal; Ambedkar et al. (1999) and Verma &

Das (1997) from India; Alam (2000) from Bangladesh; Weerasekara (1997) from Sri Lanka; Kumbi & Isehek (1999) from Ethiopia; and Adedoyin & Adetoro (1989) from Nigeria—also show that pregnancy in adolescence results in poorer obstetric outcomes compared to pregnancy during adulthood. However, studies from developed countries are not so definite. While some studies have reported poorer outcomes among younger adolescents, such as Amini et al. (1996), Brown et al. (1991) and Satin et al. (1994) from the United States of America, others have shown no difference or even better outcomes among late adolescents compared to older women. The latter includes Yoder & Young (1997) from the United States of America; Bradford & Giles (1989) from Australia; and Mukasa (1992) and Ncayiyana & ter Haar (1989) from South Africa.

Possible explanations for the difference between developing and developed country findings include the availability and quality of prenatal care and the poor nutritional status of adolescent girls in developing countries. A literature review by Kurz (1997) concluded that primiparity, continued growth during pregnancy, quality of obstetric antenatal care and poor socioeconomic status are major risk factors associated with poor outcomes of adolescent pregnancy. This was supported by a World Health Organization analysis of 25 studies, which found an association between pre-term birth and the mother's nutritional status. That analysis concluded that women with a pre-pregnancy weight and height of less than 45 kg and 145 cm, respectively, were more likely to bear low birth-weight or premature infants (World Health Organization, 1995).

A few studies—including some from developed countries—have reported that pregnant adolescents continue to grow during their pregnancy, and apparently their growth competes with the fetus for nutrients (Scholl et al., 1994). Thus, continued growth during pregnancy due to stunting may be one reason there is a higher incidence of low birth weight and pre-term birth occurs among adolescent mothers compared to adult mothers in developing countries but not in developed countries. Low gynaecological age (defined as conception within two completed years of menarche), in particular, has been reported as an important factor responsible for almost double the risk of having a preterm birth and low birth weight babies (Scholl et al., 1989). Given that large numbers of girls in Nepal are malnourished and reach menarche at an average age of 13.2 years, these research findings suggest that girls who become pregnant before age 15 are at higher risk of having a premature or low birth weight baby.

Another important explanation for poor obstetric outcomes among adolescent mothers is the lower use of prenatal care compared with use by adult women. Findings from Nepal consistently show that the percentage of adolescents seeking antenatal care is lower compared to adult mothers, even though most adolescents have children within wedlock. The reasons for this are unclear, but could include poor social status of young women in their husbands' families, or a tendency for adolescents to hide their pregnancies. It is essential to identify these factors so that obstetric services can be made more adolescent friendly.

Conclusions

Adolescent girls who delay marriage and childbearing benefit by completing their own growth first. They avoid putting themselves and their babies at risk of nutritional deprivation. This evidence points to a need for programmes such as the following:

a. Because early marriage and childbearing are associated with less education and lower future income for young mothers, programmes that keep girls in school should be promoted. The attainment of higher levels of education by young women can be expected to yield a greater use of reproductive health services and better employment prospects.

b. Parents and community members need to be informed about the adverse health and social consequences of early childbearing, as well as the benefits of delaying marriage and childbearing until at least two completed years after menarche.

c. Where marriage in adolescence continues, promoting contraceptive use can delay childbirth until the couple is physically, socially and emotionally ready to bear a child. Therefore, there is a need for reproductive health services, particularly adolescent-friendly family planning.

d. Programmes to improve the economic status of adolescent women can bring about positive change, since economic factors may lie behind early marriage and childbearing.

References

Adedoyin MA, Adetoro O (1989) Pregnancy and its outcome among teenage mother in Ilorin, Nigeria. *East African Medical Journal*, 66(7):448–452.

Adhikari N, Amatya A (1996) Outcome of adolescent pregnancy. Paper presented at *8th Congress of Pediatrics, Kathmandu, Nepal.*

Alam N (2000) Teenage motherhood and infant mortality in Bangladesh: maternal age dependent effect of parity one. *Journal of Biosocial Science*, 32(2):229–236.

Ambedkar NN et al. (1999) Teenage pregnancy outcome: a record based study. *Indian Journal of Medical Science*, 53(1):14–17.

Amini SB et al. (1996) Births to teenagers: trends and obstetric outcomes. *Obstetrics and Gynaecology*, 87(5):668–674

Bradford JA, Giles WB (1989) Teenage pregnancy in western Sydney. *Australian and New Zealand Journal of Obstetrics and Gynaecology*, 29(1):1–4.

Brown HL, Fan YD, Gonsoulin WJ (1991) Obstetric complications in young teenagers. *Southern Medical Journal,* 84(1):46–48.

Central Bureau of Statistics, Nepal (1995) *Population Monograph of Nepal*. Kathmandu, Nepal.

Dali S et al. (1989) *A Study of Low Birth Weight at TUTH*. Kathmandu, TU Institute of Medicine.

Dali SM, Pradhan N (1992) Obstetric performance of adolescent pregnancy at TUTH. *Journal of the Institute of Medicine,* 14(1):13–19.

Kumbi S, Isehek A (1999) Obstetric outcomes of teenage pregnancy in northwestern Ethiopia. *East African Medical Journal*, 76(3):138–140.

Kurz K (1996) Adolescent nutritional status in developing countries. *The Proceedings of the Nutrition Society,* 55:321–331.

Kurz K (1997) *Health Consequences of Adolescent Childbearing in Developing Countries,* ICRW working paper number 4. Washington, DC, International Center for Research on Women.

Malla DS, Shrestha PL (1996) *Adolescent Pregnancy and Its Outcome*. Mimeograph published by Maternity Hospital, Kathmandu, Nepal.

Mukasa FM (1992) Comparison of pregnancy and labour in teenagers and primigravidas aged 21–25 years in Transkai. *South African Medical Journal*, 18; 81(8):21–23.

Ncayiyana DJ, ter Haar G (1989) Pregnant adolescents in rural Transkai: age per se does not confer high-risk status. *South African Medical Journal*, March 4; 75(5):231–232.

Nepal Ministry of Health, New Era, Macro International Inc. (1996) *Nepal Family Health Survey*. Kathmandu, Nepal Ministry of Health, Department of Health Services, Family Health Division and New Era, Macro International Inc.

Population Reference Bureau (2000) *The World's Youth 2000*. Washington, DC, Population Reference Bureau.

Regmi SC, Adhikari R (1994) *A Study on the Factors Influencing Nutritional Status of Adolescent Girls in Nepal,* Research paper series number 6. Washington, DC, International Center for Research on Women.

Satin AJ et al. (1994) Maternal youth and pregnancy outcomes: middle school versus high school age groups compared with women beyond the teen years. *American Journal of Obstetrics and Gynecology*, 171(1):184–187.

Scholl TO, Hediger ML, Ances IG (1990) Maternal growth during pregnancy and decreased infant birth weight. *American Journal of Clinical Nutrition*, 51(5):790–793.

Scholl TO et al. (1989) Association between low gynaecological age and preterm birth. *Paediatric Perinatal Epidemiology*, 3(4):357–366.

Scholl TO et al. (1993) Maternal growth during pregnancy and lactation. *Hormone Research*, 39(Suppl. 3):59–67.

Scholl TO et al. (1994) Maternal growth during pregnancy and the competition for nutrients. *American Journal of Clinical Nutrition*, 60(2):183–188.

Thapa S, Acharya LB, Aryal RH (1997) Schooling, marriage, work and childbearing among the youth population of Nepal: Emerging insights and challenges. Mimeograph presented at the *1997 Workshop on Youth Across Asia, Kathmandu.*

Verma V, Das KB (1997) Teenage primigravidae: comparative study. *Indian Journal of Public Health*, 42(2):52–55.

Weerasekara DS (1997) Adolescent pregnancies—is the outcome different? *Ceylon Medical Journal,* 42(1):16–17.

Yoder BA, Young MK (1997) Neonatal outcomes of teenage pregnancy in a military population. *Obstetrics and Gynaecology*, 90(4):500–506.

World Health Organization (1995) Maternal weight gain and pregnancy outcomes. *Bulletin of the World Health Organization*, Suppl. Vol. 73.

Ramesh K. Adhikari
Professor in Child Health
Institute of Medicine
Maharajgunj Campus
Post Box No. 2533
Kathmandu
Nepal

Newly married adolescent women: experiences from case studies in urban India

Annie George

Background

Newly married women in India are, by and large, adolescent women. As Jejeebhoy (1998) noted in her review of literature on adolescents, the situation of adolescent women is particularly precarious, as they tend to have limited education, skills and opportunities for employment. They have relatively poor health and limited access to good nutrition, and many are caught in a cycle of early marriage and child- bearing. Marriage adds dramatic changes to their lives that involve their bodies, emotions, and daily life experiences. These changes often occur in unfamiliar surroundings among virtual strangers, as a large proportion of marriages in India are patrilocal and arranged by family elders. Yet, as marriage is customarily accorded central significance in the lives of Indian women, newly married adolescent women are aware that they have to "adjust" to the multiple changes in their lives. How do they deal with marriage and the changes it brings? What do they know of, and how do they handle new bodily experiences? What actions do they take to be subjects of their new bodily experiences? In this paper, in an attempt to answer some of these questions, I present and interpret adult women's recollections of their experiences as newly married adolescents.

Methods

This paper is based on two qualitative data sets with similar methods and participants. Both studies gathered information about the adult sexual lives of working class women in Mumbai, and both asked women about their early marital lives. However, this was not the focus of either study and it required recall of events that happened many years in the past. Hence, the data have certain limitations with respect to adolescent marital experiences. One study gathered data in 1991–1992, using *repeated focus group discussions* with 35 women, divided into 6 groups (George & Jaswal, 1995). The participants in the focus groups were clients or employees of various nongovernmental organizations (NGOs) that worked for poor people in Mumbai. The women's ages ranged from 20 to 40 years, and the average age at marriage was 15 years. Sixteen were illiterate; the rest had at least five years of schooling and one was a graduate. At the time of the study, 25 out of 35 women were married and the rest were widowed, deserted, separated or divorced. Nineteen women were Hindu, 11 women were Buddhist, and the rest had other religious affiliations. Twenty-two women were engaged in wage-earning activities like rag picking, cleaning homes and offices, and working as community workers for NGOs.

The second data set was gathered in 1996–1997 using *repeated in-depth interviews* with 65 women (George, 1997). Each respondent was interviewed an average of three times, with interviews lasting half an hour to two hours each. Participants in the in-depth interviews were purposively selected with the help of NGOs. The 65 participants ranged in age from 20 to 38 years. Forty-seven were literate; on average, they had five years of schooling. Thirty-six women were gainfully employed and one in three was the primary wage earner. The average age at marriage was 16 years. On average, each had been married for twelve years and had three children. Marital discord had led 22 of the 65 women to be separated from their husbands at least once during the marriage.

Key findings

In narratives of their first sexual experiences, women typically present themselves as one of four types of brides: reluctant, shy, fearful or pragmatic. Elements of each scenario overlap, and I make these distinctions merely for analytical purposes. Each of these scenarios is presented below.

Reluctant brides: "I was tricked into it." In this type of narrative, women describe themselves as innocents who were tricked into sex. In most cases, the typical story is that the woman had no knowledge about sexual relations, and had to be "tricked", usually by older kinswomen from the husband's family, into being in the room where her husband was waiting for her. In some narratives, older women are portrayed as "accomplices" of the husband, helping the eager husband consummate the marriage. In other narratives older women were presented as the decision-makers, who decided when a married couple could start cohabiting. In these cases, the newly married women had either just attained, or not yet attained puberty. These narratives can be read in multiple ways. On the one hand, the narratives suggest that if the women were knowledgeable about sex, they probably would not *consent* to it; they had to be forced into sex through trickery. On the other hand, the narratives also suggest that, following the dominant discourse on ideal womanhood, the women wanted to present themselves as good women, who had to be robbed of their innocence. However, such processes are not totally violating, and some narratives portray husbands as responsive to their wives' wishes and experiences of pain, fear and shyness.

Shy brides: "Daily sharam." In these narratives, women used the word '*sharam*' and '*laaj vatene*', translated here as 'shyness' and 'being or feeling shy' to describe their feelings about sexual relations. The word 'shy' does not capture the complexity of the term '*sharam*', which contains connotations of sexual modesty, femininity, virtue and honour. Shyness did not stem from lack of sexual knowledge alone, although most women did not know the details about sexual intercourse prior to marriage. Shyness also arose from the social situations in which newly married adolescent women found themselves. For instance, SEM[1] had her first sexual relations in the in-laws' house in the village. Everybody was around, and so she felt strange, scared and shy. Cultural practices, such as sharing the same room and having a bath after sexual activity, were means by which family members could easily know whether a couple had had sexual relations. This invasion into their privacy, along with restricted private space, and the presence of family members who were strangers to the newly married adolescent women, all added to their sense of '*sharam*'. Families often exerted pressure on the couples to be sexually active, adding to their sense of shyness.

Fearful brides: "What will happen? How will it be?" The word '*darr*' or '*bhiti*', translated as 'fear', were frequently used in the narratives to describe a newly married adolescent woman's sexual experience. One woman from the focus group discussion study described her experience by

1 All names are pseudonyms.

saying: *"I was scared. I felt he would beat me if I refused. I did not like sleeping with him, right under my mother-in-law's cot. I felt he was using force on me. There was no need to sleep so soon in front of everyone. But he never experienced any shame, and my mother-in-law would tell me that I should go to my husband, I am no longer small."* Participants in the in-depth interview study spoke about the conditions that caused newly married adolescent women to fear sexual life. As one participant described, "*When I am with some unknown person, then one is going to feel fear isn't it? I felt fear. I had pain and bleeding the first time.*" Another condition causing fear was ignorance of exactly what sexual relations entail. Even when women had information about sexual relations, however, it did not necessarily decrease their fear. Most women said that their fear vanished as sex became a 'habit'. Fear of the unknown person, bodily experience, and its consequences decreased over time with increasing familiarity.

Pragmatic brides: "This is married life." Although the sexual experiences of newly married adolescent women may or may not have been framed by fear or shyness, all the women learned that sexual intercourse was a necessary component of marriage and of their identities as married women. As one woman described, "*Many women explained to me that **if you do this, a woman has a life*** [emphasis added] *or else he will move away from you. They would all say this.*" This woman narrated clearly what many other women also learnt—that if a woman complies and provides sex whenever the man wants, then she "has a life". "*My friends and family told me (right before her first sexual experience), don't make a noise, you must bear the touch of a man. This man has married and brought you here for this.*" These narratives show the disciplining nature of early sexual experience, which enjoys social sanction and which married women learn through frequent bodily experience. Women in the focus group expressed the precarious nature of their existence, which one woman expressed as follows: "*A woman needs some support. How long will her parents support her? So, a woman like me will say, 'if I've got to have clothes to wear and food to eat, then you do whatever you want (with my body) but keep me as a wife should be kept.'*" If women do not live up to the expectations of a wife, including being sexually available, then husbands can move their attention to other women who may be more willing. So, in order to have "a life", status, esteem and honour, married woman had to submit to the demands of their husbands.

Conclusions

The broader social context of newly married women of both data sets indicates that they were dependent on their husbands for social status and economic support, although they may also have been financial contributors to the household. They had limited contact with their birth families, and may have had limited social contacts and supports in their marital home. During the early days of marriage, newly married adolescent women and their husbands may have been under the authority of the husbands' parents and other older relatives, and thus had relatively limited autonomy to make decisions about their personal lives. The women's responses to their early married lives, when seen from these overlapping frames, shows a range of responses from selective compliance to selective resistance. However, I also argue that pragmatism, resulting from the precarious, tenuous nature of their social situation may be the dominant response of these women.

In summary, theories of the body can be used to read the sexual experiences of newly married adolescent women in Mumbai and point to the following general patterns. First, newly married adolescent women are disciplined into normal adult womanhood through embodied experiences of sexual relations. Second, women tend to be pragmatic and use such regulation to fashion their identities as normal, good wives. Third, women's emotions mediate between their social contexts and their sense of control over their life situations. Finally, newly married women's bodies are sites where individual, cultural and political conditions meet and are expressed in the form of bodily experience of pleasure, pain, illness or health. Women's bodies, therefore, have the potential for personal and social transformations. These observations are all reasons for undertaking more rigorous, culturally appropriate social science investigations into the sexual behaviour, knowledge and reproductive health decision-making authority of differently situated adolescent women and men.

References

George A (1997) *Sexual Negotiation and Sexual Decision-making among Poor Women and Men in Mumbai. An Exploratory Study*. Baroda, Sahaj Society for Health Alternatives.

George A, Jaswal S (1995) *Understanding Sexuality: Ethnographic Study of Poor Women in Bombay*. Women and AIDS Program Research Report Series No. 12. Washington, DC, International Center for Research on Women.

Jejeebhoy SJ (1998) Adolescent sexual and reproductive behavior: a review of the evidence from India. *Social Science and Medicine,* 46(10):1275–1290.

Further Reading

Bourdieu P (1990) *The Logic of Practice.* (Translated by Richard Nice). Stanford, California, Stanford University Press.

Bourdieu P (1997) *Outline of a Theory of Practice.* (Translated by Richard Nice). Cambridge, Cambridge University Press.

Butler JP (1993) *Bodies that Matter: On the Discursive Limits of "Sex".* New York, Routledge.

Foucault M (1979) *Discipline and Punishment: The Birth of Prison.* (Translated by Alan Sheridan). New York, Vintage.

Foucault M (1980) *The History of Sexuality, Vol. 1.* New York, Vintage.

George A (1998) Differential perspectives of men and women in Mumbai, India, on sexual relations and negotiations within marriage. *Reproductive Health Matters,* 6(12):87–96.

Goffman E (1969) *Strategic Interaction.* Philadelphia, University of Pennsylvania Press.

Grosz EA (1994) *Volatile Bodies: Towards a Corporeal Feminism.* Bloomington, Indiana University Press.

Hochschild AR (1983) *The Managed Heart: Commercialization of Human Feeling.* Berkeley, University of California Press.

Holloway W (1984) Gender differences and the production of subjectivity. In: Henriques J, Holloway W, Urwin C, Venn C, Walkerdine V, eds. *Changing the Subject: Psychology, Social Regulation and Subjectivity.* London, Metheun:228–252.

Lock M, Kaufert P (1998) Introduction. In: Lock M, Kaufert P, eds. *Pragmatic Women and Body Politics.* Cambridge, Cambridge University Press.

Lyon L (1996) C. Wright Mills meets Prozac: the relevance of 'social emotion' to the sociology of health and illness. In: James V, Gabe J, eds. *Health and Sociology of Emotions.* Cambridge, Massachusetts, Blackwell Publishers:55–78.

Mauss M (1985) Category of the human mind: the notion of person; the notion of self. In: Carrithers M, Collins S, Lukes S, eds. *Category of the Person.* Cambridge, England, Cambridge University Press:1–25.

Riessman CK (1993) *Narrative Analysis.* Newbury Park, California, Sage.

Scheper-Hughes N, Lock M (1987) Mindful body: a prolegomenon to future work in medical anthropology. *Medical Anthropology Quarterly*, New series, 1(1):6–41.

Scheper-Hughes N, Lock M (1991) The message in the bottle: illness and the micropolitics of resistance. *Journal of Psychohistory,* 18(4):409–32.

Turner B (1996) *The Body and Society*, 2nd ed. Thousand Oaks, Sage Publications.

Annie George
Department of Social & Behavioural Sciences
University of California, San Francisco
San Francisco, CA 94143
USA

IV

Sexual risk behaviours, perceptions and norms among unmarried adolescents: evidence from case studies

Risk behaviour and misperceptions among low-income college students of Mumbai

Leena Abraham

Background

Sexual behaviour studies of unmarried youth in India estimate that 19-28% of young men and 1–9% of young women have had (penetrative) sexual experience (Family Planning Association of India, n.d.; Watsa, 1993; Goparaju, 1993; Bhende, 1994; Rangaiyan, 1996; Abraham, 1998; Jejeebhoy, 1998). These studies indicate that premarital sex among young men is not as rare as commonly believed, while it continues to be comparatively rare among young women. Gender differences in sexual behaviour are not merely the result of over-reporting by men and under-reporting by women, but rather are the outcome of a sexual ideology that promotes male sexuality and controls female sexuality in India (Abraham, 1999). Studies have reported that young people form a significant segment of those attending sexually transmitted infection (STI) clinics and those infected by HIV (AIDS Research and Control Organisation, 1995; National AIDS Control Organisation, 1994; Ramasubban, 1992; Urmil et al., 1989); it is, therefore, important to understand the risk behaviour of young men and women. This article discusses data on sexual behaviour gathered among unmarried, low-income youth attending college in Mumbai during 1996–1998.

Methods

As sexual behaviour studies tend to focus on English-speaking students of 'elite' colleges, our study aimed to gather data from low-income students. The study was conducted in and around the premises of four colleges with co-ed, low-income student bodies. The colleges included both higher secondary (Junior College) and undergraduate courses (Senior College) in the arts, science and commerce streams. The sample consisted of students in their first year of higher secondary, who had just entered college, as well as students in their third year of Senior College, who had spent a minimum of four years in college. A majority of juniors were aged 16–18, and a majority of seniors were aged 20–22. This study design was chosen to ensure coverage of students with and without sexual experience.

In the first phase, researchers gathered qualitative data through focus group discussions (FGDs) and in-depth interviews with students from two of the four colleges. In the second phase, they conducted a survey among students from the other two colleges. A total of 75 students distributed in 10 groups took part in the FGDs, and each group participated in at least two 1– 1½ hour sessions. The FGDs explored students' social interaction, views on marriage, partners and premarital sex, sexual experiences and sources of information. The FGDs were followed by in-depth interviews with 87 students to gain more detailed information about their personal views and experiences. The qualitative data gathered in the first phase were used to design the structured, self-administered questionnaire, which was applied among a representative sample of boys and girls from the two classes mentioned. The final sample consisted of 966 students (625 boys and 341 girls). Researchers made the questionnaire available in both English and Marathi, the local language.

As stated above, the students in our study belonged to families of low socioeconomic background. The families lived in poor and crowded living conditions, very often in single-room tenements located in slums. The students belonged to different religious and ethnic groups. For instance, one college had a sizeable Muslim population, while the remaining three had a majority of Hindu students from various middle and lower castes. Students from middle class families constituted a minority in all four colleges. The students did not consider themselves to be "very religious", but considered their families to be "religious".

Key findings

Mixed sex peer groups were not common, and fewer girls than boys said they were members of mixed sex peer groups. However, friendships with the opposite sex can be established in different ways. Respondents distinguished three types of friendships with opposite sex peers: *bhai-behen*, 'true love' and 'time pass'. *Bhai-behen* is said to be a platonic relationship; 'true love' is a romantic one with the intention of marriage; and 'time pass' is a transitory sexual relationship (Abraham, 2000). The boundaries of these categories are fuzzy, and there are times when partners perceive the relationship differently, as well as instances when *bhai-behen* is used as a cover for other types of friendship. The extent of physical intimacy varies between each type of relationship from minimal physical intimacy (*hath masti* — 'hitting', 'shaking hands') in *bhai-behen* to sexual intercourse in 'time pass' relationships. In general, 'true love' does not involve intercourse but includes holding hands, touching, kissing and hugging.

In our study, we used the term 'any sexual experience' to refer to any of the following acts: kissing, hugging, touching genitals, sexual intercourse, anal or oral sex. According to FGD data, however, students did not consider kissing and hugging as 'sexual acts'. For most students, sexual behaviour or 'sex' meant vaginal intercourse, or oral and anal sex. Many students also considered 'touching' sex organs or being 'touched' by the opposite sex as a sexual act.

The survey data showed that many boys and girls had engaged in sexual acts of varying degrees of physical intimacy, but there were marked gender differences. While "any sexual experience" was reported by nearly half the boys (49%), only 26% reported sexual (vaginal) intercourse. Comparatively fewer girls reported either "any sexual experience" (13%) or sexual intercourse (3%) (Table 1).

Sexual partners of girls were peers, either as 'true love' or 'time pass' partners. Girls tended to be monogamous, except in some instances of 'time pass' relationships. Boys' sexual partners included peers (as both 'time pass' and 'true love' partners), commercial sex workers (CSWs) and older women, whom they called 'aunties'. Boys not only engaged in multiple partnerships but also explored different types of sex through these partnerships (Abraham, 1999). The sexual networks of boys depended on opportunities to meet different partners, peer influence, personal income, erotic exposure and leisure time available. The qualitative data showed five sets of sexual partnerships among boys, including: 1) only CSWs; 2) only 'time pass' partners; 3) 'true love' partners and CSWs; 4) 'time pass' partners, aunties and CSWs; and 5) a 'true love' partner. Except for the last category, which was the only reported monogamous relationship, all were multiple partner relationships, either

Table 1. Sexual experience of boys and girls

	Boys (*N* =625)		Girls (*N* =341)	
	Number	Per cent	Number	Per cent
Any sexual experience*				
Never	294	47	284	83.3
Ever	308	49.3	43	12.6
No response	23	3.7	14	4
Sexual intercourse				
Never	453	72.5	323	95
Ever	165	26	10	3
No response	7	1	8	2
Oral sex				
Never	500	80	324	95
Ever	105	17	9	3
No response	20	3	8	2
Anal sex				
Never	567	91	330	97
Ever	38	6	3	1
No response	20	3	8	2

* Includes kissing, hugging, touching genitals, sexual intercourse, anal or oral sex.

serially monogamous or simultaneous partnerships.

Survey and interview data showed that most boys had basic information regarding condoms; however, this knowledge did not lead to consistent condom use. Condom use and risk perception varied depending on the type of partner, the type of sex and the circumstances of the sexual experience. Among boys who had sexual intercourse, about 52% never used condoms with their "regular" partner, and 56% never used condoms with "casual" partners. Among those with multiple partners, none reported consistent condoms use with all partners (Table 2).

During interviews, boys said that they were more likely to use condoms with CSWs than with girlfriends or 'aunties'. Survey data suggest that sex worker contacts were probably under-reported by boys. Of the 29 boys who reported a CSW contact, 13 reported condom use at least once in these contacts; however, they were — in fact — less likely to report regular condom use than boys engaging in sex with girlfriends or other casual partners. Qualitative data suggest that boys did not use condoms in the first few instances of sex with CSWs. Their first experience was often unplanned and occurred under peer pressure. At that moment, condoms were not foremost on the youth's mind as much as fear of sex itself and fear of being found out by the family. However, in a few instances, the CSW insisted on condom use, and some boys reported that the brothels supplied the condoms. Condom use reportedly increased with

Table 2. Frequency of condom use among male students who reported sexual intercourse, by type of partner (*N*=165)

Frequency of condom use	Number	Per cent
***Regular partner* (*N*=165)**		
Never	85	52
Once	24	15
Sometimes	20	12
Always	20	12
No response	16	10
***Casual partner* (*N*=165)**		
Never	94	57
Once	12	7
Sometimes	17	10
Always	21	13
No response	21	13
CSWs/Call girls (N=29)		
Never	0	0
Once	13	45
Sometimes	4	14
Always	0	0
No response	12	41

Table 3. Reasons for non use of condoms among boys (*N*=125)

Reason	Number	Per cent
Not aware of condom	20	16
Sex suddenly happened	26	21
Condom reduces pleasure	19	15
Partner married, it is her responsibility	6	5
Condom not available	6	5
Feel shy to buy	7	6
Partner insisted not to use	2	2
Do not know how to use a condom	10	8
No response	29	23

subsequent experiences with CSWs, mainly out of fear of AIDS.

The survey explored boys' reasons for not using condoms (Table 3). Of the 125 boys who reported not using condoms, just over 23% did not give any reason. Others said that "sex suddenly happened" (21%), they were "not aware of condoms" (16%), or "condom reduces pleasure" (15%). Qualitative data suggest that low use of condoms could be due to situational factors, lack of information — particularly at the time of first sexual experience — and low risk perception associated with certain kinds of sexual partners.

Young men did not fear infection from sex with peers, although they did fear pregnancy. Sexual intercourse was rare in 'true love' relationships, and if it occurred, young people generally took precautions against pregnancy. Condom use in 'time pass' relationships was inconsistent. Boys said that they generally planned sex within a 'time pass' relationship and used condoms for fear of pregnancy, unless "sex suddenly happened" or they "got an unexpected chance for sex". Boys considered sex with 'aunties' to be the least risky, since the woman initiated the relationship and — in their view — was responsible for contraception. As a result, boys did not usually use condoms, according to focus group discussion data from third-year boys. They did not report using condoms during oral or anal sex with other males (though there were very few cases reported); nor did most boys think it was necessary to use condoms during oral or anal sex. In general, students did not have information about the potential risks of HIV/AIDS from unprotected sexual relationships with another male.

More than half the students who engaged in sex did not perceive any risk of contracting STIs, including HIV. This seemed to reflect ignorance about STIs as well as different perceptions of risk from different types of relationships. Boys who were not sexually active considered those who were active to be "at risk" and those who were sexually active considered those who visited CSWs to be "at risk". Some younger students mentioned sexual abstinence before marriage and avoiding certain partners such as CSWs or 'time pass' friends as effective measures of protection against HIV. Girls seemed to believe that abstaining from premarital sex not only preserved their *izzat* (honour) and ensured marital bliss, but also provided insurance against HIV. Projecting risks onto others and believing oneself to be immune from risks could increase their vulnerability to STIs by making young people less likely to take preventive measures against possible infection.

Conclusions

About one-fourth of boys in this particular sample had engaged in risky premarital sex, and their sexual networks included multiple partners and unsafe sex. They carried misperceptions about what constituted risky behaviour and therefore did not consider themselves at risk. Although many girls were aware that some boys had sexual relations with their peers and that some went to "red light areas", they did not perceive any risk of contracting HIV from their future partner or spouse. However, as long as boys continue to have unprotected sex within multiple, transitory relationships, including relationships with 'aunties', 'time pass' friends and CSWs, they are at risk of contracting STIs, including HIV, and are likely to pass on the infection to their spouse or other partners.

Acknowledgements: This study was funded by the Rockefeller Foundation and supported by the International Center for Research on Women. I acknowledge the cooperation of the students and the sincere efforts of the research staff.

References

Abraham L (1998) *Understanding youth sexuality: A study of college students in Mumbai*. Mumbai, Tata Institute of Social Sciences (unpublished report).

Abraham L (1999) Drawing the Lakshman Rekha: Gender dimensions of youth sexuality in urban India. Paper presented at the *International Conference on Sexualities, Masculinities and Culture in South Asia: Knowledge, Practices, Popular Culture, and the State*, organized by the School of Literary and Communication Studies, Deakin University, Melbourne, Australia.

Abraham L (2000) Bhai Behen, True love, Time-pass...friendships and sexual partnerships among youth in an Indian Metropolis. Paper presented at the *Workshop on Reproductive Health in India: New Evidence and Issues. Pune, India, Feb. 28–March 1.*

Abraham L, Kumar KA (1999) Sexual experiences and their correlates among college students in Mumbai City, India. *International Family Planning Perspectives*, 25(3):139–146.

AIDS Research and Control Organization (1995) *Summary Report of HIV Positive Cases*. Bombay, ARCON.

Bhende A (1994) A study of sexuality of adolescent girls and boys in underprivileged groups in Bombay. *The Indian Journal of Social Work*, LV(4)557– 571.

Family Planning Association of India (n.d.) *Youth Sexuality: A Study of Knowledge, Attitudes, Beliefs and Practices among Urban Educated Indian Youth, 1993–94*. Bombay, FPAI and SECRT.

Goparaju L (1993) Unplanned, unsafe: Male student's sexual behaviour. Paper presented at the *Workshop on Sexual Aspects of AIDS/STD Prevention in India*. Bombay, Tata Institute of Social Sciences.

Jejeebhoy S (1998) Adolescent sexual and reproductive behaviour: A review of the evidence from India. *Social Science and Medicine*, 10:1275–1290.

National AIDS Control Organisation (1994) *Country Scenario: An Update*. New Delhi, Government of India, Ministry of Health and Family Welfare.

Ramasubban R (1992) Sexual behaviour and conditions of health care: Potential risks for HIV transmission in India. In: Dyson T, ed. *Sexual Behaviour and Networking: Anthropological and Socio-Cultural Studies on Transmission of HIV*. Belgium, Deronaux – ordine:75–201.

Rangaiyan R (1996) *Sexuality and sexual behaviour in the age of AIDS: A study among college youth in Mumbai* [Doctoral Dissertation]. Mumbai, International Institute of Population Sciences.

Urmil AC, Dutta PK, Sharma KK, Ganguly SS (1989) Medico-social profile of male teenager STD patients attending a clinic in Pune. *Indian Journal of Public Health*, 33(4):176–182.

Watsa MC (1993) Premarital sexual behaviour of urban educated youth in India. Paper presented at the *Workshop on Sexual Aspects of AIDS/STD Prevention in India*. Bombay, Tata Institute of Social Sciences.

Leena Abraham
Tata Institute of Social Sciences, Mumbai
Post Box No. 8313
Sion-Trombay Highway
Deonar
Mumbai 400 088
India

Adolescent reproductive health in Pakistan

Yasmeen Sabeeh Qazi

Background

Adolescence is a formative time of transition to adulthood, roughly concurrent with the second decade of life. What happens between ages 10 and 19 shapes how girls and boys live out their lives as women and men—not only in the reproductive arena, but also in the social and economic realms. Throughout the world, girls and boys are treated differently from birth onward, but at puberty this gender divide widens. Boys enjoy new privileges, while girls endure new restrictions (Mensch, Bruce & Greene, 1998). In Pakistan, boys gain autonomy, freedom of movement, opportunity, and power (including power over sexual and reproductive lives of girls), while girls are systematically deprived of freedom and independent action. Only recently have the sexual and reproductive health needs of adolescents received attention in Pakistan. As part of an initial situation analysis, investigators conducted a study to explore unmarried adolescents' knowledge, attitudes and sources of information about sexual and reproductive health, as well as to assess levels of physical and sexual abuse.

Methods

Researchers conducted a pilot survey using face-to-face interviews among 310 unmarried young people aged 13 to 21 years. In addition to applying a structured questionnaire, interviewers were encouraged to discuss a series of issues with young respondents, and they recorded qualitative notes on these in-depth discussions. Respondents included 177 girls and 133 boys who were attending school, working or doing neither. Respondents were selected with the help of NGO (nongovernmental organization) staff working in the communities. In addition, researchers interviewed 110 parents and guardians about their perceptions of adolescents' behaviour and their suggestions for helping adolescents become responsible adults. To allow for regional comparisons, researchers gathered data in four provincial cities, including Karachi, Quetta, Swabi and Gujranwala, as well as from urban, periurban and rural areas.

Key findings

A majority of girls and boys reported that they had discussed "bodily changes" during puberty and menstruation with friends or family members. Those who did not tended to be younger respondents. More boys than girls seemed to know about changes during puberty among the opposite sex. One finding with implications for hygiene education was that girls reported feeling "dirty" during menstruation, which may reflect the common practice of refraining from washing during this time.

A majority of boys and girls reported having heard about or discussed pregnancy. Despite the fact that unmarried girls are not expected to talk about pregnancy in Pakistani culture, 81% of girls reported having done so. Not surprisingly, older girls were better informed. Fewer female respondents reported knowing ***how*** a woman becomes pregnant: 66% of girls versus 77% of boys. However, an awareness of the connection between pregnancy and menstruation did not necessarily mean that they understood the actual mechanics of pregnancy. For example, only half the boys knew that, after puberty, girls could get pregnant through a sexual relationship, and younger girls reported misconceptions such as the belief that kissing could cause pregnancy. In fact, only 58% of girls surveyed had discussed sexual intercourse, although researchers considered this figure relatively high given that sex is not often discussed openly in Pakistani society. A much higher percentage of boys (72%) than girls reported having discussed sexual intercourse (Table 1).

A majority of both boys and girls had discussed contraceptive methods, but twice as many boys (32%) as girls (15%) had ***not*** heard about or discussed contraceptive methods. The gender difference may reflect girls being told about the importance of marriage or having heard women in the family talk about contraceptives. However, girls and boys who had heard about contraceptives may not necessarily know how to use them. Contraceptive use (mainly condoms and pills) was extremely low—reported by about 5% of both girls and boys.

The young people were also asked about their knowledge of HIV/AIDS. Probably due to mass awareness campaigns, most respondents had heard of AIDS in a general sense, but they reported many misconceptions. For example, they thought that touching, kissing, holding hands, and using common washrooms could transmit HIV/AIDS.

When asked about information sources, about half (51%) of the girls stated that information about sex could be "most" effectively provided by a mother, father or guardian, while 40% said the same about a sister or brother. In contrast, only 30% of boys considered parents to be among the most informative sources, and a large proportion (41%) considered them to be among the least informative. Even fewer boys (21%) felt that siblings are among the most informative sources of information. This gender difference may reflect girls' tendency to discuss intimate matters with their mothers, while boys look outside their families for information. One finding that has relevance for sex education in the schools was that many young people (43% of girls and 36% of boys) perceived teachers to be the least informative about sex.

The survey also asked adolescents about physical and sexual abuse. About 66% of boys and 28% of girls said that they had experienced physical abuse, either by a family member or someone else. Of those who reported physical abuse, a majority said that their abuser was someone living with them—an adult, sibling or another teenager. More boys than girls reported physical abuse, but a higher proportion of cases among girls (65%) were perpetrated by adults living in the house, compared to 33% of the cases among boys. About 19% of girls and 14% of boys reported some kind of sexual

Table 1. Knowledge among young people of selected reproductive health topics

Health topic	Boys (N = 133)	Girls (N = 177)
Had discussed pregnancy (%)	86	81
Had discussed sexual intercourse (%)	72	58
Had discussed contraceptive use (%)	61	80
Said they knew how a woman becomes pregnant (%)	77	66

abuse. Given the sensitivity of the topic, this is probably an underestimate.

Conclusion

These study findings suggest that both male and female adolescents in Pakistan often lack knowledge about sexuality and reproduction, and are unprepared for the physical and emotional changes that take place during this period of life. During what is already a vulnerable time of transition, many young people experience physical and sexual abuse. Ideally, parents should provide information and guidance about sexual matters. However, given the social and cultural context in Pakistan, parents are often reluctant to discuss "sensitive" issues with their children. Policies and programmes could take several approaches to address the need for more education on sexuality and reproductive health. One way to do this may be to provide counselling to parents, to help them communicate more effectively with their children. Second, they can prepare other responsible persons such as teachers and health care providers to understand adolescent development and be able to provide appropriate information about sexuality and reproduction to adolescents.

Reference

Mensch BS, Bruce J, Greene ME (1998) *The Uncharted Passage: Girls' Adolescence in the Developing World.* New York, Population Council.

Yasmeen Sabeeh Qazi
Executive Director
PAVHNA (Pakistan Voluntary Health & Nutrition Association)
9C, 18th Commercial Street
Defence Phase II Extension, D.H.A.
Karachi-75500
Pakistan

The Influence of gender norms on the reproductive health of adolescents in Nepal—perspectives of youth

Cynthia Waszak, Shyam Thapa and Jessica Davey

Background

Gender norms are social rules for how females and males are supposed to behave within a given culture. In Nepal, as in other South Asian countries, these norms perpetuate a cycle in which many girls leave school early to become young wives. The 1996 Nepal Family Health Survey found that only 50% of girls had ever been enrolled in school, compared to over 80% of boys. Among the girls who did not complete secondary education, 57% cited marriage or pregnancy as reason for leaving school. In Nepal, 50% of girls marry before age 18, and early childbearing follows early marriage, usually within 18 months (Pradhan et al., 1997).

The effect of gender norms on reproductive health emerged as an important theme in focus group discussions (FGDs) conducted in 1999 as one component of the Nepal Adolescent and Young Adult (NAYA) study. The study focused on the effect of gender norms on access to schooling, work and familial expectations related to marriage and parenthood. This paper describes these norms and their effects from the perspective of Nepali youth.

Methods

Researchers held 72 focus group discussions in 11 districts with married and unmarried youth aged 14–22. FGDs were stratified by gender and marital status. In rural settings, researchers stratified the groups further by literacy/education level, whereas for urban settings, they stratified the sample by age group (14–17 and 18–22). Researchers purposively selected the 11 districts to encompass two major ecological regions (Hill and Terai), five development regions and urban–rural settings. The study districts represented diverse ethnic groups with Brahman and Chhetri having the largest shares (about 17% each). During FGDs, participants discussed issues relevant to the reproductive health of young people, including schooling, work, love, marriage, pregnancy, childbirth and their need for services (Thapa, Davey & Waszak, 2000). Researchers held the FGDs in school classrooms, hotel rooms and private homes. The FGDs were conducted in Nepali and generally lasted about one hour. Every effort was made to capture the essence of the young people's perspectives and to preserve the flavour of their expressions, proverbs and idiomatic phrases.

Key findings

Both girls and boys reported gender inequalities in decisions about schooling. They explained that parents were more likely to educate sons than daughters and often kept girls home to help with domestic chores or to look after younger siblings.

Girls were often kept at home to ensure that they remain chaste until marriage. Even when families had the economic means to educate both sons and daughters, they often sent boys to "good boarding schools" and kept daughters in local schools. One respondent explained why parents preferred to invest in sons' educations as follows:

> *People have the idea that if they educate a son, he will earn money and look after them later. Some parents feel that there is no use educating a girl, because one day she has to go off to her husband's place.* (Uneducated woman from urban Baitadi)

Some respondents suggested that attitudes may be changing in communities where girls were not "allowed to go to school" in the past. Many parents may actually want their daughters to go to school, but economic and social pressures are often too great. Female FGD participants spoke about the value of education for girls, saying for example:

> *We believe that if girls are educated, then they can support themselves and be independent. Also, if they are mistreated by their husbands, they will know about their rights and can seek help from them from the law. Likewise, they will be able to take care of their families properly.* (Married woman from rural Dhanusa)

Girls with no education were wistful about their lack of opportunity. A young woman with limited education from Dhankuta said, "*We could have learned many things if we were given the chance to study. Then we would not have to cut grass and collect firewood. We could teach others as well.*"

According to FGD participants, many parents took their daughters out of school in order for them to marry. Even when girls were not compelled to leave school upon marriage, increased household work and responsibilities inherent in early marriage and motherhood often made it difficult for girls to continue in school. In contrast, when boys discussed reasons for having to leave school, they were more likely to mention economic reasons rather than marriage. In fact, they suggested boys in poor circumstances were more likely to marry late, because they were expected to be financially independent before marriage.

Many parents experienced anxiety about getting their daughters married, according to the FGD respondents. In some cases, parents believed that they would fulfil their religious duties (*dharma kamaiencha)* by marrying their daughters early (*kanyadaan).* Others worried that if girls delayed marriage, it would become "hard to find a suitable bridegroom". In addition, much pressure for early marriage came from concern over a girl's **'character'**. The longer girls remained unmarried, the more chances there were of ruining their character and of reducing their chances of marriage. As one respondent described, many "*parents fear that she might run away with a man or have a love marriage, which will lead to their dishonour in the society.*" There is a proverb about why daughters should marry early:

> *Chori lai dherai rakhnu bhaneko dhoka ma pani bharnu jastai ho. Spilled water on the doorstep is very dangerous: anything can happen. Likewise, keeping daughters at home too long is very risky and dangerous.* (Young uneducated woman from Kapilbastu)

The young people in this study acknowledged a double standard in expectations for girls and boys, not only on the part of parents, but also of their peers. One participant explained why boys wanted to marry young girls, saying:

> *The boys do not want to get married to girls older than that as they think that older girls are not virgins. There is a greater chance of older girls having premarital sex. The boys always want to marry virgin* [chokho] *girls whether or not they are virgins themselves.* (Young man from urban Chitwan)

Because few parents allowed open courtship prior to choosing a spouse, adolescents who spent time with members of the opposite sex did so clandestinely. Girls "caught" talking to boys in public were criticized and sometimes punished by parents and the community for being characterless or "*randi*". An educated young woman from Bataidi said, "*If the boy and girl meet in an isolated place, then society blames the girl and says she has a bad character.*" Adolescents reported that premarital sex did take place, but out of the view of parents and the community. During the FGDs, more boys than girls discussed sex in the context of premarital romances. As one young man from Jhapa said, "*After the youth fall in love, they do everything married couples do. After they meet, they have sexual relationships and feel good when they meet each other.*"

Girls who engaged in a sexual relationship before marriage were unlikely to know how to protect themselves against pregnancy or sexually transmitted infections (STIs), since such information was considered inappropriate for unmarried girls. The consequences of unprotected premarital sex for girls in Nepal were often severe, especially if they got pregnant. The respondents said that a boy who fathered a premarital pregnancy was normally asked to marry the girl, and if he did not, "*... the girl's life is ruined. The news will spread fast in the village and the girl is helpless. It is hard for her to get married.*" In some cases, girls who get pregnant before marriage were "*married off to a widower or old man. Those men are given money to marry such girls.*"

Opinions varied among the focus group participants about the "ideal" age for marriage, but there was consensus that girls and boys needed to be older at marriage than they typically were. Regardless of the age at marriage, adolescents described the situation in Nepal as one in which girls and women were often powerless to make reproductive decisions. The participants explained that, unlike boys, girls did not generally have any choice about whom they would marry. More educated parents were more likely to give their daughters a say in marital decisions. Moreover, girls had little to say in decisions regarding sex or childbearing. As one educated woman from Dhankuta explained:

> *... if a woman does not feel like having sex, she has to do it anyhow if the man feels like it. Similarly, if the husband or the in-laws want a son, the woman has to keep giving birth until she has one. The decision depends entirely upon the family.*

When girls got married, they were often pressured to begin childbearing right away and were criticized if they did not. As a young woman in Jhapa described:

> *If the couples do not have children for a few years, the girl is called tharangi* [infertile] *and is considered unlucky. The community members will not even look at such a woman before doing something important for fear she will cause misfortune.*

The FGD participants described how early motherhood brought physical and social difficulties. They expressed particular concern about the treatment of young pregnant wives. While most adolescents in our study understood the need for good nutrition during the prenatal period, they noted that young pregnant wives from poor families suffered from a lack of food and mistreatment by their in-laws, especially mothers-in-law. As one unmarried woman from Dhankuta said:

> *Pregnant women are not cared for during their pregnancies as they are daughters-in-law. It is believed that the daughter-in-law should eat only after she feeds all the family members... The pregnant women have to go through a lot of hardships and sometimes sleep without having anything to eat.*

The participants described practices that contributed to poor health for pregnant girls, including the belief that "*the more you work, the lighter your body becomes and the easier it is in delivery*".

Though marriage practices and arrangements had more disadvantages for girls, marital expectations also posed challenges for boys. Boys faced difficulties in establishing their financial independence, considered necessary preparation for marriage. The need to find work before marriage resulted in longer periods of remaining single for boys than for girls. Financial pressures could result in boys having to migrate out of the area, even after marriage. The longer boys remained single, the more likely they were to engage in sex outside of marriage, placing themselves at risk of STIs in an environment that lacked adequate STI prevention education.

Conclusion

Worldwide data show a clear relationship between education and age at marriage (Singh & Samara, 1996), but the direction of causation is not clear. The findings of this study suggest that the causal relationships between lack of education, early marriage, low social status and poverty may be circular rather than linear. The family economic situation determines which families send children to school; gender norms then may determine which, if any, children in the family go to school. Even when schooling is available for girls, parents fear that more education will reduce their daughters' chances of finding suitable husbands. And for many, the well-being of the family is dependent on the marriage of their daughters according to local norms.

Regardless of the precise causal relationships, the consequences of early childbirth exacerbated by poverty include poor health outcomes for both the mother and the child (Hobcraft, 1987; Mensch, Bruce & Greene, 1998; Senderowitz, 1995). There also are health risks for girls who do not marry early (Singh & Samara, 1996). A longer period of being single may create risks of premarital pregnancy and STIs, especially in an environment in which information and services are not available to unmarried girls and boys, and in which there are severe social sanctions for girls who experience premarital pregnancy. Greater access to education for girls is a logical step towards delaying childbearing and creating better lives for girls.

Acknowledgements: Financial support for the Nepal Adolescent and Young Adult study was provided by the United States Agency for International Development (USAID) through Family Health International headquarters. The conclusions reached in this paper do not necessarily represent the views of USAID, the reviewers or the organizations with which the authors are affiliated.

References

Hobcraft J (1987) Does family planning save lives? Technical background paper prepared for the *International Conference on Better Health for Women and Children through Family Planning, Nairobi, Kenya*.

Mensch B, Bruce J, Greene M (1998) *The Uncharted Passage: Girls' Adolescence in the Developing World.* New York, The Population Council.

Pradhan A, Aryal Ram H, Regmi G, Ban B, Govindasamy P (1997) *Nepal Family Health Survey 1996,* Kathmandu, Nepal and Calverton, Maryland, Ministry of Health [Nepal], New ERA and Macro International Inc.

Senderowitz J (1995) Adolescent health: reassessing the passage to adulthood. World Bank Discussion Paper No. 272. Washington, DC, World Bank.

Singh S, Samara R (1996) Early marriage among women in developing countries. *International Family Planning Perspectives,* 22:148–157.

Thapa S, Davey J, Waszak C (2000) *Reproductive Health Needs of Adolescents and Youth in Nepal: Results from a Focus Group Study.* Kathmandu, Family Health International.

Further reading

Amin S, Sedgh G (1998) *Incentive Schemes for School Attendance in Rural Bangladesh.* Working Paper No. 106. New York, The Population Council.

Assaad M, Bruce J (1997) Empowering the next generation: girls of the Maqattam garbage settlement. *Seeds*, 119.

Barnett B, Stein J (1998) *Women's Voices, Women's Lives: The Impact of Family Planning.* Research Triangle Park, NC, Family Health International.

Jejeebhoy S (1998) Adolescent sexual and reproductive behavior: a review of the evidence from India. *Social Science and Medicine,* 46:1275–1290.

Luther N, Thapa S (1999) *Infant and Child Mortality in Nepal.* Kathmandu, Nepal, Family Health International.

Thapa S (1996) Girl child marriage in Nepal: Its prevalence and correlates. *Contributions to Nepalese Studies,* 23:361–375.

Thapa S, Acharya LB, Aryal RH (1997) Schooling, marriage, work, and childbearing among the youth population of Nepal: Emerging insights and challenges. Report prepared for the *Workshop on Youth Across Asia, Kathmandu, Nepal, 23–25 September 1997.*

Thapa S, Chhetry D, Aryal R (1996) Poverty, literacy and child labour in Nepal: A district-level analysis. *Asia-Pacific Population Journal,* 11:3–12.

Shyam Thapa, PhD
Director and Senior Scientist
Population and Reproductive Health
Family Health International
GPO Box 20520
Kathmandu
Nepal

Differences in male and female attitudes towards premarital sex in a sample of Sri Lankan youth

Kalinga Tudor Silva and Stephen Schensul

Background

In Sri Lanka, as in other societies in this region, strong norms persist that prohibit premarital sexual contact between young men and women. The taboo on sex has been particularly rigid for young women who are traditionally expected to maintain virginity until marriage and even to prove it as part of the marriage ceremony. However, this taboo has come under severe strain due to increasing age at marriage, increased opportunities for male–female contact in educational institutions, workplaces, etc. and greater exposure to new ideas about love and sex transmitted through the media.

Sri Lanka is characterized by relatively late age at marriage and has witnessed a considerable increase in marital age over the last 50 years, especially among women. At present, age at marriage is typically around 29 years for men and 27 years for women (Dissanayake, 2000*).* Along with this evidence of marital postponement, there is some indication of a decline in age at sexual debut (Silva et al., 1997). This study explored the ways in which young unmarried youth in Sri Lanka reconcile new ideas about love and premarital sex with traditional norms that disallow these behaviours. Specifically, the study explored the ways in which young unmarried people perceive love and sex, the extent to which young men and women hold different attitudes with regard to premarital sex, and the implications of these attitudes and behaviours for sexual health programmes targeted at youth.

Methods

To compare differences in the perceptions of low- and middle-income, and poorly and well educated young people, this study gathered data among respondents from two groups: youth from a low-income urban community, and university students from faculties of liberal arts and medicine. The sample consisted entirely of never-married youth and adults aged 17 to 28. The mean age for the urban community sample was 21 years, compared to 25 years for the university sample. Researchers chose this study design to ensure that the sample included respondents from a broad range of socioeconomic backgrounds. As education was considered an important factor leading to the postponement of marriage (Caldwell et al., 1989), the inclusion of community and university samples allowed researchers to study the impact of higher education on perceptions about sexuality and marriage.

The study used a mix of qualitative and quantitative research techniques. In the first phase, researchers gathered qualitative data through key informant interviews, open-ended interviews and pile sorting. The open-ended interviews involved a total of 156 youth including 93 university students (42 males and 51 females) and 63 community youth (30 males and 33 females). In the second phase, a larger and randomly chosen sample of youth participated in a self-administered survey. The survey sample consisted of 615 respondents, including 303 from the community (151 males and 152 female respondents) and 312 from the university (163 males and 149 females). Following the survey, a peer education intervention programme was implemented with a view to addressing the problems identified through qualitative and quantitative investigations. Findings of the larger study are presented in Silva et al. (1997) and Silva, Sivayoganathan & Lewis (1998). The results of the intervention programme have been discussed in Nastasi et al. (1999). Using survey findings and results of qualitative investigations, the present paper explores the attitudes of male and female respondents with regard to premarital sex.

Key findings

The study inquired of young respondents whether they were currently "in love". This group included those who were sexually active as well as those who were not. While 50% of the sample reported having a current love partner, this proportion varied from 30% and 49% among female and male university students respectively, to 51% and 63% among low-income female and male youth from the community.

While gender differences in the proportions of youth reporting a current love partner were apparent, they were not statistically significant. In contrast, attitudes towards premarital sexual activity differed significantly by gender even more widely than by class. For example, compared to female respondents, male respondents reported more favourable attitudes towards premarital sex (Table 1), and nearly half (46%) of male respondents agreed that it is acceptable to have sex if it does not destroy a girl's virginity, compared to only 14% of female respondents.

These findings clearly illustrate the intensity with which gender double standards persist. Virginity at marriage continues to be highly valued. It is therefore not surprising that young women—for whom the consequences of premarital sex are most profound—are more likely than young men to adhere to these norms. As revealed in key informant and semi-structured interviews, young men, on the other hand, while refraining from penetrative sex with their "love" partners, are indeed engaging in penetrative sex with casual partners, including older women and commercial sex workers.

Observed differences between the attitudes of university students and those of low-income youth were somewhat unexpected, although they were narrower than gender differences. The hypothesis that highly educated youth are less likely to hold traditional attitudes towards the acceptability of premarital sex than less educated youth is not

Table 1. Attitudes towards premarital sexual activity, by sex and study group

Per cent who agree or strongly agree with the following statements	Sex		Study group	
	Female *(N=301)*	Male *(N=314)*	Low-income *(N=303)*	University *(N=312)*
I would like to marry/be a virgin at marriage (%)	82**	57	68	70
It is wrong to destroy virginity before marriage (%)	76**	65	67*	73
It is acceptable to have sex if it does not destroy the virginity of a girl (%)	14**	46	33*	28

* Difference between the two groups is significant at the 0.05 level.

**Difference between the two groups is significant at the 0.01 level.

borne out in these data. Indeed, the data suggest that low-income and less educated young people are somewhat more likely than university students to approve of premarital sexual activity.

Finally, the study findings suggest that young people stop short of approving penetrative sexual activity with a committed or "love" partner. Even among those who approved of premarital sex, the vast majority was in favour of non-penetrative sexual practices that preserve female virginity.

Conclusions

Evidence from the study suggests that while young people in Sri Lanka do indeed engage in dating and establish committed "love" relationships, they also remain ambivalent about the nature of these relationships and the acceptability of premarital sex. Double standards persist and premarital sex among women continues to be considered unacceptable, especially by young women. Typically, young people resolve this conflict in two ways—either by engaging in non-penetrative sexual relations with "love" partners, or, in the case of young men, resorting to penetrative sexual activity with casual partners, including older women and sex workers. The extent to which these sexual behaviours are risky or protected remains an open question. Relations with casual partners and/or sex workers must certainly put young men at risk of infection and in a position to transmit infection to their "love" partners and future spouses. Sexual health programmes targeted at youth in Sri Lanka need to pay greater attention to issues such as non-penetrative sex, risks of sex with casual partners and the implications of the concept of female virginity in relation to sexual risks.

Acknowledgements: This study was supported by a grant from the International Centre for Research on Women. It was implemented by a multidisciplinary and international team from the Universities of Peradeniya (Sri Lanka) and Connecticut (USA).

References

Caldwell J et al. (1989) Is marriage delay a multiphasic response to pressures for fertility decline? The case of Sri Lanka. *Journal of Marriage and Family,* 51:327–335.

Dissanayake L (2000) Factors influencing stabilization of women's age at marriage. In: *Demography of Sri Lanka.* Colombo, Sri Lanka, Department of Demography, University of Colombo:45–58.

Nastasi BK et al. (1999) Community-based sexual risk prevention program for Sri Lankan youth: influencing sexual decision making. *International Quarterly of Community Health Education* 18(1):139–155.

Silva KT, Sivayoganathan C, Lewis J (1998) Love, sex and peer activity in a sample of youth in Sri Lanka. In: Hettige S, ed., *Globalization, Social Change and Youth.* Colombo, Sri Lanka, German Cultural Institute:34–52.

Silva KT et al. (1997) *Youth and Sexual Risk in Sri Lanka.* Women and AIDS Research Program Phase 11: Research Report Series No. 3. Washington, DC, International Center for Research on Women.

Dr Kalinga Tudor Silva
Professor of Sociology
University of Peradeniya
Peradeniya
Sri Lanka

Dr Stephen Schensul
Associate Professor
Department of Community Medicine
Center for International Community Health Studies
University of Connecticut
270 Farmington Avenue, Suite 260 MC 6330
Farmington, CT 06030-6330
USA

V

Unwanted sex: sexual violence and coercion

Sexual coercion among unmarried adolescents of an urban slum in India

Geeta Sodhi and Manish Verma

Background

While carrying out programmes in the Tigri area of Delhi, Swaasthya, a nongovernmental organization, identified adolescents as a particularly vulnerable group in terms of sexual and reproductive health (SRH). In order to design appropriate programmes, Swaasthya recognized the need to understand better the social context that influences adolescent sexual behaviour. Therefore, in 1996–1997, they conducted a qualitative study in an urban resettlement colony called Shantibaug (a pseudonym). The research objectives were to study unmarried adolescents' sexual behaviour, information needs and networks. In the course of the research, sexual coercion emerged as an important issue, even though this was not the original focus of the research. This paper describes the kinds of coercion faced by adolescents and the sociocultural factors that lead to coercion.

Methods

The sensitive topic of sexuality demanded a study with an 'emic' perspective, that is, from the point of view of adolescents themselves. To do this, researchers recruited adolescents from the community to collect ethnographic data from their peers. The study began with 5 – 10 key informant interviews, and researchers used these findings to develop in-depth interview and focus group discussion guidelines. They then conducted 71 in-depth interviews, 11 case studies (detailed life histories), and 15 follow-up interviews with boys and girls, most of whom were unmarried. Finally, researchers held eight focus groups to gather information on normative behaviour: four with boys and four with girls. Researchers translated the data from Hindi into English and coded the issues that emerged at the time of translation.

Key findings

The Shantibaug colony is home to about 15 000 people, generally from the lower socioeconomic bracket. A majority are Hindus with some Muslims, Christians and Sikhs. The prevailing culture is patriarchal, in which girls are seen as the family's *izzat* (honour) and are sometimes referred to as '*paraya dhan*' or someone else's property (i.e. their future husband's). Arranged marriages are the norm, and any perceived 'misdemeanour' on the girls' part may compromise their prospects of a 'good' marriage. As a result, families restrict girls' mobility and limit interactions with boys who are not part of the family.

Researchers chose the term "coercion" to encompass not only physical violation of individuals but also lesser (but often traumatic) manifestations such as teasing and harassment. During 71 in-depth interviews, respondents mentioned teasing 198 times and described 32 separate instances of more serious kinds of sexual coercion. Typically, groups of two to four boys tease girls who pass on the street. Teasing includes comments, singing film songs, whistling, shouting, waving, and making lewd sounds, suggestive hand gestures and facial expressions. Boys who lack other opportunities use teasing as a way to interact with girls. While teasing is mild compared to other issues discussed in this paper, it may reinforce attitudes about male dominance as boys become aware that society tolerates this behaviour. Most teasing goes 'unrewarded', but in a few cases it leads to friendships between boys and girls.

Girls in the study described matrimony and the desire for "true love", not sex, as reasons for entering relationships. A 14 year-old girl who had a boyfriend who was interested in her since she was 12 years old said, "*when one loves somebody from childhood and later marries that person then it is called true love and in false love everything is done (have sex) and then he leaves her...*" Another 19 year-old girl had a relationship with a boy who she says had loved her since she was young. When he asked her to have sex, she said, "*It doesn't look good, doing all this before marriage. My didi* [older sister] *says that those who do true love they never ask from a girl for all this.*" In contrast, most boys interviewed felt that boys befriend girls with physical relationships foremost in their minds. An 18 year-old boy remarked, "*mostly, boys do friendship for the sake of physical relations...some boys keep friendship till friendship, but mostly boys want...*[to] *establish physical relations as early as possible.*" An 18 year-old boy remarked, "*Boys mostly...do ashiqui* [romance] *to have chut* [female genitals]."

The interviews suggested that cinema plays a major role in adolescents' lives and serves to perpetuate gender stereotypes. Girls embrace the notions of romantic love and "happily-living-after" scenarios from Hindi films, while boys watch pornographic films that objectify women and reinforce boys' desire to seek sexual satisfaction. Respondents described a number of relationships that began as consensual but led to sexual coercion, ranging from forced kissing to forced sexual intercourse. In some cases coercion became progressively more violent. For example, one 15 year-old girl described how her boyfriend "*kissed me forcefully on top in my bhabhi's* [sister-in-law's] *room. He took me there on the pretext that he had to talk to me.*" Subjugation at the start of the relationship led to more severe violence. This girl explained:

> *...he gets angry if I talk to anyone in the lane. One day he saw me talking to my brother...he came in the evening and beat me up. He was saying that boy was my year* [friend]*...he beat me so much even then I did not say anything to him because I love him so much.*

An important factor that places girls at risk is that revelation of a relationship may lead to severe repercussions. Armed with this knowledge, boys can use blackmail to demand sex. A 19 year-old boy told of his sexual relationship with a married girl during which he became violent. He said, "*She was feeling the pain. I did this till I was satisfied.*" When the girl tried to get out of the relationship, coercion progressed to blackmail. In his own words, he:

> *...gave her Dhamki* [threat] *that if she will not do then I will tell everybody. Then I started taking money for each sexual intercourse. I used to threaten her that I will tell everybody. She used to give me Rs 20, sometimes Rs 50 or 100.*

Sometimes boys use the threat of defamation to demand sex for their friends. A 19 year-old student remarked, "*...friends also help in establishing physical relations with his girlfriend.... And if the girl says no then boys defame her in her gali* [lane] *and colony. Because there is no effect on boy's character.*"

This situation does not necessarily improve after the girl is married. The cultural context condones sexual coercion within marriage. An 18 year-old girl described her sister's wedding night, saying, "*She did not want to celebrate first night but her husband was annoyed...he didn't agree and did it forcefully. She was having a lot of pain so her Bhabhi took her to the dispensary the next morning.*" This non-consensual sex/rape is considered part of a girl's life. When asked what happens on a wedding night one 18 year-old girl said, "*the girl knows that on first night the boy will have sex with her. Even if the girl refuses, he will do sex forcefully.*" A 19 year-old painter spoke of how he overrode the will of his new wife "*...At night, I asked her to take off her clothes. She refused. When I asked her two–three times, she started crying. I made her keep quiet, and after that I took her clothes off and did my work.*" Older women tell girls to accept this situation as normal. According to one girl, they say, "*If you won't give him then he would force and you will have pain.*"

Male respondents also described using violence with commercial sex workers (CSWs). A 16 year-old boy related an incident in which his friend held a CSW down while he had anal sex with her. He described how, "*she said it was paining and refused to do it...she started screaming and tried to move away... I asked my friend to hold her and not to let her move forward. She screamed and bit my hand.*"

Respondents described other acts of sexual violence, including threats, rape and attempted rape. One respondent described a friend who experienced incest by a brother. She spoke of her friend's helplessness saying, "*She feels like running away. But where could she go?*" One 16 year-old boy described raping a girl who had run away from home because her parents wanted to marry her off. When he met her in the street, he lured her to a friend's home, saying, "*'Where would you sleep—on the road? You come with me to my home and sleep. You could leave in the morning.'... I talked to her for some time and then I kissed her, pressed her breasts, that girl was refusing. But I did it forcefully. I f—-ed her a lot.*"

Girls are not the only ones coerced. Interviews revealed two instances in which older boys forced 12 and 13 year-old boys to have anal sex. One 16 year-old boy described how, "*elder boys used to ask me for Gandh* [anal sex]. *At that time, we used to feel very bad, but after some time, we also started asking from our age boys for anal sex.*" A 19 year-old married adolescent said, "*...when we were young, we used to have anal sex with large numbers of boys.... We all together used to go to the latrines. Whosoever we would see there, we used to snatch his container and f— him. We couldn't put it inside but used to touch it on the skin only.*"

These encounters are straightforward cases of rape or molestation, which carry harsh legal penalties. However, society often tolerates coercion and places blame squarely on the victim, as the following instance illustrates. A 14-year-old girl narrated how a boy on the street assaulted her. "*Once I was coming through the street...and this boy came from the front, pressed my breasts, and ran away. I had not wrapped a chunni* [scarf]." *Chunni* is a symbol of modesty in the Indian social context, and without it, women are often said to have loose morals for exhibiting their breasts. The girl's mother beat up the boy, but the neighbour commented, "*fault lies in your daughter who did not wear a chunni.*" The neighbour's comment reflected tolerance of the boy's behaviour, by placing blame on the girl's lack of character.

Conclusions

These research findings suggest that boys and girls are at polar opposites regarding what they want from relationships. Boys are outspoken about their desire for sex, while girls speak about romantic and matrimonial aspirations in a relationship. Cinema plays a role in perpetuating gender stereotypes, by encouraging girls to idealize the notion of 'true love' and encouraging boys to seek sexual gratification. Society perpetuates abuse by tolerating certain kinds of coercion, which emboldens boys to become even more aggressive and violent. While boys have license from society to take advantage of sexual opportunities, girls risk defamation.

These research findings suggested a number of implications for interventions and programming that Swaasthya incorporated into their work. First, it was clear that there was a need for perspective building and sensitization about coercion and gender stereotypes. Because cinema has such a strong influence on young people, Swaasthya helped young people from the community to develop video programmes on these topics, which it screens on street corners and local cable programmes. Second, because girls who experience coercion often lack social support, Swaasthya created opportunities within its programmes for greater interaction between adolescent girls and gatekeepers, including parents. In addition, it organized girls' groups for peer support and collective action. Third, given that girls' lack of life skills increases their vulnerability, Swaasthya established a skill-building programme that addressed decision-making, problem-solving and communication and negotiation skills. The preliminary evaluation of these programmes indicates that they appear to be achieving some success.

Further reading

Heise L, Moore K, Toubia N (1995) *Sexual Coercion and Reproductive Health: A Focus on Research*, New York, Population Council.

Jejeebhoy S (1996) *Adolescent Sexual and Reproductive Behaviour: A Review of the Evidence from India. Working Paper No. 3.* Washington, DC, International Center for Research on Women.

Mehta S, Groenen R, Roque F (1998) Adolescents in changing times: issues and perspectives for adolescent reproductive health in the ESCAP region. Background paper for *High-level Meeting to Review the Implementation of the Programme of Action of the International Conference on Population and Development and Bali Declaration on Population and Sustainable Development and to Make Recommendations for Further Action.* Bangkok, United Nations Economic and Social Commission for the Asia and the Pacific.

Segala UA (1999) Family violence: A focus on India. *Aggression and Violent Behaviour* 4(2) (Summer). [Available at: www.asiamedia.ucla.edu]

Zillmann D (1998) *Sexual Behaviour Research among Adolescents in Tigri.* Report submitted to the Rockefeller Foundation, New Delhi, Swaasthya.

Zillmann D (2000) Influence of unrestrained access to erotica on adolescents' and young adults' dispositions toward sexuality. *Journal of Adolescent Health* 27(2, Suppl. 1):41–44.

Dr Geeta Sodhi
Founder and Director
SWAASTHYA
Lower ground floor G1323
Chittaranjan Park
New Delhi
India

Experiences of sexual coercion among street boys in Bangalore, India

Jayashree Ramakrishna, Mani Karott and Radha Srinivasa Murthy

Background

There are an estimated 100 million street children worldwide, including 40 million in Latin America, 30 million in Asia and 10 million in Africa. Street children as a group can be hard to define, but may include children who are "of" the street and those who live "on" the street (de la Barra, 1998). By some estimates, India has over 414 700 street children, mainly in big cities (Pinto, 1993). Many are homeless and must fend for themselves without adult care. In such situations, children are often forced into "survival sex", i.e. sex for protection, food, drugs and shelter (Inciardi & Surratt, 1998; Swart-Kruger & Richter, 1997). Street life is hierarchical, with well-developed power structures, and sexual coercion is a common way of exercising power. Sexual coercion encompasses behaviours that range from physical and mental coercion to enticement with economic and psychological rewards.

BOSCO, a nongovernmental organization, has worked with street children in Bangalore since 1980. An estimated 85 000–100 000 street children live in Bangalore alone (BOSCO, 1998; Reddy, 1992). After a study for developing a drug prevention programme (BOSCO, 1999) found that more than 50% of children with a drug habit also practised unsafe sex, BOSCO carried out a study to examine high-risk sexual behaviour among street children in Bangalore. The research did not specifically aim to study coercive sexual behaviours, but this emerged as a dominant theme during data analysis.

Methods

The study employed a combination of qualitative and quantitative research methods. Using social mapping, free listing, pile sorting and rating, researchers gathered information on boys' perceptions of sexual behaviour and coercion. They conducted in-depth interviews with children and key informants. In addition to qualitative data, researchers gathered quantitative information from 121 boys on socio-demographic profiles, family history, sleeping arrangements, alcohol/drug use and sexual activity. Study participants came from four of seven areas where BOSCO has outreach programmes. All members of the research team had more than five years experience working with street children, and their rapport with respondents was essential to the success of the study.

Key findings

Boys in the study ranged from age 9 to 23. A majority (45%) were 14–17 years old, and the median age was 16 years. On average, boys had been on the street for five to six years. Boys cited poverty as the major reason for leaving home. Nearly one-fourth did not have a father or mother, and a large per cent had an alcoholic parent. One-fourth never went home, and 40% went home only for festivals, even though their parents lived in the same town. Most boys did not have close associations with adults.

Life on the street is fraught with danger. Police and local hoodlums (*goondas*) are feared by all. Living in a gang offers some protection from outsiders, though older gang members may take advantage of younger boys. Groups of boys work, sleep and play together. Drug and alcohol use is common. Half the boys inhaled "solution" (typewriter correcting whitener), and nearly half (46%) consumed alcohol. Street boys are extremely mobile; they change jobs and sleeping places frequently. Apart from a group of 16 boys in the study who lived at home, the other boys slept at the BOSCO shelter, in the streets, parks and workplaces. In the social stratification of street boys, rag pickers are at the bottom, coolies are higher up, and parking attendants or those who sell cinema tickets are at the top. Although some boys earn a good wage, they do not have a way to save money and are often robbed.

The boys in the study were quite comfortable talking about sex with a trusted adult. Children on the street use the English word "sex" or "*sexu*" when talking of sex-related themes. Twenty-three boys free-listed words that came to mind when they heard the term "*sexu*". Sex was commonly seen as "work" (*khelsa*). For instance, masturbation is referred to as "hand work" (*kai khelsa*), oral sex as "mouth work" (*bai khelsa*) and anal intercourse as "back work" (*hinde khelsa*). Street boys have a negative attitude towards sex and often refer to it as "bad work" (*ketta khelsa*) and "dirty work" (*galeej khelsa*). Anal sex and oral sex between same-sex partners were clearly distinguished as "doing" and "getting done". Boys did not use the term "rape" in regards to boys, but the English word "force" (force *madduvadu*).

Sixty-one boys rated 26 items according to how pleasurable and how dangerous they considered each sexual act. Overall, they rated consensual sex with girls as the most pleasurable activity, followed by raping a girl. When asked how they knew that rape was pleasurable, they replied that men in movies seemed to enjoy it. Forcing boys to have anal sex was not thought to be as pleasurable as coercing girls, nevertheless they said that it gives some pleasure.

The major reasons boys cited for having sex included pleasure (*maja*), excitement/arousal (*udhvega/choolu*), desire (*asé*), and feeling depressed/bored (*béjaar*). Two spoke of falling in love. Some street boys expressed fond feelings for "girl friends", such as vendors or girls involved in casual sex work. During the study period a boy committed suicide because he thought a girl who sold peanuts had rejected him. Many boys said that they had a lot of "feeling" towards the sex worker with whom they had had their first sexual experience. They had wanted to have a long-term relationship, and many said they intended to marry them. But these women told them to just finish their "work" quickly and were not interested in "talk" or feelings. After several such encounters, street boys began to view women on the street in a negative light. They referred to sex workers as prostitutes (*sulé*), vehicle/carts (*gaadi/vandi*) and things or goods (*maal*).

Sexual coercion needs to be viewed in the broader context of street life. According to the quantitative data gathered in this study, 74 (61%) out of 121 boys were sexually active. Four were initiated at age nine or younger. Most (36) were initiated between ages 10 and 12; twenty-one were 13–14 years old. Anal sex, which is usually a boy-to-boy activity, was the most commonly reported sexual behaviour, followed by vaginal sex. Few (8) practised solely vaginal or solely anal sex; the majority mentioned at least two behaviours. Older boys tend to have sex with girls as well as anal sex with boys. At times friends have anal sex, oral sex or practise mutual masturbation (Table 1).

Table 1. Number and per cent of sexually active street boys reporting selected sexual behaviours (*N*=74)

Sexual behaviours	Number	Per cent
Anal intercourse	46	62
Vaginal intercourse	42	57
Self masturbation	30	41
Mutual masturbation	24	32
Oral sex	10	14
Sex with eunuchs (Hijra)	4	5

Older boys, 15 years and above, often force or entice younger boys, some as young as 6 years old, to have anal sex. Younger boys are afraid and upset when they are "forced", but do not see how they can avoid the older boys. The older boys threaten to beat them or ostracize them. In many cases the younger boys are dependent on the older boys for protection. Older boys also entice younger boys with money, food or empty bottles that can be sold. They may also take them to a movie or give them "solution". Street boys hesitated to express fear, and some said that over time they had become used to the idea of being forced. In one narrative, a 12 year-old boy described how he is no longer afraid when boys "force" him. In his own words:

> *...older boys come and force us, when we refuse they beat us. They tell me that they will give money. Initially when others "call" us we are afraid. They also did it from the back* [anal sex]. *Initially it was a little painful, but afterwards there was no pain. Now, I have no fear.*

Later, however, he said that when he thinks of boys forcing him, he is afraid. Perhaps the denial of fear is a way of coping with pain and trauma. This boy also described having relations with adult porters who give him food and money and beat other boys who trouble him. The porters show affection but at the same time they have sex with him. He said, "*I don't like any of them.*"

Younger boys perceive that the older boys must be getting pleasure (*maja*) from "forcing" them, and they are eager to experience this *maja*. They are not averse to forcing younger boys, so there are no clear distinctions between coercers and the coerced. The younger boys said they wanted to have sex with girls, but were too afraid and shy to approach women. One uneducated 16 year-old said that he and other youngsters felt ashamed to visit sex workers, as they are very young. They were more comfortable with young street girls or drunken sleeping women. Drunken sleeping women are easy targets. They may wake up and scold the boys, or they may cooperate. Others show no reaction, or appear "dead", as one boy remarked. Young street girls are sometimes willing to exchange sex for money and food. According to one informant, young girls call them saying, "*give us food and money and you can sleep with us.*" So he and some young boys have had sexual relationship with girls who are 8–12 years old.

Conclusions

In summary, social conditions, poverty and drug use shape concepts of sexuality and coercion among street boys. Pleasure or *maja* is a dominant theme associated with sex. Sex with girls is deemed to be most pleasurable, even if it is rape. Sex with boys also gives pleasure, although "doing" anal sex is much more pleasurable than having it "done". All things being equal, however, boys prefer consensual sex. Despite the pleasure boys derive from sex, they hold a negative view of sex: that it is bad, dirty and shameful. Nevertheless, they are willing to talk about sexual matters.

Sexual coercion on the street is an exercise of power, a way to maintain status and subdue a subordinate. Boys who have been forced, in turn want to be in positions of command. Just as sex may express power, it may also be interpreted as an expression of affection and protection. Boys who are "forced" may feel they will receive protection from hazards of street life. The nature of street life—including the lack of food, shelter, protection and emotional support combined with strong power structures—sustains sexually coercive behaviours.

Programmes must consider multiple risk factors when carrying out interventions (Richter, 1997). BOSCO is drawing upon these research findings to modify the street boys' environment by providing safe places to sleep, healthy recreation options, safe ways to save money and opportunities to build relationships with caring adults. In addition, BOSCO is providing life-skills training, counselling and health education to help street boys adopt safer sex behaviours.

Acknowledgements: We gratefully acknowledge the contributions of street educators Mr Basavaraju, Mr Ramaswamy, Mr Ramesh, Ms Sheeba Thomas and Mr Shivamallu, and the support of Fr K.D. Varghese Kootungal, Executive Director, BOSCO, Bangalore, and Fr Varghese Pallipuram, Project Holder, BOSCO; and the research guides, Dr Shekhar Sheshadri, and Dr Vivek Benegal; Dr Pushpinder Pelia Lubana, and Professor Pertti Pelto, NIMHANS Small Grants Programme for Research on Sexuality and Sexual Behaviour.

References

BOSCO (1998) *Annual Report 1997–1998.* Bangalore, BOSCO.

BOSCO (1999) *Report of the Drug Abuse Prevention Programme*. Bangalore, BOSCO.

de la Barra X (1998) Poverty: the main cause of ill-health in urban children. *Health Education and Behavior*, 25(1):46–59.

Inciardi JA, Surratt HL (1998) Children in the streets of Brazil: drug use, crime, violence, and HIV risks. *Substance Use & Misuse*, 33(7):1461–1480.

Pinto G (1993) Street children an urban phenomenon. In: Kanth A, Verma RM, eds. *Neglected Child—Changing Perspectives.* Delhi, Prayas.

Reddy N (1992) *Situational Analysis of Street Children in Bangalore*. NOIDA, Delhi, National Labour Institute.

Richter L (1997) Street children and HIV/AIDS. *AIDS Bulletin*, 6(4):4–6.

Swart-Kruger J, Richter LM (1997) AIDS-related knowledge, attitudes and behaviour among South African street youth: reflections on power, sexuality and the autonomous self. *Social Science and Medicine*, 45(6):957–966.

Jayashree Ramakrishna, PhD MPH
Additional Professor
Department of Health Education
National Institute of Mental Health and Neuro Sciences
Post Bag 2900
Bangalore 560 029
India

Gender, sexual abuse and risk behaviours in adolescents: a cross-sectional survey in schools in Goa, India

Vikram Patel, Gracy Andrews, Tereze Pierre and Nimisha Kamat

Background

There is growing evidence that the broader context of reproductive health pertaining to adolescence needs attention. For example, in developing countries, mental disorders such as depression and substance abuse are among the most important causes of morbidity and disability in adolescents. Attempted suicide is the single most important cause of death and hospitalization among adolescents in South Asia (Eddleston et al., 1998). Girls are more likely to attempt suicide than boys, and this seems to be linked with their lack of control over reproductive decision-making. Studies show that violence against women is a serious social and public health issue in India (Jejeebhoy, 1998). Sexual abuse of adolescents may also be a widespread problem with serious implications for their mental health. This paper describes findings from a survey focusing on the prevalence and correlates of abuse among school-going adolescents in Goa, India. The researchers examined numerous issues related to abuse, drawn from the broader context of adolescent development, including sexual behaviour, mental health, parental relationships and educational achievements.

Methods

The project had two stages. The first stage gathered qualitative data on adolescents' needs among adolescents and adult key informants. The second stage involved a cross-sectional survey conducted in eight Goan schools. All students in the survey sample were in their first year of higher secondary school (i.e. their 11th year of schooling). Researchers collected data through self-administered questionnaires in classroom settings. The questionnaire was developed using qualitative data from the first phase of the project and existing instruments, such as the 12-item General Health Questionnaire (used to measure mental health).

The study defined sexual abuse as being any verbal or physical sexual experience in the previous 12 months that was forced or against the wishes of the individual. Five key aspects of abuse were measured using the following questions: Have you experienced any of these in the past 12 months: Someone talking to you about sex in a manner that made you uncomfortable? Someone purposely brushing their private parts against you? Someone forcing you to touch their body parts against your wishes? Someone touching you in a sexual manner without your permission? Someone forcing you to have sex with them?

Figure 1. Per cent of adolescents who reported sexual abuse during prior 12 months, by type of abuse

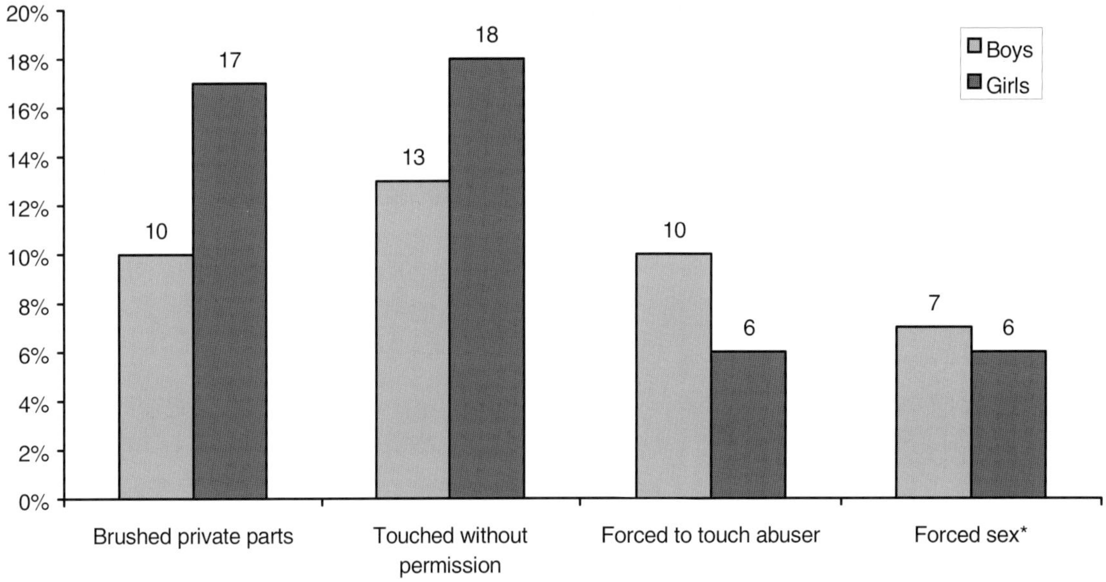

* Forced sex refers to forced intercourse, including vaginal, oral or anal.

Key findings

On the day of the study, 811 eligible students were present in the eight schools, and none refused to participate. The average age was 16 years, and just over half the sample (53%) were boys. About half were Catholic (49%), and most of the remainder (46%) were Hindu.

One-third of the students (266) had experienced at least one type of sexual abuse in the previous 12 months. Six per cent of adolescents reported that they had been forced to have sex. There was no statistical difference between boys and girls in the overall prevalence of sexual abuse or in the per cent who reported forced sexual intercourse. Notable gender differences were observed, however. Boys were more likely to report that someone had talked to them about sex or forced them to touch the perpetrator, while girls were more likely to report that the perpetrator had touched them or brushed his private parts against them (Figure 1). Of the 266 adolescents who reported abuse, nearly half (47%) had experienced abuse more than once, and those who reported sexual abuse were far more likely to have also experienced other kinds of physical and verbal violence in the previous 12 months.

The most common perpetrators (53%) were older students or friends (see Table 1). Parents or relatives accounted for 8% and teachers for 4% of perpetrators. A large proportion (27%) of the perpetrators fell into the category "miscellaneous",

Table 1. Type of perpetrator and action taken by victim among adolescents who reported experience of sexual abuse within the past 12 months, as a per cent (*N* = 266)

	Per cent
Type of perpetrator	
Student/ friend	53
Other person (e.g. stranger, neighbour, bus passenger, priest)	27
Parent or relative	8
Teacher	4
Action taken by victim	
Nothing	35
Verbal retaliation	17
Ran away	12
Avoided perpetrator/ended friendship	10
Physical retaliation	6
Told parents/friends	7

Table 2. Mental and physical health and risk behaviours among adolescents: comparison of those who reported forced sex compared to those who did not report abuse

	Experienced forced sex	Did not experience forced sex	Adjusted P value
	(N = 51)	(N = 760)	
Measures of mental health			
General Health Questionnaire score	5.1	3.6	<0.001
"Life not worth living" (%)	46	27	0.01
Regular alcohol use (%)	19	5	0.001
Physical health and health-seeking			
Visited doctor (%)	43	25	0.005
Aches (%)	29	9	<0.001
Stomach upset (%)	14	5	0.01
Risk behaviour			
Vaginal sex (girls) (%)	23	2	0.001
Vaginal sex (boys) (%)	38	6	<0.001
Anal sex (girls) (%)	14	1	<0.00
Anal sex (boys) (%)	24	2	0.001

which included strangers, neighbours and others. The most common response to abuse was to do nothing (35%). Seventeen per cent responded to the abuse with verbal retaliation and 6% responded with physical retaliation. Seven per cent told a parent or friend. However, these findings mask the considerable gender disparity: none of the boys and only 15% of girls had told a parent or friend about the abuse.

While sexual abuse takes many forms, the researchers did an in-depth analysis of the correlates of forced sexual intercourse. The 6% of adolescents who experienced forced sexual intercourse had significantly poorer scores in their board examinations than did those who had not experienced forced sexual intercourse (53.2 versus 58.2, P=0.04). Their physical and mental health was significantly worse, as measured by self-reported complaints and General Health Questionnaire scores (Table 2). Parental relationships were also significantly poorer among these adolescents, especially among girls. Adolescents of both genders who had experienced forced sex were far more likely to engage in consensual sexual intercourses, both vaginal and anal (Table 2).

Conclusions

The major findings of this study indicate that sexual abuse and violence are common among this population. They also suggest that school is not necessarily a safe place for young people. Students or friends were the most common perpetrators of sexual abuse, especially for boys. Most victims suffer in silence. Many adolescents experienced multiple types of sexual abuse, and there was a strong association between experience of sexual abuse and experience of other forms of violence. Gender differences emerged in the type of abuse and the type of perpetrator. Whereas boys were typically abused by friends or older boys in their school, girls were more often abused by strangers. The study findings suggest that there is a constellation of risk behaviours and poor mental health outcomes associated with sexual abuse. Those who experienced forced sexual intercourse had poorer educational performance and physical and mental health. They also had greater levels of suicidal ideation, higher rates of substance abuse and gambling behaviour. They had poorer relationship with their parents, especially the girls, and more active consensual sexual behaviour.

The implications for policy and programmes are clear. Health workers who care for adolescents must be trained in the assessment of abuse and mental health, communication skills and psychosocial interventions. Interventions aimed at improving reproductive health must address issues such as personal safety and prevention of abuse, mental health and self-esteem, substance abuse and communication skills (e.g. with parents). Gender-sensitive programmes for boys and girls are needed, and programmes should focus on teachers and parents. Given the limitations of the cross-sectional study design, it was not possible to identify which correlates were possible causal factors and which were consequences of the abuse. Cohort studies are needed to examine causal associations and outcomes of abuse, as well as to evaluate possible interventions. These should be priorities for future research.

This summary has been adapted from the full article by Patel V and Andrew G (2001) entitled "Gender, sexual abuse and risk behaviours in adolescents: a cross-sectional survey in schools in Goa", published in *The National Medical Journal of India*, 14:263–267.

References

Eddleston M, Rezvi Sheriff MH, Hawton K (1998) Deliberate self-harm in Sri Lanka: an overlooked tragedy in the developing world. *British Medical Journal*, 317:133–135.

Jejeebhoy S (1998) Associations between wife-beating and foetal and infant death: impressions from rural India. *Studies in Family Planning,* 29(3):300–308.

Vikram Patel, MRCPsych, PhD
Senior Lecturer
London School of Hygiene & Tropical Medicine
United Kingdom

Sangath Centre
841/1 Alto Porvorim
Goa 403521
India

VI

Meeting adolescents' needs for contraception

Adolescence and safety of contraceptives

Olav Meirik

Most studies of safety and efficacy of contraceptives have been done in adult women, and equivalent data for adolescents are scarce. While much of the information from studies in adults is also valid for adolescents, there are particular concerns about the clinical performance of specific contraceptives in adolescents and their possible effects on development and maturation. Moreover, user-dependent methods that require consistency of use (e.g. contraceptive pills, condom) may be less effective when used by adolescents.

One specific concern for hormonal contraceptives has been that these methods might interfere with the maturation of the hypothalamic-pituitary-ovarian system of postmenarchial adolescents. Rey-Stocker et al. (1981) examined healthy adolescent women 1–6 years after menarche for the secretion of gonadotropins, thyrotropin, prolactin, estradiol, progesterone and thyroid hormones in the follicular and luteal phase of the menstrual cycle. They also studied the same hormones in adolescent women of similar postmenarchial age who had taken combined oral contraceptive pills continuously for 3–24 months. There were no differences in the endocrine profiles of never users and past users of oral contraceptives. The authors concluded that combined oral contraceptives do not adversely affect the maturation of the hypothalamic-pituitary-ovarian system in adolescents.

Another recent concern is the effect of suppression by hormonal contraceptives of ovarian function including estradiol, and the effect of this suppression on bone mass in adolescent women. More than 90% of bone mass of the skeleton is acquired before age 20 (Theintz et al.,1992); and estrogens are essential for bone acquisition (Rizzoli & Bonjour, 1997). Depot-medroxyprogesterone acetate (DMPA) suppresses the excretion of estradiol by the ovary to low levels (Ortiz et al., 1977). Combined oral contraceptives and combined monthly injectables also suppress ovarian estradiol, but contain estrogens that compensate for the suppression. The implantable contraceptive Norplant suppresses ovarian estradiol to a lesser extent than other hormonal methods (Croxatto et al., 1988). It is established that the use of DMPA reduces bone mass, albeit reversibly, in adult women (Meirik, 2000). Two relatively small studies indicate that use of DMPA during adolescence is associated with a lower rate of bone accumulation or even reduction of bone mass (Cromer et al., 1996; Scholes et al., 1999). For adolescents, who are still at a stage when they are accumulating bone mass, this is of concern since it is not known whether low bone mass in early adult life is associated with increased risk of fracture later in life. For these reasons DMPA should not be a first contraceptive choice for adolescent women.

Concerns about increased risk of cancer, and in particular breast cancer, have negatively influenced the acceptability of combined oral contraceptives. Recent data illustrate that, for women younger than 20 years, the excess risk of breast cancer associated with use of combined oral contraceptives is in the order of 1 per 1 000 000 woman-years and that the excess risk disappears 10 years after stopping use (Collaborative Group on Hormonal Factors in Breast Cancer, 1996).

Use of intrauterine devices (IUDs) among adolescents is controversial. The main concern is the increased risk of pelvic inflammatory disease (PID) associated with IUD use (World Health Organization, 1987), although modern IUDs and current clinical practice attenuate the risk (Grimes, 2000). Young women are at higher risk of PID than adult women; Bell & Holmes (1984) estimated age-specific incidence rates of PID in sexually active women and reported that the rate was highest in adolescent women and declined exponentially with increasing age. Relatively small clinical studies found high rates of expulsion of IUDs among nulliparous adolescent women (Weiner, Berg & Johansson, 1978; Kulig et al, 1980), and indications of an increased risk of PID among them (Weiner, Berg & Johansson, 1978). However, a study of IUD use in parous adolescent women found that the clinical performance of the method was similar to that in adult women (Diaz et al., 1993). Until more evidence is available on the safety of IUD use in nulliparous adolescents, this method should not be a first choice for them.

Hormonal contraceptive methods have high contraceptive efficacy, but do not protect against sexually transmitted infections including human immunodeficiency virus (STI/HIV). Only for the male condom is there good documentation of STI/HIV prevention (Hatcher et al., 1994; World Health Organization, 2000). Sexually active adolescents have behavioural patterns that place them at higher risk of STI/HIV than the average adult, and their naïve immunological system probably contributes to the higher risk. The male condom is a good choice for contraception and STI/HIV prevention, but requires consistent and correct use to achieve effective prevention against pregnancy and STI/HIV (Hatcher et al., 1994; World Health Organization, 2000). To provide adolescents with knowledge, skills and motivation to protect themselves from unwanted pregnancy and STI/HIV is a challenge to which communities and health services are obliged to respond.

References

Bell T, Holmes KK (1984) Age-specific risks of syphilis, gonorrhoea, and hospitalised pelvic inflammatory disease in sexually experienced U.S. women. *Sexually Transmitted Diseases*, 11:291–295.

Collaborative Group on Hormonal Factors in Breast Cancer (1996) Breast cancer and hormonal contraceptives: collaborative reanalysis of individual data on 53 297 women with breast cancer and 100 239 women without breast cancer from 54 epidemiological studies. *Lancet*, 347:1713–1727.

Cromer BA, MacArdle Blair J, Mahan JD, Zibners L, Naumovski Z (1996) A prospective comparison of bone density in adolescent girls receiving depot medroxyprogesterone acetate (Depo-Provera), levonorgestrel (Norplant), or oral contraceptives. *The Journal of Pediatrics,* 129:671–676.

Croxatto HB, Diaz S, Pavez M, Brandeis A (1988) Estradiol plasma levels during long-term treatment with Norplant subdermal implants. *Contraception,* 38:465–475.

Diaz J, Pinto Neta AM, Bahamondes L, Diaz M. Arce XE, Castro S (1993) Performance of the Copper T 200 in parous adolescents: are copper IUDs suitable for these women? *Contraception,* 48:23–28.

Grimes D (2000) Intrauterine device and upper-genital-tract infection. *Lancet*, 356:1013–1019.

Hatcher RA, Trussel J, Stewart F et al. (1994) *Contraceptive Technology,* 16th revised ed. New York, Irvington Publishers Inc.

Kulig JW, Rauh JL, Burket RL, Cabot HM, Brookman RR (1980) Experience with the copper 7 intrauterine device in an adolescent population. *Journal of Pediatrics*, 96:746–759.

Meirik O (2000) Hormonal contraceptives and bone mass. *IPPF Medical Bulletin*, 34:1–3.

Ortiz H, Hirol M, Stancyk FZ, Goebelsman U, Mishell DR (1977) Serum medroxyprogesterone acetate (MPA) concentrations and ovarian function following intramuscular injection of depo-MPA. *Journal of Clinical Endocrinology and Metabolism*, 44:32–38.

Rey-Stocker I, Zufferey MM, Lemarchand MT, Rais M (1981) The sensibility of the hypophysis, the gonads and the thyroid of adolescents before and after the administration of oral contraceptives. A resume. *Pediatric Annals,* 10:480–485.

Rizzoli R, Bonjour JP (1997) Hormones and bones. *Lancet,* 349 (Suppl. 1):SI 20–23.

Scholes D, Lacroix AZ, Ott SM, Ichikawa LE, Barlow WE (1999) Bone mineral density in women using depot medroxyprogesterone acetate for contraception. *Obstetrics and Gynecology,* 93:233–238.

Theintz G, Buchs B, Rizzoli R, Solsman D, Clavien H, Sizonenko PC, Bonjour JP (1992) Longitudinal monitoring of bonemass in healthy adolescents: Evidence for a marked reduction after 16 years of age at the level of lumbar spine and femoral neck in female subjects. *Journal of Clinical Endocrinology and Metabolism,* 75:1060–1065.

Weiner E, Berg AA, Johansson I (1978) Copper intrauterine contraceptive devices in adolescent nulliparae. *British Journal of Obstetrics and Gynaecology*, 85:204–206.

World Health Organization (1987) *Mechanism of action, safety and efficacy of intrauterine devices.* Geneva, World Health Organization (WHO Technical Report Series No. 753).

World Health Organization (2000) *Improving access to quality care in family planning; medical eligibility criteria for contraceptive use,* 2nd ed. Geneva, World Health Organization (WHO/RHR/00.02).

Olav Meirik, MD, PhD
Instituto Chileno de Medicina Reproductiva
Ave Luis Thayer Ojeda 1303
Dto 402
Providencia, Santiago
Chile

Contraceptive behaviours of adolescents in Asia: issues and challenges

Saroj Pachauri and K.G. Santhya

Background

With the widespread acceptance of family planning, nearly every Asian country has experienced a drop in birth rates. However, national populations are expected to continue to grow for some years because of population momentum—a consequence of the large number of adolescents and young people in Asia. Of the 1.15 billion adolescents in the world, over 700 million live in Asia (United Nations, 2000). Although adolescents in Asia have several common concerns, there is tremendous diversity in this region. This diversity, coupled with the paucity of data on adolescents, makes it difficult to carry out a comprehensive analysis of the challenges faced by adolescents in Asia and the nature and scope of efforts required to address them.

Adolescents form one of the largest groups with unmet needs for reproductive health services. One of the most important challenges facing reproductive health programmes in Asia is to address the needs of adolescents as they initiate sexual activity and are exposed to the risk of unwanted pregnancy and infection. Understanding the extent to which young people know about and use contraceptives is, therefore, a significant issue for research and policy.

This paper examines contraceptive behaviours of adolescents in Asia. The analysis is limited to Bangladesh, India, Nepal, Pakistan and Sri Lanka in South Asia and to Indonesia, the Philippines, Thailand and Viet Nam in South-East Asia. We have drawn data from Demographic and Health Surveys, several national surveys conducted during the past decade and some small-scale studies. It is important to bear in mind that, as these surveys have a number of drawbacks, it is difficult to present a truly representative and comprehensive picture of adolescent behaviours, and results have to be interpreted with caution.

An understanding of the context that determines reproductive attitudes and behaviours is important for analysing contraceptive behaviours of adolescents. First, it is important to note that male and female gender roles typically create an imbalance in negotiating positions between partners in Asian cultures. Such imbalances are exacerbated for younger women since they are more vulnerable. Second, adolescents do not constitute a homogeneous entity. There are significant social, economic and gender differences. For example, girls do not have the same education and employment opportunities as boys, and they face family and societal pressures for early marriage and early childbearing. Sexual coercion within and outside marriage is the norm (Pachauri, 1996). Third, there has been a significant shift towards delayed marriage among adolescent women in all the countries discussed in this paper. However, early marriage continues to be the norm in Bangladesh, India and Nepal where between one-third and one-half of girls aged 15–19 years are married (National Institute of Population Research and Training, Mitra & Associates, 1997; Pradhan et al., 1997; International Institute for Population Sciences & Macro International, 2000).

Consistent with early marriage, early childbearing is the norm in these countries. For example, in Bangladesh more than three out of five (63%), in India nearly one-half (48%), and in Nepal more than two out of five (43%) of currently married 15–19 year-old girls had a child (National Institute of Population Research and Training, Mitra and Associates, 1997; Pradhan et al., 1997; International Institute for Population Sciences & Macro International, 2000).

Finally, available evidence from these countries suggests that an increasing proportion of unmarried adolescent boys and girls are becoming sexually active. A review in India showed that between 20% and 30% of boys and up to 10% of girls were sexually active before marriage (Jejeebhoy, 1996). A study in rural Bangladesh showed that by age 18, 38% of unmarried boys and 6% of unmarried girls were sexually active (United Nations Population Fund, 1998a). Thus, contraceptive behaviours of adolescents in these countries must be examined against this backdrop of prevailing gender power differentials, early marriage and childbearing among adolescent girls in some countries, and rising premarital sexual activity among adolescent boys and girls in almost all countries.

Knowledge and use of contraceptives among adolescents

In all the countries discussed in this paper, almost all married adolescents had knowledge of contraception (Pradhan et al., 1997; International Institute for Population Sciences & Macro International, 2000; Macro International, 2001). Pakistan is an exception as only 75% of currently married adolescent girls reported knowledge of at least one modern contraceptive method (Population Council et al., 1998). However, knowledge about specific modern spacing methods, such as oral contraceptives, injectables, intrauterine devices (IUDs), and implants, is low among married adolescent girls— 59% in Pakistan and 63% in India. It is, however, very high (99%) in Bangladesh and Thailand (Alan Guttmacher Institute, 1998). Knowledge of condoms among adolescent girls is even lower in many countries (Figure 1).

In addition, knowledge of the sources of supply of contraceptive methods is not universal in many of these countries (Alan Guttmacher Institute, 1998; Population Council et al., 1998; United Nations Population Fund, 1998b).

There is a large gap between knowledge and use of contraception among 15–19 year-old married adolescents in these countries. While contraceptive use among currently married adolescents has increased in many of these countries, less than 10% report using a traditional or modern contraceptive method in India (8%), Nepal (7%) and Pakistan (6%) (International Institute for Population Sciences & Macro International, 2000; Pradhan et al., 1997; Hakim, Cleland & Bhatti, 1998). In comparison, between one-fifth and two-fifths of married adolescent girls report using a contraceptive method in Viet Nam (18%), Sri Lanka (20%), the Philippines (22%), Bangladesh (33%), Thailand (43%), and Indonesia (45%) (National Institute of Population Research and Training, Mitra and Associates, 1997; Pradhan et al., 1997; Hakim, Cleland & Bhatti, 1998; International Institute for Population Sciences & Macro International, 2000; Macro International, 2001) (Figure 2).

Married adolescents use modern contraceptive methods more frequently than traditional methods, although the specific methods most commonly used vary among countries. Oral contraceptives are most commonly used in Bangladesh (18%),

Figure 1. Awareness of condoms among married adolescent girls in selected countries of South Asia and South-East Asia

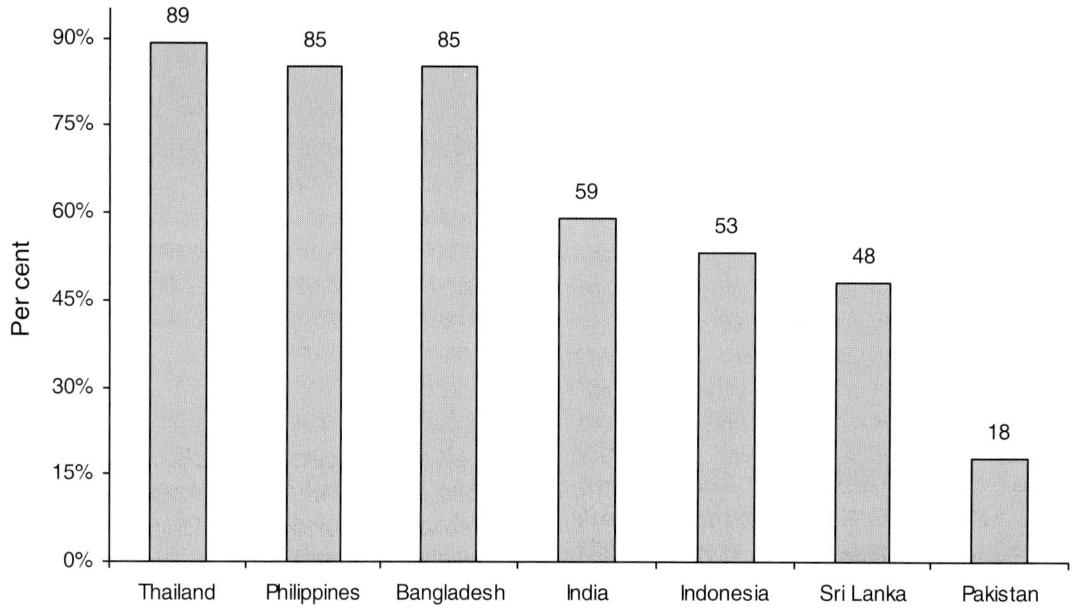

Sources: ***India:*** National Family Health Survey 1998–99 (International Institute for Population Sciences & Macro International, 2000); ***All other countries***: Alan Guttmacher Institute (1998).

Figure 2. Contraceptive use among married adolescent girls in selected countries of South Asia and South-East Asia

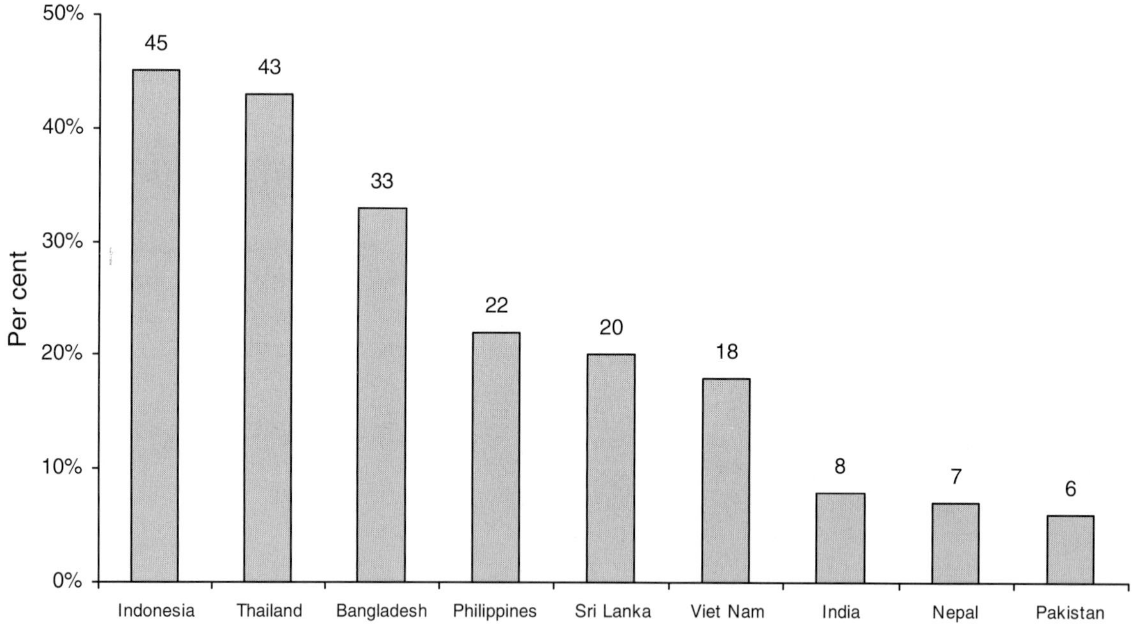

Sources: ***India***: National Family Health Survey 1998–99 (IIPS & Macro Int., 2000); ***Nepal:*** Family Health Survey 1996 (Pradhan et al, 1997); ***Pakistan:*** Pakistan Fertility and Family Planning Survey 1996–97 (Hakim, Cleland & Bhatti, 1998); ***All other countries***: Demographic and Health Survey for various years (Macro International).

the Philippines (6%), Sri Lanka (7%), and Thailand (25%). In comparison, the most frequently used method is the condom in Nepal (2%) and Pakistan (1%), injectables in Indonesia (24%), and the IUD in Viet Nam (34%). Although used by only a small minority (2%), tubal ligation is the most commonly used method among married adolescents in India (National Institute of Population Research and Training, Mitra and Associates, 1997; Pradhan et al., 1997; Hakim, Cleland & Bhatti, 1998; International Institute for Population Sciences & Macro International, 2000; Macro International, 2001).

It is important to understand continuation rates and the reasons why adolescents discontinue using contraceptive methods, but data on discontinuation are scarce. In countries that have relatively high levels of contraceptive prevalence, such as Indonesia and Bangladesh, adolescents are more likely to discontinue use of contraception within the first year than are older women. Furthermore, failure rates are higher in all countries for adolescents than for adult women (Singh, 1998).

A large proportion of births to adolescents in all these countries are unplanned, and this clearly underscores the huge unmet need for contraception among adolescents (Figure 3).

The magnitude of unmet need among married adolescents varies among countries. While one-tenth of currently married adolescent girls in Indonesia and Viet Nam had an unmet need, close to one-third and two-fifths of those in the Philippines and Nepal, respectively, had an unmet need for contraception (Pradhan et al., 1997; Macro International, 2001).

Abortion practices among adolescents

Reliable information on abortion among adolescents is lacking in all these countries. National surveys conducted in India, Nepal, Pakistan and Viet Nam report low abortion rates among married adolescents; however small-scale studies report higher rates. For instance, in a study of 2588 abortions in Indonesia, 58% of the abortions were

Figure 3. Percentage of births to married adolescent girls that are unplanned in selected countries of South Asia and South-East Asia

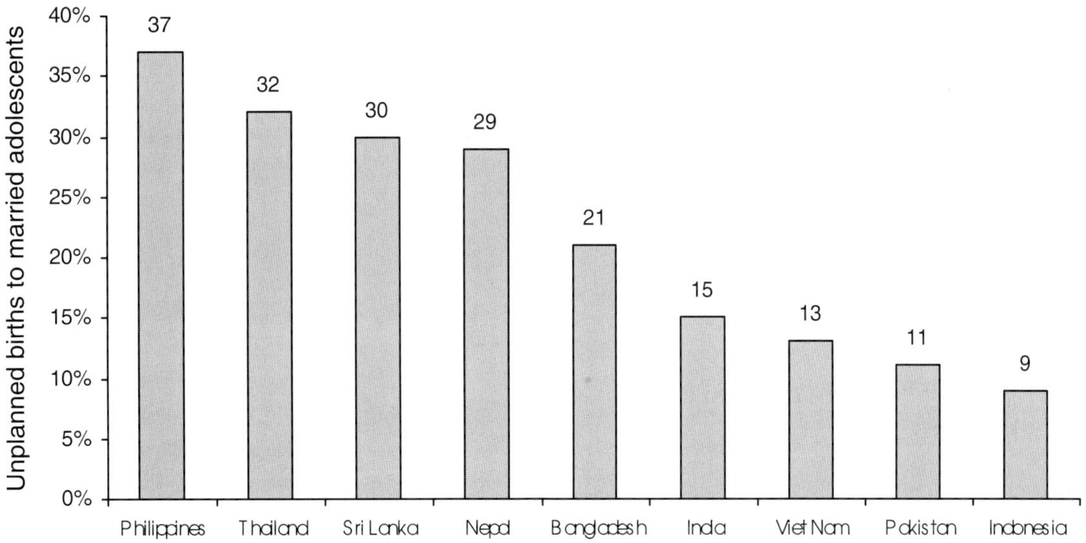

Sources: ***Bangladesh:*** National Institute of Population Research and Training, Mitra and Associates (1997); ***India:*** International Institute for Population Sciences (IIPS), Macro International (2000); ***Indonesia:*** Central Bureau of Statistics (CBS), Indonesia et al. (1998); ***Nepal:*** Pradhan A et al. (1997); ***Philippines:*** National Statistics Office (NSO), Philippines et al. (1999); ***Sri Lanka:*** Department of Census and Statistics, Sri Lanka et al. (1998); ***Thailand and Pakistan:*** Alan Guttmacher Institute (1998); ***Viet Nam:*** National Committee for Population and Family Planning (NCPFP), Viet Nam et al. (1999).

among young women aged 15–24, and as many as 38% of those women were married (Rosdiana, 1998). Far less is known about the prevalence of abortion among unmarried adolescents. Findings from a number of small-scale studies in rural and urban settings in India suggest that unmarried adolescents constitute a disproportionately large percentage of those who seek abortion. These studies also suggest that at least one-half of unmarried women seeking abortions are adolescents, many of whom are below age 15 (Jejeebhoy, 1996).

Conclusions

The results of our analysis show that while knowledge of contraception is almost universal among married adolescents, understanding of specific methods and their sources is limited. Although rates vary among countries, there has been a significant increase in contraceptive use among married adolescents, but a large unmet need for contraceptives remains. Data on contraceptive use by unmarried adolescents are rare, but suggest even lower rates of use than among their married counterparts.

Discussions in Asian countries are beginning to focus on how reproductive health programmes for adolescents should be designed and implemented. A few studies are under way to test interventions. At present there is a poor fit between the design of reproductive health programmes and the needs of adolescents. Strategies should be designed to address the needs of subgroups of adolescents, disaggregated by their distinct characteristics. Policy prescriptions need to challenge social norms that devalue girls. The answers lie in finding routes to economic and social survival for girls, and providing information that is honest and timely. In addition, there is a need to recognize the power differentials in relationships that prevent information and services from reaching adolescents.

Although the availability of data on adolescents has increased in recent years, there are several gaps in knowledge. Available evidence suggests that an increasing proportion of unmarried adolescent boys and girls are becoming sexually active. However, data on contraceptive behaviours of unmarried adolescents are grossly inadequate and much less is known about the behaviours of adolescent boys than adolescent girls. An understanding of contraceptive discontinuation could provide important information for the design of services for adolescents, but these data are not currently available. Data on abortion among adolescents, especially unmarried adolescents, are lacking. Finally, a better understanding about the circumstances surrounding sexual initiation and the decision to practise contraception is needed to design user-friendly programmes for adolescents.

References

Alan Guttmacher Institute (1998) *Into the New World: Young Women's Sexual and Reproductive Lives.* New York, Alan Guttmacher Institute.

Boyd A, Haub C, Cornelius D (2000) *The World's Youth 2000 Data Sheet.* Washington, DC, Population Reference Bureau.

Central Bureau of Statistics (CBS), Indonesia et al. (1998) *Indonesia Demographic and Health Survey, 1997.* Calverton, MD, CBS and Macro International.

Department of Census and Statistics, Sri Lanka, Ministry of Plan Implementation, Sri Lanka, Institute for Resource Development (1988) *Sri Lanka Demographic and Health Survey, 1987.* Columbia, MD, Institute for Resource Development.

Hakim A, Cleland J, Bhatti MH (1998) *Pakistan Fertility and Family Planning Survey 1996–1997, Preliminary Report.* Islamabad, National Institute of Population Studies and the London School of Hygiene and Tropical Medicine.

International Institute for Population Sciences, Macro International (2000) *National Family Health Survey-2 India, 1998–1999.* Mumbai, International Institute for Population Sciences.

Jejeebhoy SJ (1996) *Adolescent Sexual and Reproductive Behaviour—A Review of the Evidence from India*. Working Paper No. 3. Washington, DC, International Center for Research on Women.

Macro International (2001) *Demographic Health Surveys*. [Available at: http//www.measuredhs.com]

National Committee for Population and Family Planning (NCPFP), Viet Nam, Population and Family Health Project and Macro International (1999) *Viet Nam Demographic and Health Survey, 1997*. Hanoi, NCPFP.

National Institute of Population Research and Training, Mitra and Associates (1997) *Bangladesh Demographic and Health Survey 1996–1997*. Dhaka, Bangladesh, NIPORT, Macro International Inc.

National Statistics Office (NSO), Philippines, Department of Health, Philippines, Macro International (1999) *Philippines National Demographic and Health Survey, 1998.* Manila, NSO and Macro International.

Pachauri S (1996) Reproductive health: the concept, ideology and operational issues. In: Sengupta J, Ghosh D, eds. *Perspectives in Reproductive Health*. New Delhi, New Age Publishers Ltd.

Population Council, Ministry of Population Welfare, Pakistan, and UNFPA (1998) *Pakistan Contraceptive Prevalence Survey 1994–1995. Final Report*. Islamabad, Population Council.

Pradhan A, Aryal RH, Regmi G, Ban B, Pavalavalli G (1997) *Nepal Family Health Survey 1996*. Kathmandu, Nepal and Calverton, Maryland, Ministry of Health (Nepal), New ERA, and Macro International Inc.

Rosdiana D (1998) Pokok-Pokok Pikiran Pendidikaan Pendidikan Seks untuk Remaja. In: Kollman N, ed. *Kesehatan Reproduksi Remaja*. Jakarta, Indonesia, Yayasan Lembaga Konsumen.

Singh S (1998) Adolescent childbearing. *Studies in Family Planning,* 29(2):117–136.

United Nations (2000) *The World's Women 2000 Trends and Statistics*. New York, United Nations.

United Nations Population Fund (1998a) Adolescent health and development: Issues and strategies. Country Paper, Bangladesh. *UNFPA South Asia Conference on the Adolescent, New Delhi, 21–23 July*.

United Nations Population Fund (1998b) Socioeconomic, demographic and reproductive health profiles of adolescents in SAARC countries. *UNFPA South Asia Conference on the Adolescent, New Delhi, 21–23 July.*

Saroj Pachauri, PhD
Regional Director, South and East Asia
The Population Council
Zone 5A, Ground Floor
India Habitat Centre
Lodi Road
New Delhi 110003
India

Constraints on condom use among young men in border towns of Nepal

Anand Tamang and Binod Nepal

Background

Over 1500 AIDS cases have been reported in Nepal, and the numbers are rising, particularly among young people aged 14–29. As of May 2000, 1077 (70%) of all reported human immunodeficiency virus (HIV) infections were among adolescents and young adults between ages 14 and 29 (National Centre for AIDS and STD Control, 2000). Given the hidden nature of the problem, the actual size of the infected population is likely to be considerably larger. Heterosexual sex, including commercial sex, is a major route of HIV transmission. Little research has been done on the sexual behaviour of young men in border towns, despite the fact that commercial sex is common in those areas. To address this gap in knowledge, we carried out a qualitative and quantitative study in five border towns between 1997 and 1999. The research questions included: (1) To what extent do sexually active young men residing in border towns engage in casual sexual relations, use condoms and consider themselves to be at risk of contracting sexually transmitted infections (STIs), including HIV? (2) What factors constrain young men who engage in risky sex from wearing condoms? This paper presents data from the subsample of study participants who fell into the age group 18–24 years.

Methods

The study involved a survey among men residing in border towns. The subsample of young men between the ages of 18 and 24 included 242 respondents, of whom 40% were 18 or 19 years old. Most (80%) were unmarried. We used multivariate analysis to identify variables correlated with casual sex, such as alcohol consumption. In addition, we calculated odds ratios for having had casual sex, according to education, occupation and other variables. The quantitative data were supplemented with qualitative, in-depth case studies.

Key findings

A majority of unmarried young men reported sexual experience, including 54% who said that they were sexually active. Nearly one-third (30%) of all men in the subsample had their first sexual experience before age 18. Casual sex among respondents was common; over one-fourth (27%) of all respondents reported having casual sex within the previous 12 months. This proportion was slightly lower (20%) among 18–19 year-old respondents than in the subsample as a whole. Of those who reported having casual sex in the past year, about one-third (31%) also reported having sex with a commercial sex worker.

Over half the young men surveyed said that they consumed alcohol. Out of 133 alcohol users (55%), nearly three-quarters (74% or 98 men) were sexually active. The multivariate analysis found that young men who drank were almost four times more likely to be involved in casual sex than those who did not drink. Many young men reported consuming alcohol before having sex as a way to overcome shame and fear. As one 19 year-old explained, "*Without a drink, I feel ashamed to talk to a girl. But after drinking, I can do anything in mood.*"

All respondents in the sample knew about condoms. However, nearly half (62) of the 131 sexually active young men had never used one, and even those who had used condoms reported inconsistent use with non-regular sex partners (Table 1).

Table 1. Condom use by men in border towns who had engaged in casual sex during the previous 12 months (*N* = 65)

	Number
Number who had ever used a condom with a casual sex partner	39
Number who had used a condom during last sex with a casual sex partner	31

In the survey, young men cited a number of reasons for not using condoms with non-regular sex partners, including that they did not carry a condom with them, that there was no time for a condom, that their partners did not have sex with others or were not infected with HIV, that sex with condoms was less enjoyable, or simply that they did not feel like using one.

In-depth interviews with young men provided more detail about their attitudes towards condoms and their perceptions of their own risk. As the following quote exemplifies, most (58 out of 65) young men involved in casual sex did not perceive themselves to be at risk of contracting STIs, including HIV. One 21 year-old unmarried policemen explained, "*I did not use condom during last time I had sex, since I did not carry one. Since my partners are not carrying any diseases, how can I be at risk of getting AIDS?*" Even those who perceive themselves to be at risk may not use condoms for various reasons. For example, a 19 year-old unmarried man who reported having sex with commercial sex workers explained, "*There is no enjoyment in using condoms. Someday a man has to die, so why not enjoy and die?*"

Conclusions

In summary, casual sex is common in border towns of Nepal. Alcohol consumption is associated with increased involvement in casual sex. There is a large gap between knowledge, attitudes and practice regarding condom use among young men. Most young men surveyed who reported having casual sex did not perceive themselves to be at risk of contracting STIs, including HIV. These research findings suggest that more HIV/STI prevention efforts are needed among young men in border towns. Programme planners and policy-makers need to find ways to improve risk perception and increase preventive behaviour.

Reference

National Centre for AIDS and STD Control (2000) *Cumulative HIV/AIDS Situation of Nepal (monthly bulletin)*. National Centre for AIDS and STD Control, Ministry of Health, Nepal.

Anand Tamang
Centre for Research on Environment
Health and Population Activities (CREHPA)
P.O. Box 9626
Kathmandu
Nepal

Situation analysis of emergency contraceptive use among young people in Thailand

Wanapa Naravage and Siriporn Yongpanichkul

Background

In Thailand, studies estimate that one out of three pregnancies is unwanted (Chayovan & Knodel, 1991) and 200 000–300 000 women terminate their pregnancies each year (Koetsawang, 1993). Adolescents are more likely than adults to hide a pregnancy, seek late-term abortion, and have the procedure performed by untrained providers under unsafe conditions, which often leads to permanent disability or death (Sertthapongkul & Phonprasert, 1993; Koetsawang, 1993; Griensven, 2000).

Emergency contraception (EC) first became available in Thailand in the form of two Ovral® or Eugynon® pills taken within 48–72 hours after sexual intercourse. Because of side-effects, this regimen was not popular. An alternative form of EC became available in 1984 when a dedicated product, Postinor® (and later Madonna®), was introduced. Few studies have assessed patterns of EC use in Thailand; so in 1999, PATH (Program for Appropriate Technology in Health) conducted a study to assess users' knowledge, attitudes and use patterns, drugstore delivery of EC and stakeholders' opinions.

Methods

This study gathered qualitative and quantitative data among purchasers and users, drugstore personnel, stakeholders and potential providers in Bangkok. First, data were gathered on purchaser and user attitudes, perceptions and experiences. Focus group discussions (FGDs) and in-depth interviews were conducted with community members who had used or purchased EC within the previous six months, including three FGDs with men, and one FGD and four in-depth interviews with women. In addition, men and women who purchased EC at six drugstores were asked to complete anonymous, self-administered questionnaires on a voluntary basis. All selected drugstores were located in business areas, close to factory dormitories and entertainment areas in Bangkok. During a 6-week period, 36 men and 33 women completed questionnaires. Most were working adults, but young people aged 18–24 made up about one-third (22) of those who filled out questionnaires. Drugstore personnel reported that some adolescents did not want to participate in the purchaser survey even though it was anonymous, so these data may not be representative.

Second, data were gathered on the perceptions and experiences of providers and stakeholders through a survey, in-depth interviews and the use of simulated clients. Self-administered questionnaires were distributed among 106 drugstore personnel attending a meeting. This questionnaire asked whether their drugstores sold dedicated packages of EC, how frequently they made such sales, and their perceptions of EC clients. In addition, researchers conducted 10 in-depth interviews with drugstore personnel to gather more in-depth information about their attitudes towards young people seeking EC and their practices related to dispensing EC. Simulated clients were also used to assess the practices of dispensing EC in 20 stores. Finally, 18 in-depth interviews were conducted with stakeholders, including policy-makers, family planning experts, representatives from women's nongovernmental organizations (NGOs) and family planning providers.

Key findings

FGD respondents offered several common local names for EC, including *ya kum chua crow*, meaning temporary control of pregnancy, *ya kum lang rum,* meaning control of pregnancy after unprotected sex, *ya ka asuji* meaning pills that kill sperm, and *ya kum dheb plan,* meaning pills that have an immediate effect protecting from pregnancy. All these meanings reflect the perception that the pills are used as a post-coital method, but none specifically refers to emergency situations.

According to FGD respondents and drugstore personnel, the majority of purchasers are men buying EC for women, and it is generally men who select the method for their girlfriends. Women, especially adolescents, said that they feel ashamed to purchase EC themselves. Women often lack information about the pill, and during the discussions, women raised many questions about short-term and long-term effects.

The majority of young people who filled out the purchaser questionnaire learned about EC through friends (17 of 22) or drugstore personnel (5 of 22), similar to reports from the FGDs. Among the 22 young purchasers, more men than women had made the decision to choose EC (13 versus 9). When asked why they used EC, the most common reason was that they had sex infrequently (8 out of 22). The majority said that if EC failed, they would keep the baby; less than half said they would seek an abortion. Most young people had purchased EC more than once (17 out of 22). When asked whether they would keep using EC, the majority (15 of 22) said that they would. In terms of past contraceptive use, the majority of young people or their partners (12 out of 22) had used oral contraceptives or condoms before switching to EC. Nearly half (10 out of 22) the young people said they had used EC in combination with other methods. In FGDs, some men mentioned that they used EC with temporary partners whom they believed were free of STDs/HIV, but used condoms with women who might have more than one partner, such as prostitutes. In general, married men said that their wives did not use EC.

Few respondents reported knowledge of the correct use of EC. The majority (12 out of 22) said that they planned to take only one tablet after having sex. Four of the 22 said that they planned to take one tablet ***before*** sex. Only two reported planning to take two tablets after sex, the correct use of EC. This practice was confirmed in FGDs with men and women, who said that they or their partner did not consider taking the second tablet. Nine out of 17 respondents who had purchased EC in the past reported that they or their partners used more than two tablets of EC per month, which suggests that they may use it regularly, contrary to its intended purpose (Table 1).

A majority of purchasers said that they had received some information from drugstore personnel. However, more than half of purchasers felt that the information was inadequate, and they wanted to know more about side-effects, contraindications and long-term consequences. The information they received consisted mainly of instructions on how to take the pills and a warning not to take more than four tablets per month. Purchasers did not mention receiving important messages such as efficacy of the pills, not to use EC regularly, that the pills cannot prevent STIs/HIV, or information

Table 1. EC use patterns among young purchasers (aged 18–24) surveyed in Bangkok drugstores (*N*=22)

	Number
Frequency of EC purchase	
First time purchase	5
Had purchased EC more than once	17
EC use per month (among those who had purchased EC in the past)	
1 tablet per month	1
2 tablets per month	6
3 tablets per month	1
4 tablets per month	6
5 tablets per month	1
6 tablets or more per month	1
Don't know	1
How taken	
One tablet after having sex	12
One tablet before having sex	4
Two tablets after having sex	2

about side-effects. It is noteworthy that nothing in the package mentions the importance of taking the second pill. Furthermore, drugstore staff were aware of the study's subject matter, and may have given more information than usual. This was confirmed through the use of simulated clients, who found that less than half of the drugstore personnel provided any information to purchasers.

Stakeholders were generally aware of the growing use of EC among young people. They felt that EC is needed as an alternative choice for women; however, they felt that both the general public and service providers lack adequate knowledge about the method. Medical and family planning experts said that provision of EC through drugstores is appropriate and ensures easy access, but some stakeholders felt that this encourages irresponsible sexual behaviour and/or incorrect use of EC. Many stakeholders mentioned the need to integrate sex education in schools and the need to train health personnel at every level about EC.

Conclusions

These study findings suggest that both purchasers and providers lack adequate information about EC, which points to a number of policy and programme implications. First, there is an urgent need to formulate standard guidelines for EC use that mirror those of the World Health Organization and other international bodies. Instructions in the insert leaflet should include key messages such as: (a) EC is for emergency use only, and should not be used as a regular method; (b) EC cannot prevent STI/HIV infection; and (c) users should complete the two-tablet dose.

Public and private health professionals, drugstore personnel and representatives from women's nongovernmental organizations need additional training on EC. For example, academic institutes that train health professionals should include EC in their curriculum. Manuals and other educational materials on EC should be produced for family planning providers, particularly drugstore personnel. And drugstore networks, such as Pharmacist Associations and the Drugstore Club of Thailand, should promote awareness of EC among their members.

Finally, young people need to be convinced to use other contraceptive methods rather than EC as their regular method. They should be informed that EC is for "emergency" use only. Counselling services should provide accurate information on EC and related topics to young people. In the long run, sex education for young people needs to be integrated into formal education. Such programmes should aim to give young people a comprehensive understanding of contraceptive methods, including EC, as well as to produce attitude changes on gender issues.

References

Chayovan N, Knodel J (1991) *Coital activity among married Thai women: evidence from the 1987 Thailand Demographic and Health Survey*. Population Studies Center Research Report No. 91-221 (translated into Thai). Ann Arbor, Michigan, University of Michigan, Population Studies Center.

Griensven F (2000) Sex, drugs and HIV/STD among adolescents in Northern Thailand: an innovative, rapid, biological and behavioural assessment. Paper presented at the *XIII International AIDS Conference, Durban, South Africa, 9–14 July*.

Koetsawang S (1993) Illegally induced abortion in Thailand, Paper presented at the *IPPF SEARO Regional Programme Advisory Panel Meeting on Abortion, Bali, Indonesia, 29–30 October.*

Sertthapongkul S, Phonprasert P (1993) Causes of unplanned pregnancy and decision process for abortion: a case study at Bangkok private clinic. *Journal of Development Administration*, Bangkok, Thailand.

Wanapa Naravage and Siriporn Yongpanichkul
PATH (Program for Appropriate Technology in Health)
37/1 Soi Petchburi15, Petchburi Road
Bangkok 10400
Thailand

VII

The context of abortion among adolescents

Menstrual regulation among adolescents in Bangladesh: risks and experiences

Halida Hanum Akhter

Background

Under the Penal Code dating back to 1860, induced abortion is permitted in Bangladesh only to save the life of the mother. Legalization of first-trimester abortion on broad medical and social grounds was proposed in 1979, but legislators did not take action. In 1979, however, the Bangladesh Government included menstrual regulation (MR) in the national family planning programme and encouraged doctors and paramedics to provide MR in all government hospitals and health and family planning complexes (Bangladesh, Population Control and Family Planning Division, 1979). The Government considers menstrual regulation to be an "interim method of establishing non-pregnancy for a woman at risk of being pregnant, whether or not she actually is pregnant" (Ali, Zahir & Hasan,1978). Nearly 8000 doctors and 6500 paramedics now provide MR services in government clinics throughout the country, in addition to those providers who work in private MR clinics. Despite the widespread availability of legal and safe MR services, however, many young women resort to illegal and unsafe abortion. This report describes some aspects of the sexual and reproductive health situation of adolescent women in Bangladesh and summarizes the available data on young women's experiences with menstrual regulation and induced abortion.

Aspects of the sexual and reproductive health situation of adolescents

Studies suggest that many adolescent women in Bangladesh lack adequate knowledge about reproductive health. Recent studies from both rural and urban areas (Akhter et al., 1998a; Akhter et al., 2000) found that nearly half of the adolescent women in the studies had no information about menstruation before it began. A recent large-scale study (Barkat et al., 2000) found that over half of the married adolescents in the study were unaware of the causes of menstruation (58%) or the consequences of unprotected sex (57%). More than half (57%) of the unmarried adolescents and over 40% of the married adolescents had not heard of menstrual regulation (Table 1).

Table 1. Knowledge of selected reproductive health topics among young people in Bangladesh, 2000

Health topic	Unmarried adolescents	Married adolescents
Unaware of cause of menstruation (%)	55.4	58.4
Unaware of consequences of unprotected sex (%)	41.5	57
Never heard of abortion (%)	35.4	24
Never heard of menstrual regulation (%)	56.7	42

Source: Barkat et al., 2000.

About half of all women in Bangladesh marry before age 20, and on average, women become pregnant within 13 months after marriage (Khan et al., 1997). According to the 1997 Demographic and Health Survey (DHS), nearly 15% of all 16–19 year-old married women were pregnant at the time of the survey, and 58% had begun childbearing by age 19 (NIPORT et al., 1997). At 31%, the contraceptive prevalence rate among married adolescents is much lower than the national average for married women of 51%. Contraceptive use is increasing among married adolescents, but estimates of unmet need remain high. According to the Centre for Health and Population Research, unmet need among married women aged 10–14 and 15–19 is 33% and 22% respectively (Quamrun et al., 1999).

Use of menstrual regulation among adolescents

Several large- and small-scale studies have measured the magnitude of MR use among adolescent women. The 1997 DHS found that 1.6% of currently married adolescents reported undergoing menstrual regulation. Some evidence suggests that about 19% of women who undergo MR are aged 15–19 (Koenig et al, 1988).

One study (Akhter et al., 1998b) collected data among women hospitalized for delivery of an unwanted pregnancy or complications of induced abortion, as well as those who sought MR. Women who had no knowledge of MR were more likely to be hospitalized for complications of unsafe abortion than those who knew about MR. The study found that adolescents constituted 6% of women giving birth to an unwanted child, 8% of women hospitalized for complications of induced abortion, 9% of those who received MR services and 15% of women rejected by MR providers (Table 2).

It is noteworthy that adolescents constituted a larger proportion of women rejected by MR clinics than of those accepted. Typically, providers reject women for two main reasons. In some cases providers reject women who are pregnant for the first time because they are concerned about infection or future infertility. In other cases, providers reject women who are too far along in their pregnancy to undergo the procedure. Adolescents — particularly unmarried adolescents — may be more likely to be too late in recognizing their pregnancy and/or seeking services.

This study found that a majority of adolescent women seeking to terminate a pregnancy did so for their first pregnancy, including 81% hospitalized for complications of induced abortion, 46% of those who underwent MR, and 67% of those rejected by MR services. The majority of adolescents had not used a contraceptive method in the six months prior to seeking pregnancy termination (Table 2). When adolescents were asked why they had not

Table 2. Proportion of adolescents among women with unwanted pregnancy, and their history of contraceptive use

	Hospitalized for:		Sought services at an MR clinic:	
	Delivery of an unwanted pregnancy (*N* = 726)	Complications of induced abortion (*N* = 628)	Accepted (*N* = 1288)	Rejected (*N* = 175)
Per cent of women <20 years old	5.5	8.4	8.8	15.4
Per cent of women <20 years old reporting no contraceptive use within the six months prior to becoming pregnant	85	75.5	69	63

Source: Akhter et al., 1998b.

Table 3. Method used to induce abortion that led to complications (*N* = 38)

Type of method used	Number of cases
MR procedure/syringe	18
Rubber catheter	4
Solid stick inserted	7
Taking medicine	6
Other	3

Source: Akhter et al., 1998b.

used contraception, approximately one-third said that they were unaware of contraceptive methods or did not know where to obtain them. An additional one-third mentioned that their husband did not want them to use contraception.

When 38 young women hospitalized for abortion complications were asked what kind of provider had induced the abortion, respondents mentioned physicians (7), nurses (7), traditional birth attendants (7), the woman herself (5), family planning workers (3), and allopathic village doctors (2). Seven women did not respond. The most frequently used methods of inducing abortion included MR syringes (18), insertion of solid sticks (7), insertion of rubber catheters (4), and ingestion of medicine (6) (Table 3).

Health consequences of abortion among adolescents

A national study (Akhter et al., submitted for publication) investigated abortion-related morbidity and mortality in 1996–1997 and found that of 30 668 reported cases of complicated induced abortion, 1415 (5%) resulted in death. Adolescents constituted 7% of those who experienced complications and 8.1% of those who died. Nearly 1% of women who died and 0.2% of those who experienced a reported complication were unmarried. Using medical records from five hospitals, Rochat & Akhter (1999) documented 52 abortion-related tetanus deaths occurring in 1996 and found that 10 cases were in women aged 10–19. The study by Akhter et al. (1998b) found that 13% of adolescents hospitalized for induced abortion had life-threatening complications. Half had symptoms of severe infection. Over 21% had mechanical injury to the cervix or vagina. About 16% had evidence of a foreign body having been inserted into the vagina, cervix or uterus.

Conclusions

These research findings highlight numerous issues. First, studies suggest that adolescents lack an adequate understanding about the maturation process, fertile periods, and the risks of unprotected sex. The majority do not use contraceptives to prevent unwanted pregnancies. Adolescents lack knowledge about the risks and consequences of pregnancy termination, and many are unaware that menstrual regulation services are available. Because they do not have the information needed to recognize their pregnancy and seek MR quickly, they are often rejected by MR clinics because their pregnancy is too far advanced. In many cases, these factors lead young women to resort to unsafe methods of abortion.

To address this situation, adolescents need to be provided with better information and services to help them understand their sexuality and protect them from unwanted pregnancy. Greater awareness of the availability of MR services could reduce the numbers of young women who resort to unsafe abortion. Policy-makers could also address barriers that influence the numbers of adolescents who are rejected by MR clinics. Finally, social barriers such as the need to have a male escort need to be addressed to facilitate adolescent women's access to reproductive health care.

References

Akhter HH, Rochat R, Chowdhury M, Shah R, Yusuf H (submitted for publication) Complications from induced abortion in Bangladesh and impact on mortality related to types of practitioner and method in 1996.

Akhter HH, Karim F, Chowdhury ME, Rahman MH

(1998a) *A study to identify the risk factors affecting nutritional status of adolescent girls in Bangladesh.*. Dhaka, Bangladesh, BIRPERHT (BIRPERHT Publication No. 119, Technical Report No. 67).

Akhter HH, Ahmed YH, Chowdhury ME, Rahman MH, Khan AR (1998b) *A study to assess the determinants and consequences of abortion in Bangladesh,* Dhaka, Bangladesh, Development Assistance Council and BIRPERHT (BIRPERHT Publication No. 118, Technical Report No. 66).

Akhter HH, Hossain MM, Akhter M, Desai SN, Rahman MH (2000) *Report on needs assessments on reproductive health information and care among adolescents in Paurashava schools and colleges.* Dhaka, BIRPERHT (BIRPERHT Publication No. 123; Technical Report No. 71).

Ali MS, Zahir M, Hasan KM (1978) *Report on Legal Aspects of Population Planning in Bangladesh.* Dhaka, The Bangladesh Institute of Law and International Affairs.

Bangladesh, Population Control and Family Planning Division (1979) Circular No. FP/Misc-26/79/278 (600), issued on 31 May 1979. Government of People's Republic of Bangladesh, Population Control and Family Planning Division Memo No. 5-14/MCH-FP/Trg/79.

Barkat A, Khan SH, Majid H, Sabina N (2000) *Adolescent Sexual and Reproductive Health in Bangladesh: A Needs Assessment.* Dhaka, Bangladesh, Human Development Research Centre, prepared for Family Planning Association of Bangladesh .

Khan MA, Rahman M, Khanam PA, Barkat-e-Khuda, Kane TT, Ashraf A (1997) Awareness of sexually transmitted diseases among women and service providers in rural Bangladesh. In: Kane TT, Barkat-e-Khuda, Phillips JF, eds. *Reproductive Health in Rural Bangladesh, Policy and Programmatic Implications, Volume 1.* Dhaka, MCH-FP Extension Project (Rural), International Centre for Diarrhoeal Disease Research, Bangladesh:1–20.

Koenig MA, Fauveau V, Chowdhury AI, Chakraborty J, Khan MA (1988) Maternal mortality in Matlab, Bangladesh: 1976–1985. *Studies in Family Planning* 19(2):69–80.

Quamrun N et al. (1999) *Strategies to Meet the Health Needs of Adolescents: A Review.* Special Publication. Bangladesh, Operations Research Project, Health and Population Extension Division, Centre for Health and Population Research, International Centre for Diarrhoeal Disease Research, Bangladesh.

National Institute of Population Research and Training, et al. (1997) *Bangladesh Demographic and Health Survey 1996–1997.* Dhaka, NIPORT, Calverton, Maryland, Mitra and Associates, Macro International Inc.

Rochat R, Akhter HH (1999) Tetanus and pregnancy-related mortality in Bangladesh. *Lancet,* 354(9178):565 (letter).

Halida Hanum Akhter, MBBS, MCPS, MPH, Dr PH
Director
Bangladesh Institute of Research for Promotion of Essential & Reproductive Health and Technologies (BIRPERHT)
House # 105, Road # 9/A, Dhanmondi R/A
Dhaka-1209
Bangladesh

Induced abortions: decision-making, provider choice and morbidity experience among rural adolescents in India

Bela Ganatra and S.S. Hirve

Background

An estimated six million abortions take place in India each year. However, gaps remain in our understanding of the context of abortion, the decision-making process, the reasons why women seek abortion and choose different types of providers, and the extent to which abortions result in complications. The information that is available is drawn largely from urban hospital populations or secondary analysis of case records. During 1996–1998, researchers with the KEM Hospital Research Centre in Pune, India carried out a community-based study on induced abortion in a predefined rural area of western Maharashtra. This paper presents the research findings that relate to adolescent abortion-seekers from that study.

Methods

Exploring such a sensitive issue through community-based research posed complex challenges (Ganatra & Hirve, 2001). To identify women who had an induced abortion in an 18-month reference period, the abortion study used a multiple-source community and provider-based case-finding process. Of the 1717 married women identified, 1409 acknowledged that their abortion was induced and agreed to talk about it, including 197 (14%) aged 20 or less, and 570 (41%) between the ages of 21 and 24. In addition, researchers identified 43 unmarried adolescent abortion-seekers, including 25 who had never married, 18 who were separated and 2 who were widowed. Finally, researchers interviewed 159 abortion providers in and around the study area.

Information on abortion-related mortality came from a separate population-based study on maternal mortality, also done by the KEM Hospital Research Centre in the same general region and in the same villages that were part of the induced abortion study. That study screened all post-childhood female deaths in order to determine those that were pregnancy-related (Ganatra, Coyaji & Rao, 1998; Ganatra, 2001).

Key findings

As seen in Table 1, despite having a higher level of education, young married women in the abortion study had a lower status in the household than older women. Younger women had significantly lower decision-making powers, less mobility and less likelihood of having an independent source of income or control over money earned (Table 1).

Young women's lower status was reflected in the abortion decision-making process. Married adolescents were less likely to have played a major

Table 1. Profile of married adolescent abortion-seekers compared with youth and adult abortion-seekers

	Adolescents ≤ 20 years old (N=197)	Youth 21–24 years old (N=570)	Adults ≥ 25 years old (N=642)
Woman's education (years)	6.89 (SD 3.31)	6.66 (SD 4.31)	5.64 (SD 4.91)
Cohabiting with mother-in-law	OR 2.13 (1.52–2.48)	OR 1.44 (1.13–1.83)	OR 1.0
Economic independence of woman			
own independent income (%)	11.7	20.5	26.9
able to keep/spend their own salary (%)	20.0	33.7	38.7
Autonomy			
permission needed to go to market (%)	66.1	58.6	52.9
permission needed to go to health centre (%)	81.4	71.3	64.1
permission needed to go to natal home (%)	99.4	96.6	92.7
Decision-making by women			
cooking, market purchases (%)	14.6	28.4	34.6
purchase of major items (TV etc.) (%)	15.7	22.2	30.1
seeking care for own illness (%)	39.0	44.4	47.4
Discussion / communication with husband on issues relating to contraception (%)	74.0	87.9	81.8

role in the decision, more likely to have been coerced into an abortion, and, conversely, more likely to have faced opposition from their families than older women (Table 2).

Spacing between children was the main reason that adolescents underwent an abortion (53.3% of all abortions). Although less common than in other groups, sex selection to avert the birth of a girl child accounted for nearly one of every eight abortions among adolescents. Despite the cultural premium placed on producing a child as soon after marriage as possible, 7% of abortions among these rural adolescents were done to postpone the birth of the first child. Contraceptive use between the last pregnancy/marriage and the index abortion was significantly lower among adolescents (13%) than among young women (23%) or adults (31%). The gestational age at which the three groups terminated their pregnancies was similar, and, contrary to expectations, married adolescents did not come in for later abortions than older women.

Women across the age groups chose similar providers and showed a marked preference for the private sector. Few married women opted for traditional providers in this setting where other services were available. Although they chose similar providers, the actual abortion experience varied with age. For example, both public and private sector providers were more likely to insist on spousal consent for younger abortion-seekers, even though

Table 2. Married women's role in the decision to terminate a pregnancy

	Adolescents ≤ 20 years old (N=199)*	Youth 21–24 years old (N=593)*	Adults ≥ 25 years old (N=676)*
Woman reported playing a major role in decision to terminate the pregnancy (%)	75.8	86.1	91.1
Woman herself opposed the abortion (%)	4.5	1.9	1.5
Woman faced opposition from her family for her decision to have an abortion (%)	18.9	16	12.3

*N refers to abortion episodes. Many women had more than one induced abortion during the reference period; hence N is higher in this table than in Table 1.

it is not a legal requirement. Adolescents were significantly less likely to be counselled about contraceptive use and were subsequently less likely than older women to adopt a contraceptive after abortion (36% of adolescents compared with 58% of women aged 25 or older). Perceived post-abortion morbidity was higher among adolescents; however, life-threatening complications were similarly low across all age groups and were related to provider type and gestational age rather than the woman's age.

Unmarried adolescent abortion-seekers reported a markedly higher use of traditional providers than married women, despite the availability of other abortion services (Table 3). The principal factors influencing provider choice were the level of support from the family and/or the concerned man, need for anonymity and provider attitudes. Cost may play a role as well, since the mean cost of a second-trimester private-sector abortion for an unmarried adolescent was three times that of a similar abortion for a married adolescent. In-depth case studies revealed that providers charged higher prices for unmarried clients. It is noteworthy that nearly 60% of adolescents who had undergone an abortion were unaware that abortions among unmarried women were legal. Similarly, of the 159 abortion providers interviewed, 40% selectively refused services to unmarried or separated women.

The population-based study on maternal mortality from the same region found that abortion-related mortality accounted for only four of the 140 pregnancy-related deaths identified during a 35-month reference period. However, three of these four deaths were among adolescents. In addition, four unmarried pregnant adolescents committed suicide in order to preserve family honour and died without accessing any sort of abortion services. Thus, deaths related to abortions and unwanted pregnancies accounted for 18% of pregnancy-related deaths among adolescents as compared with 2% of deaths among older women.

Conclusions

While the state of Maharashtra has better geographic access to abortion services than many other parts of India, these study findings suggest that for adolescents, access is impeded by their low autonomy, mobility and status within the household. These findings clearly demonstrate the need for existing family planning programmes to focus on the needs of young, recently married women, especially those who wish to delay the birth of the first child or postpone a subsequent birth. Post-abortion contraceptive counselling currently targets older women who have finished childbearing. Such counselling needs to expand to both married as well as unmarried adolescents.

Being unmarried compounds the vulnerability of being young and poses strong cultural, provider

Table 3. Choice of provider, gestational age and perceived morbidity among unmarried and married adolescent abortion-seekers

	Married adolescents (*N*=199)*			Unmarried adolescents (*N*=46)*		
	Number		Per cent	Number		Per cent
Choice of provider						
Traditional provider	2		1	12		26.1
Private practitioner	161		80.5	30		65.2
Public hospital	37		18.5	4		8.7
Mean gestational age at abortion (weeks)		10.8			12.7	
Morbidity experienced	143		71.9	33		72.2**

* *N*: number of abortion episodes in reference period.

**Includes one death.

and legal barriers. The most telling indicator of this vulnerability is the substantial contribution of suicides due to unwanted pregnancies to maternal deaths in the area. There is a compelling need to spread legal awareness among adolescents and providers to ensure that barriers such as spousal consent and higher costs do not make access to services more difficult than it already is. The finding that lower costs, provider sensitivity and concerns about confidentiality led unmarried adolescents to use traditional providers even where safer options were available argues for technically sound services to improve quality of care and, in particular, provider attitudes. Abortion providers need to explore ways to make their services more anonymous, perhaps by mainstreaming them with other medical services. This would reduce the extent to which the stigma associated with illegitimate pregnancies becomes a barrier to the ability to respond to women's needs.

Acknowledgements: This study was funded by a grant from the Ford Foundation to the KEM Hospital Research Centre, Pune. The study on Maternal Mortality was funded by a WHO grant (No.M/183/263 Safe Motherhood Research, Div. of Family Health) to the KEM Hospital Research Centre, Pune. A grant from the Institute of Reproductive Health, Department of Population and Family Health, Johns Hopkins School of Public Health, provided the opportunity for preparation of this paper.

References

Ganatra BR (2001) Induced abortions: programmatic and policy implications of data emerging from an ongoing study in rural Maharashtra. In: Puri C, Van Look P, eds. *Sexual and Reproductive Health: Recent Advances, Future Directions.* New Delhi, New Age International Limited Publishers:249–261.

Ganatra BR, Coyaji KJ, Rao VN (1998) Too little, too far, too late: a community-based case control study on maternal mortality. *Bulletin of the World Health Organization*, 76(6):591–598.

Ganatra BR, Hirve SS (2001) Ethical dilemmas in social science research — a field study on induced abortion. *Issues in Medical Ethics*, January, 9(1).

Bela Ganatra and S.S. Hirve
Research Fellows
Department of Population and Family Health
Johns Hopkins School of Public Health
615 N Wolfe Street
Baltimore, MD 21205
USA

VIII

Reproductive tract and sexually transmitted infections

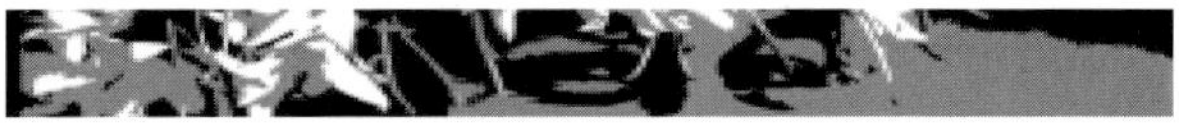

Impact of sexually transmitted infections including AIDS on adolescents: a global perspective

Purnima Mane and Ann P. McCauley

Background

In recent years, the reproductive and sexual health of adolescents has drawn increasing attention. Rates of sexually transmitted infections (STIs) are soaring among young people, with one-third of the 333 million new STI infections each year occurring among young people under the age of 25 (World Health Organization, 1999). Each year, more than one out of 20 adolescents contracts a curable STI, not including viral infections (World Health Organization, 1997). Most importantly, younger age groups are hardest hit by the pandemic of acquired immunodeficiency syndrome (AIDS). More than half of all new human immunodeficiency virus (HIV) infections today occur in young people between the ages of 15 and 24. This situation persists in a policy climate that continues to deny adolescents information and services that they need to make informed choices about their sexual and reproductive health, despite evidence that adolescents show a remarkable capacity to adopt safer behaviours when given access to such knowledge, skills and services (Aggleton et al., 2000b; Joint United Nations Programme on HIV/AIDS, 1997). This paper describes the physiological, behavioural and social factors that make adolescents more vulnerable than adults to STIs, the consequences of STIs, including HIV, and the policy implications that follow.

Vulnerability of adolescents to STIs and HIV

Physiology is the first factor that makes adolescents—particularly girls—more vulnerable than adults to STIs. Because girls have a large mucosal surface area exposed to infection and have not developed mature mucosal defence systems, the cells that line the opening of the cervix are more susceptible to chlamydia, gonorrhoea and HIV than those of adult women (Population Council, 1999; Van Dam, 1995). This fact argues for later sexual initiation for girls. Yet, research carried out by the International Center for Research on Women (ICRW) partners in Brazil, Malawi and Papua New Guinea indicates that many girls have intercourse before menarche (Weiss, Whelan, & Rao Gupta, 1996). Not surprisingly, in some countries infection rates among girls are higher than among boys. In Kenya, for instance, nearly one girl in four between the ages of 15 and 19 is believed to be living with HIV compared with one boy in 25; in Zambia, in the same age group, 16% of girls versus 1% of boys are HIV-infected (Joint United Nations Programme on HIV/AIDS, 1998).

Social powerlessness, poverty and economic dependence contribute to the vulnerability of youth. Many young people lack control over who their sexual partners are, how many partners they have, or the circumstances and nature of sexual activity. Immediate needs for shelter, food, lodging, clothes, or even school fees may prevent young people from choosing safe sex, which increases the likelihood of infection. Research indicates that young people worldwide suffer from sexual abuse and exploitation. Although this is more common for girls, many boys are also sexually abused or coerced (Heise, Moore & Toubia, 1995). Adolescents in situations such as armed conflict, social upheaval, refugee and migrant situations, and those who are homeless, drug users, orphans, or living with HIV may be highly vulnerable to infection resulting from sexual exploitation. Unfortunately, they are often outside the reach of government programmes and policies. Their needs must therefore be given special attention.

In some cases, social norms put young people at risk by encouraging them to have sex in unsafe circumstances. For example, social approval of early marriage forces girls into early sexual activity. Unmarried girls often face pressures to have sex, such as in Zimbabwe, where girls report that they have to have sex with their boyfriend in order not to lose him (Bassett & Sherman, 1994). Social norms often push boys into early sexual initiation and risky behaviour. Deprived of reliable information and access to preventive methods, boys are often ill-equipped to protect themselves from STIs (Joint United Nations Programme on HIV/AIDS, 1999c). Young gay men face even more difficulties in a world that favours heterosexuality (Aggleton et al., 2000a).

Social norms often forbid discussion of sex, despite evidence that information prevents unwanted pregnancies, lowers rates of STI transmission and delays sexual initiation (Joint United Nations Programme on HIV/AIDS, 1997). In focus group discussions with low-income Indian adolescents, researchers found that no one had explained to any of the girls about menstruation, sexual intercourse, or childbearing (Bhende, 1995). Adults often justify this harmful refusal to inform young people about sexuality as a way to maintain their "purity". For girls in particular, just knowing or asking about sex may cause others to criticize them because it is interpreted as a sign of being sexually active. This social norm cuts girls off from accurate and useful information and the ability to protect themselves (Weiss, Whelan & Rao Gupta, 1996). To maintain the image of innocence, girls in Thai factories said that, even if they knew about sex, they pretended they did not, so that they were seen as virgins. This was the reason that they could not carry condoms or suggest condom use (Cash & Anasuchatkul, 1995). In some ways the HIV pandemic has increased the amount of information that adults give young people about sex. However, the Population Council's Horizons studies among school youth in Mexico, South Africa and Thailand indicate that many young people have only superficial knowledge about HIV. The young people in those studies knew basic information about HIV, but they also believed that mosquitoes and toilet seats could transmit HIV.

In all these factors, gender acts as a major differential. Data show that more girls than boys are uninformed about their bodies and STIs. Many are not in a position to negotiate safer sex and are more susceptible to rape or coerced sex. Clearly the impact of STIs and HIV on girls is likely to be more significant (Bassett & Sherman, 1994).

Consequences of STIs and HIV for young people

Many STIs can be cured or treated. However, the consequences of untreated or incurable STIs include infertility, illness and death—both for those young people who are infected and their children. The social and emotional costs of infertility are especially high for women in contexts where parenthood is highly valued. Failure to produce children can result in emotional trauma, family neglect, abuse or abandonment. STIs can also lead to the illness or death of a young person or a neonate. STIs cause many young people to suffer chronic morbidity, including painful ulcers or warts, and skin lesions. STIs such as HIV, human papillomavirus (HPV), and hepatitis B may all eventually lead to death. Shame and fear of reprisal often prevent young people from getting timely treatment for an STI, thus worsening the situation. One serious consequence of STIs is that they may facilitate HIV infection. Evidence suggests that STIs, including syphilis, herpes and gonorrhoea, can increase the risk of HIV transmission 2–9-fold (Population Council, 1999). While shame adds to the misery of having a curable STI, the stigma of HIV can drastically affect young people's mental and emotional health.

As the global HIV pandemic spreads, growing numbers of young people who are not infected suffer consequences because people close to them have either died or are ill with AIDS. The Joint United Nations Programme on HIV/AIDS (UNAIDS) estimates that 16 million young people have already been orphaned by AIDS (Joint United Nations Programme on HIV/AIDS, 2000b). For many, the loss of a parent was preceded by years of living with an ill parent. These children experience not only the grief of losing a parent and the possibility of being stigmatized by others in the community, but also a high likelihood of having a series of caregivers, receiving less food to eat and having to end their education (United Nations Children's Fund, 1999). Studies from Côte d'Ivoire, Haiti, India, and Thailand found that children were taken out of school as one means through which affected families reduced expenditures (Joint United Nations Programme on HIV/AIDS, 1999d). The first to leave school are likely to be the older children who can earn income or care for others, particularly girls. A study in Mumbai found that in families with an HIV-positive member, income fell, children were taken from school and put into the labour market, and the burden of care fell on the women. Because of the stigma associated with HIV, households were careful to keep secret the HIV status of the family member, thus cutting them off from community resources (Joint United Nations Programme on HIV/AIDS, 1999d). In these settings, adolescents have been compelled to take on adult roles prematurely and the period of transition to adulthood disappears. They care for ill parents, and many eventually become the head of the household (Foster et al., 1997).

Long-term structural changes in high prevalence countries will also affect adolescents. In areas of high HIV prevalence, AIDS affects the whole educational system. As teachers become ill, class sizes grow and the quality of the education diminishes. In 1998, for example, Zambia lost 1300 teachers—about 70% of the number of new teachers who finished training and started to teach that year (Joint United Nations Programme on HIV/AIDS, 2000a). Demographers who used to talk about population pyramids now talk about population chimneys, because of the lack of adults in the most productive years between 35 and 60. This loss will weaken institutions such as governments and inhibit the growth of private-sector enterprises. As a result, poverty will become more widespread (Joint United Nations Programme on HIV/AIDS, 2000c), further threatening the economic and social security of young people. In sum, adolescents in regions greatly affected by HIV face a bleak future if action is not taken. Researchers have noted the changes in adolescent opportunities and expectations, and have advocated policies and programmes that will assist them to face some of the challenges, but little is known or said about the psychological impact of HIV on these young people.

Conclusions

To address the impact of STIs on adolescents, we need to ensure access to information and services, and protection from discrimination. The examples of Switzerland and Uganda demonstrate that, where governments acknowledge the problem of HIV and provide access to information, services and protection from discrimination, they can reduce the rate of new infections among young people. We also need to ensure that young people have access to new technologies now being developed.

Scientists are working on new treatments, microbicides and vaccines for STIs including HIV. If we continue to deny young people access to information and services, however, these will do little good.

To address long-term structural changes in society, new approaches must be multisectoral and include planning for continuity in education, public safety, health care and other institutions that are likely to be impaired by high morbidity and mortality rates. In addition, policies and programmes need to recognize the heterogeneity of adolescents' lives. Finally, both rhetoric and action should emphasize positive aspects of sexual health. Adolescents need to appreciate that reproduction and sexuality are not just about unpleasant aspects of pregnancy, disease and death, but about pleasure, fulfilment and living a full life. We need an approach that is understanding without being condescending, acknowledges their potential, provides access to what is needed for a healthy transition to adulthood, and prepares them to creatively face a challenging future.

In 1993, the Director of the STD and AIDS Control Program of a state in India visited an industrial township where he talked to local sex workers about their experiences with STIs. The sex workers told him that insisting on condoms was particularly difficult during seasons when their business was down. When asked what these seasons were, they identified the period when thousands of 15 year-olds take the 10th standard All-State examinations. Policy-makers need to accept and deal with this reality, not in a moralistic fashion, but in an open manner that gives adolescents the means and social environment to ensure that they can enjoy a safe and healthy future.

References

Aggleton P, Ball A, Mane P (2000a) Young people, sexuality and relationships. *Sexual and Marital Relationship Therapy*, Special Issue, 15(3):213–220 (editorial).

Aggleton P, Chase E, Rivers K, Tyler P (2000b) *Innovative Approaches to HIV Prevention: Selected Case Studies Prepared for the Joint United Nations Programme on HIV/AIDS.* Geneva, UNAIDS.

Bassett M, Sherman J (1994) *Female Sexual Behavior and the Risk of HIV Infection: An Ethnographic Study in Harare, Zimbabwe. Women and AIDS Program Research Report Series.* Washington, DC, International Center for Research on Women.

Bhende A (1995) *Evolving a Model for AIDS Prevention Education among Underprivileged Adolescent Girls in Urban India.* Women and AIDS Program Research Report Series. Washington, DC, International Center for Research on Women.

Cash K, Anasuchatkul B (1995) *Experimental Educational Interventions for AIDS Prevention among Northern Thai Single Female Migratory Adolescents.* Women and AIDS Program Research Report Series. Washington, DC, International Center for Research on Women.

Foster G, Makufa C, Drew R, Kralovec E (1997) Factors leading to the establishment of child-headed households: the case of Zimbabwe. *Health Transition Supplement*, 2(7):155–168.

Heise L, Moore K, Toubia N (1995) *Sexual Coercion and Reproductive Health: A Focus on Research.* New York, Population Council.

Joint United Nations Programme on HIV/AIDS (1997) *Impact of HIV and Sexual Health Education on the Sexual Behaviour of Young People: A Review Update.* Geneva, UNAIDS.

Joint United Nations Programme on HIV/AIDS (1998) *Report on the Global HIV/AIDS Epidemic*. Geneva, UNAIDS.

Joint United Nations Programme on HIV/AIDS (1999a) *AIDS Epidemic Update: December 1999*. Geneva, UNAIDS.

Joint United Nations Programme on HIV/AIDS (1999b) *A Review of Household and Community Responses to the HIV/AIDS Epidemic in the Rural Areas of Sub-Saharan Africa*. Geneva, UNAIDS.

Joint United Nations Programme on HIV/AIDS (1999c) *Sex and Youth: Contextual Factors affecting Risk for HIV/AIDS.* Geneva, UNAIDS.

Joint United Nations Programme on HIV/AIDS (1999d) *Report on a Consultation on the Socio-Economic Impact of HIV/AIDS on Households, Chiang Mai, Thailand.* Geneva, UNAIDS.

Joint United Nations Programme on HIV/AIDS (2000a) *HIV/AIDS and Development.* Geneva, UNAIDS.

Joint United Nations Programme on HIV/AIDS (2000b) *Report on the Global HIV/AIDS Epidemic.* Geneva, UNAIDS.

Joint United Nations Programme on HIV/AIDS (2000c) *Socio-Economic Impact of HIV/AIDS in Africa.* Geneva, UNAIDS.

Population Council (1999) *Reproductive Tract Infections: A Set of Fact Sheets.* Bangkok, Population Council, South and East Asia—Thailand Office.

United Nations Children's Fund (1999) *The Progress of Nations 1999.* New York, UNICEF.

Van Dam CJ (1995) HIV, STD and their current impact on reproductive health: the need for control of sexually transmitted diseases. *International Journal of Gynecology & Obstetrics*, Suppl. 2:S121–S129.

Weiss E, Whelan D, Rao Gupta G (1996) *Vulnerability and Opportunity: Adolescents and HIV/AIDS in the Developing World.* Washington, DC, International Center for Research on Women.

World Health Organization (1997) *Young People and Sexually Transmitted Diseases, Fact Sheet #186.* Geneva, World Health Organization.

World Health Organization (1999) *Programming for Adolescent Health and Development.*. Geneva, World Health Organization (WHO Technical Report Series No. 886).

Purnima Mane, PhD
Vice President and Director
International Programs Division
Population Council
One Dag Hammarskjold Plaza
New York, NY 10017
USA

Ann P. McCauley, PhD
Horizons Project/International Center for Research on Women
Population Council
4301 Connecticut Avenue, # 280
Washington, DC 20008
USA

Gynaecological problems among young married women in Tamil Nadu, India

Abraham Joseph, Jasmin Prasad and Sulochana Abraham

Background

It is increasingly accepted that adolescent reproductive health deserves special attention. While a few studies have been done (Bang et al., 1989; Brabin et al., 1995), little is known about the prevalence of reproductive tract infections (RTIs) or sexually transmitted infections (STIs) among adolescents in the developing world. Because laboratory facilities are not available in many resource-poor settings, the World Health Organization (WHO) has developed clinical algorithms (called the Syndromic Approach) to diagnose and treat RTIs based on easily recognizable signs and symptoms (WHO, 2000; WHO, 2001). To determine the nature and extent of gynaecological morbidity in young married women and to test the validity of the syndromic approach, researchers from the Community Health and Development Program (CHAD) of Christian Medical College undertook a population-based, cross-sectional study in 13 South Indian villages.

Methods

The study was conducted in 13 villages of Kaniyambadi Block, a rural area of Vellore District in south India. Because of the communities' trust in CHAD's work, almost all (92%) eligible women living in the villages agreed to participate in the study. Researchers enrolled 451 non-pregnant married women aged 16–22 (mean age of 20.7 years). Information was collected on the women's menstrual and obstetric histories, perceived gynaecological symptoms, health care-seeking behaviour and contraceptive practices. All women gave blood and urine samples and underwent a medical (speculum) examination for RTI. If the laboratory tests or clinical examination detected any signs suggestive of infection, then the women were asked a second round of questions about symptoms they might have experienced.

Key findings

Among all young women in the study, 240 (53%) reported a symptom suggestive of an RTI, including white discharge (44%), burning sensation while passing urine (19%) and vaginal itch (12%). Among those reporting symptoms, 171 women (38%) had one symptom, 45 women (10%) had two symptoms and 23 women (5%) had all three.

Clinical and laboratory diagnoses indicated that 59% (265) of respondents had one or more gynaecological problem. This included 48.5% who suffered from an RTI, 9% with infertility (defined as inability to conceive after two years of married life without contraception), and 7% with a urinary tract infection. The prevalence of STIs in this study group

Table 1. Prevalence of various RTIs among married (non-pregnant) women aged 16–22 in 13 villages in Vellore District of Tamil Nadu, south India (*N* = 451)

Diagnosis	Number	Per cent
One or more gynaecological problem	**265**	**59**
Infertility	40	9
Urinary tract infection	31	7
History of genital prolapse	3	0.7
Any reproductive tract infection	**219**	**48.5**
Candidiasis	45	10
Bacterial vaginosis	82	18
Cervicitis	38	8
Pelvic inflammatory disease	28	6
Any sexually transmitted infection	**82**	**18**
Trichomoniasis	58	13
Syphilis – RPR	1	0.2
Syphilis – TPPA	7	1.5
Chlamydia trachomatis	8	1.8
Hepatitis B	8	1.8

was 18% (82 women), while 19 women had a history of genital ulcers (Table 1). No women were diagnosed with warts, molluscum, herpes, or gonorrhoea.

An analysis of possible factors affecting prevalence revealed that RTIs were more common among women who had had a greater number of pregnancies, had two or more children, had been married for a greater number of years, or had had a tubectomy. RTIs were also more common among women whose husbands were transport workers or in the armed forces. However, multivariate analysis showed that the only significant variable was duration of marriage. These findings could suggest that young married women —generally thought to be at low risk for STIs— may be exposed to STIs via their husbands (Table 2).

Confirming the findings of RTI studies among adult women, this study found a weak association

Table 2. Possible factors affecting prevalence of RTIs in young women

	N	Per cent with an RTI	OR	Chi^2	*P* value
Age of respondent					
16–18	37	35	1		
19–20	138	46	1.6	1.07	0.29
21–22	276	51	1.96	2.85	0.09
Number of years married					
<1	35	34	1		
1–4	278	46	1.6	1.3	0.26
>5	138	57	2.6	5.05	0.03
Husband's occupation					
Farmer	82	46	1		
Farm labourer	164	51	1.2	0.34	0.56
Salaried or small business	53	34	0.6	1.55	0.21
Armed forces	68	56	1.5	0.98	0.32
Transport worker	70	64	2.1	0.91	0.34
Other	14	46	0.97	0.01	0.94

N = number; OR = Odds ratio.

between self-reported symptoms and clinical/laboratory diagnosis among young women. Of the 240 young women who reported symptoms suggestive of an RTI, only 58% (138) were diagnosed with an infection. At the same time, among women who reported no symptoms, 38% (81) were diagnosed with an RTI.[1] The study found a stronger association between laboratory diagnosis and the WHO algorithms for diagnosing RTIs on the basis of clinic signs (using a speculum examination).[2] This finding suggests that even without sophisticated laboratory facilities, primary health centres could do more to diagnose and treat RTIs.

Data on health-seeking behaviour revealed that only 35% of women who reported gynaecological symptoms had ever sought treatment. Most women (78%) who did so tried home remedies or sought help from traditional medicine or unqualified private practitioners. Only 9% of women who reported symptoms had sought medical care at the government primary health centres. It is noteworthy that most (50 out of 81) "asymptomatic" women diagnosed with an RTI were in fact aware of symptoms but had not reported them during the first round of questions because they regarded these symptoms as normal or of trivial importance.

Conclusions

Women face many barriers to accessing RTI services. In this area, laboratory facilities to diagnose and treat RTIs and STIs are currently available only in District and *Taluk* hospitals or perhaps private facilities. To access these services, many women from these villages would have to travel long distances.

The high prevalence of RTIs (48.5%) and STIs (18%) and the poor utilization of health services among young married women, hitherto considered to be at low risk of infection, should be of great concern. Not only do RTIs pose a threat to health, but they also impose an economic and social burden due to the stigma associated with these infections. These study findings highlight the need to raise awareness of RTIs and STIs and to expand services for prevention and treatment for young women. To do this effectively, however, it may be necessary to improve the quality of care provided at the community level.

References

Bang RA, Bang AT, Baitule M, Choudhary T, Sarumukadda S, Tale O (1989) High prevalence of gynaecological diseases in rural Indian women. *Lancet,* 1:85–88.

Brabin L et al. (1995) Reproductive tract infections and abortion among adolescent girls in rural Nigeria. *The Lancet,* 345:300–304.

WHO (2000) *Women and sexually transmitted diseases.* Geneva, World Health Organization (WHO initiative on HIV/AIDS and Sexually Transmitted Infections. Division of AIDS and STD. Fact Sheet No. 249).

WHO (2001) *Guidelines for the management of sexually transmitted infections.* Geneva, World Health Organization (Document No. WHO/RHR/01.10).

Further reading

Amsel R, Totten PA, Spigel CA, Chen KCS, Eschenbach D, Holmes KK (1983) Non specific vaginitis: Diagnostic criteria and microbial and epidemiologic association. *American Journal of Medicine*, 74:14–22.

Bhatia CJ, Cleland J (1995) Self-reported symptoms

1 The study found that the WHO algorithms based on reported vaginal discharge alone also had poor sensitivity (50%), specificity (60%) and predictive value (47%).

2 The WHO algorithm using clinical signs for diagnosis of RTIs (including speculum examination) had a high sensitivity (95%) and specificity (93%).

of gynaecological morbidity and their treatment in South India. *Studies in Family Planning*, 26(4):203–216.

Chakraborty S, Munni M (1989) Serological surveys for syphilis amongst antenatal cases in selected hospitals of Delhi. *Indian Journal of Public Health*, 33.

Dhall K, Sarkar A, Sokhey C, Dhall CL, Ganguly NK (1990) Incidence of gonococcal infection and its clinico-pathological correlation in patients attending gynaecological outpatient department. *Journal of Obstetrics and Gynaecology of India*:410–414.

Heine P, McGregor JA (1993) Trichomonas vaginalis: A re-emerging pathogen. *Clinical Obstetrics and Gynaecology,* 36(1):137–143.

La Ruche G, Lorougnon F, Digbeu N (1995) Therapeutic algorithms for the management of sexually transmitted diseases at the peripheral level in Cote d'Ivoire: assessment of efficacy and cost. *Bulletin of the World Health Organization,* 73:305–313.

Lee HH et al. (1995) Diagnosis of Chlamydia trachomatis genito-urinary infection in women by ligase chain reaction assay of urine. *Lancet*, 345:213–216.

Ndinya-Achola JO, Kihara AN, Fisher LD, Krone MR, Plummer FA, Ronald A, Holmes KK (1996) Presumptive specific clinical diagnosis of genital ulcer disease in a primary health care setting in Nairobi. *International Journal of STD and AIDS*, 7:201–205.

Nugent RP, Krohn MA, Hillier SL (1991) Reliability of diagnosing bacterial vaginosis is improved by a standardised method of gram staining interpretation. *Journal of Clinical Microbiology,* 29(2):297–301.

Pels RJ et al. (1985) Dipstick urinalysis screening of adults for urinary tract disorders. *JAMA*, 254:240–245.

Ridgway GL et al. (1996) Comparison of the ligase chain reaction with cell culture for the diagnosis of *Chlamydia trachomatis* infection in women. *Journal of Clinical Pathology*, 49:116–119.

Sobar JD (1993) Candidal vulvovaginitis. *Clinical Obstetrics and Gynaecology*, 36(1):153–165.

Tramont EC (1995) Treponema pallidum. In: Mandell, Douglas, Bennett, eds. *Principles and Practices of Infectious Diseases.* New York, Churchill Livingstone:2117–2132.

Wasserheit JN (1992) Epidemiological synergy. Interrelationships between human immunodeficiency virus infection and other sexually transmitted diseases. *Sexually Transmitted Diseases*, March–April; 19(2):61–77.

Wasserheit JN, Harris JR, Chakraborty J, Kay BA, Mason KJ (1989) Reproductive tract infections in a family planning population in rural Bangladesh. *Studies in Family Planning*, 20(2):69–80.

World Health Organization (1985a) *Program of research, development and research training in human reproduction, 1985, Annual Technical Report.* Geneva, World Health Organization.

World Health Organization (1985b) *Neisseria gonorrhoea and gonococcal infections: Report of a WHO scientific group.* Geneva, World Health Organization:65—75 (Technical Report Series No. 616).

Younis N, Khattab H, Zurayk H, El-muethy M, Amin MF, Faraq M (1993) A community study of gynaecological and related morbidity in rural Egypt. *Studies in Family Planning* 24(3):175–176.

Dr Abraham Joseph
Community Health Department
Christian Medical College
Vellore 632002
Tamil Nadu
India

Developing an interactive STI-prevention programme for young men: lessons from a north Indian slum

Shally Awasthi, Mark Nichter and V.K. Pande

Background

India has a pressing need for education programmes that address sexually transmitted infections (STIs) among adolescents. According to a literature review by Ramasubban (1995), as many as 25% of patients attending government STI clinics in India are younger than 18 years old. Data on STI prevalence are particularly troubling in light of the rapid escalation of human immunodeficiency virus (HIV) infection in India. An estimated four to five million people are currently infected (AIDS Alert, 1999; Joint United Nations Programme on HIV/AIDS & World Health Organization, 1998), and epidemiologists speculate that India may soon have the largest HIV-infected population in the world (Bollinger et al., 1995; Kant, 1992). Although the cultural and social mores of India complicate forthright discussion of sexual activity, particularly among the young and unmarried, rising rates of STIs, including HIV/AIDS, demand that young people be educated about the dangers of unsafe sex and STI symptoms, as well as prevention and treatment of STIs.

While school-based programmes are clearly important in India, many young people at risk for STIs do not remain in school beyond seventh grade when sex-education classes are typically given. Community-based programmes are clearly needed to reach these groups. The challenge is how to develop relevant and acceptable community-based STI prevention programmes. In 1996 and 1997, researchers carried out a project in urban slums of Lucknow, Uttar Pradesh, to address this challenge. The project aimed to document sexual practices and ideas about STIs and acquired immunodeficiency syndrome (AIDS) among adolescent males and to use these data to develop and evaluate a community-based STI education programme. This paper describes the study findings and makes some recommendations for future STI programmes.

Methods

Lucknow neighbourhoods are designated as slums on the basis of lack of amenities such as electricity, safe drinking-water, and sewage and garbage disposal. Researchers selected 28 of 261 slums and assigned half to the control group and half to the study group. Between 25 and 30 young men aged 15–21 from each slum agreed to participate, giving a total of 343 in the control group and 377 in the study group. Researchers took care to recruit youths who belonged to social networks associated with both schools and sources of employment. The baseline data revealed that participants in the intervention and control groups were well matched, with a slightly higher proportion of married youths in the intervention slums. Loss to follow-up was 14 boys (4%) in the intervention group and 0% in the control group.

During the formative stage of the project, 47 adolescents were interviewed individually or as part of focus group discussions (FGDs) about their knowledge of STIs and sexual behaviour of young people in their slums. These data were used to develop both the survey and the intervention. Following the pilot research, male project staff administered the pretested questionnaire to young men in each intervention and control slum. Staff filled out questionnaires for the youth after assuring them of confidentiality. These pre-intervention data were compared with post-intervention data collected 6–8 weeks later using the same survey instrument.

The intervention consisted of three educational sessions held at two-week intervals. Facilitators presented scientific information as well as commonly held beliefs identified during the formative research phase, and then opened up the session for questions. Facilitators invited participants to write questions and place them in a locked box marked with a sign that read, "Tell your problems and get rid of the hidden disease". The programme provided basic information about: (a) reproductive physiology, fertility and conception; (b) STI transmission, types and symptoms, *gupt roga* (a local name for STIs meaning "hidden disease"), and the nature of asymptomatic infections; (c) the link between STIs and HIV infection; (d) HIV tests; and (e) STI prevention and "harm reduction"—meaning local practices meant to reduce negative effects of risky sex before, during, or after sex.

Facilitators employed and evaluated different communication strategies, including teaching by analogy. For example, to illustrate how AIDS harms the body gradually rather than all at once, facilitators compared it to termites eating a tree slowly from within. Only when the tree falls does one realize that the roots have been devoured. Each hour-long session was prepared in Hindi and pretested among young men of the same age in a slum not included in the project. The session facilitator was supported by three male assistants, who made themselves available to participants for individual private consultations about sensitive issues. During the last 15 minutes, facilitators played a taped set of educational messages that repeated key points made in the live session. Some participants listened to these messages while others discussed issues related to the session with friends or staff. At the end of the project, three FGDs were held to evaluate the programme from the perspective of the young men.

Key findings

During the project, participants placed more than 150 questions in the question box. One-third focused on HIV/AIDS, including questions such as: could one get AIDS from kissing, sharing a cigarette, or mosquito bites? And, does AIDS always end in death? One-quarter of all questions related to *gupt roga*. Some wanted to know how one could tell if girls they were about to marry had a condition that could give them *gupt roga*. Follow-up ethnographic research revealed that young men imagined causes of STIs unrelated to contagion in a biomedical sense, including having sex with a girl who has a "heaty" body (referring to body temperature in a humoral sense) or with a girl whose blood is not complementary. Youths wanted to know whether a man could get *gupt roga* if a woman was menstruating or had discharge. They also wanted to know if someone could develop STIs from too much sex. Youths wanted to know how to protect themselves before, during and after sex, including whether there were medicines one could take, or measures one could adopt, such as washing the penis after sex. They also wanted to know how a condom prevents sickness—is it just by enclosing the penis or is there some chemical in the condom? A few sought advice on how to treat "male" symptoms such as cloudy or coloured urine.

Many questions concerned masturbation. Is masturbation a sickness or addiction? How often can the body lose semen without becoming sick or weak? Does masturbation alter the size of one's penis or cause it to hang to one side? Does it affect one's virility or ability to impregnate one's wife later in life? Can one develop *gupt roga* or some other illness from excessive masturbation? Boys also asked about the causes of nocturnal ejaculation and how to prevent it. They wanted to know whether it was a sign of sickness. They asked more than a dozen questions about the effect of smoking or chewing *pan masala* (betel leaf and nut), including whether smoking affects sex drive or performance.

Although the study did not aim to establish levels of adolescent sexual activity, it did provide crude data on sexual activity. At baseline, approximately 15–17% of youths reported intercourse outside of marriage, including about 3% (22 youths) who reported intercourse with a prostitute and 3% (20 youths) who reported oral or anal sex with another male. When asked whether they anticipated having a sexual encounter in the next six months, 18% of unmarried youths stated that the likelihood was very high, 20% stated that they probably would, and 62% replied that they would not. Of the 22 youths who said they had visited a prostitute, seven (32%) reported having used a condom, whereas 42 (56%) of those who said they had had intercourse with a friend or relative reported having used a condom. Protection against pregnancy seemed to motivate most condom use. Ten out of 20 youths who reported sex with another male stated that they had a condom at least once, and all these young men also reported using a condom with a woman.

Two issues related to sexual behaviour invite further research. First, the analysis suggests a possible relationship between sex with prostitutes and sex with another male, given that eight out of 22 youths who visited prostitutes also reported sex with another male. Second, youths who engaged in weekly or daily alcohol use were significantly more likely to engage in unsafe sex than were light or non-drinkers (OR: 3.53; 95% CI: 1.64–7.61; P value < 0.0002). Eighteen per cent of the intervention group and 13% of the control group defined themselves as weekly drinkers, and 1–2% defined themselves as daily drinkers.

Before the intervention, between 59% and 66% of youths in both study and control groups reported knowing that there is more than one type of STI, but few participants were able to describe symptom clusters. In the follow-up survey, knowledge that multiple STIs exist had increased in both groups, but the increase was statistically significant only in the intervention group (from 66% to 83%). At baseline, between 30% and 40% of youths believed that women and men with an STI always show symptoms of their illness. Young men in the intervention group scored a statistically significant increase in the knowledge that symptoms may not always appear. They also registered significant increases in their knowledge of STI symptoms and in their knowledge about how long symptoms of AIDS (and associated diseases) take to become apparent. However, a majority of youths continued to be confused about how long other STIs took to become symptomatic (Table 1).

After the intervention, awareness that STIs including HIV/AIDS could be acquired from women other than prostitutes jumped significantly from 50% to 76% in the intervention group. However, young men's awareness that they were personally at risk of acquiring STIs changed little during the intervention. Population-based data about STI risk did not translate into increased recognition that their immediate environment rendered them vulnerable to STIs. Fewer than 25% of those surveyed before or after the intervention thought that STIs were a big problem where they lived. Perhaps due to secrecy surrounding the "hidden disease", few said that they knew anyone who had experienced such an illness.

The intervention made moderate headway in educating youth about ineffective "harm-reduction" practices. A statistically significant decrease was found in the proportion of the intervention group who thought that taking medicines before or after sex could prevent STIs (from 58% to 21%) or that

Table 1. Changes in knowledge about STIs in the intervention and control groups, pre- and post-intervention

		Intervention group (*N*=377)			Control group (*N*=343)			
		Baseline	**Follow-up**	**Change**	**Baseline**	**Follow-up**	**Change**	***P* value**
Knew that one can get		N=377	N=363					
STIs from women who	No.	177	276	**99**	175	201	**26**	
are not prostitutes	%	46.9	76.0	**29.1**	51.0	58.5	**7.5**	<0.001
Knew that there is more than one	No.	250	301	**51**	203	236	**33**	
type of STI	%	66.3	82.9	**16.6**	59.2	68.8	**9.6**	<0.001
Knew that STIs are not always symptomatic	No.	229	316	**87**	232	249	**17**	
in women	%	60.7	87.1	**26.4**	67.6	72.6	**5.0**	<0.001
Knew that STIs are not always symptomatic	No.	230	302	**72**	227	237	**10**	
in men	%	61.0	83.2	**22.2**	66.2	69.1	**2.9**	<0.001
Did not know how long it takes for symptoms	No.	307	295	**–12**	283	258	**–25**	
of STIs to manifest	%	81.4	81.3	**–0.1**	82.5	75.2	**–7.3**	0.9
Did not know how long it takes for symptoms	No.	377	232	**–145**	264	210	**–54**	
of HIV/AIDS to manifest	%	100.0	63.9	**–36.1**	76.9	61.2	**–15.7**	<0.001
Knew when during a woman's cycle she is least likely to	No.	90	155	**65**	93	81	**–12**	
become pregnant	%	23.9	42.7	**18.8**	27.1	23.6	**–3.5**	<0.001

using a vaginal birth control or antifungal tablet reduced the chance of disease (from 45% to 26%). The proportion of the intervention group who thought that these behaviours prevented HIV/AIDS decreased significantly from 63% to 21%. However, nearly half the youths continued to believe that washing the penis with disinfectant after sex helped prevent disease, and 30–40% continued to believe that urinating after sex greatly reduced their chances of developing STIs.

During FGDs at the end of the project, researchers asked participants what they would advise a friend to do if he had already engaged in risky sex. They indicated that they had heard about "tests", but were uncertain about what such tests revealed, or how long one should wait before being tested. Some questioned why a person shouldn't just take medicine. The test might be a waste of money or might not be evaluated correctly. They considered medicine to be a sure cure. Several youths pointed out that the sessions had not prepared them to choose a good practitioner, should it become necessary to obtain treatment. They wanted to know how they could tell if diagnostic tests or medicines were effective or reasonably priced, and wanted to know more about the cost of treatment.

Conclusions

This research project highlighted several challenges for future STI education programmes. First, communicating the message that STIs can be asymptomatic proved difficult. Teaching by analogy was somewhat successful, but project staff felt that better messages should be developed, taking into account popular notions of STIs and the need for gender sensitivity. Gender sensitivity is an important issue as it became apparent in an FGD with young Hindu men that some men associated STIs with women's impurity and inherent dangerousness. As a result, researchers decided not to explain that women tend to be asymptomatic more often than men to avoid supporting negative stereotypes of women as primary disseminators of STIs. Another future challenge is the need to address sexual behaviours other than coitus. The finding that many youths who engaged in high-risk sex with prostitutes also engaged in sex with other males highlights the need for more research on male-to-male sex in India, and the need to develop new educational messages. The challenge is how to prepare communities for frank discussions about hidden sexual behaviours. Finally, because researchers had not investigated the medicines that local practitioners prescribed, the team felt at a loss to offer advice to participants about locally available STI treatment. In the future, researchers need to investigate what young men do and whom they consult when they think they might be developing an STI. Future programmes must offer practical, reality-based recommendations about where to turn for testing and treatment.

Despite these challenges, however, the study demonstrated that STI education could be introduced to young people in a community setting using innovative approaches grounded in an understanding of local realities. Community acceptance of STI education may increase if educators address cultural as well as medical concerns, and the study demonstrated the usefulness of programmes that are informed by anthropological research.

This summary has been adapted from the full article entitled "Developing an interactive STD-prevention programme for youth: Lessons from a north Indian slum", published in *Studies in Family Planning*, 2000, 31(2):138–150.

Acknowledgements: The authors acknowledge the technical inputs of Professor Gail Slap. The study was funded by the International Clinical Epidemiology Network (INCLEN)—Institute for Research on Women and Gender, Small Grants Program.

References

AIDS Alert (1999) AIDS hits Indian population with monsoon force. *AIDS Alert-International Supplement*, 14(5):1.

Awasthi S, Nichter M, Pande VK (2000) Developing an interactive STD-prevention programme for youth: Lessons from a north Indian slum. *Studies in Family Planning*, 31(2):138–150.

Bollinger RC, Tripathy SP, Quinn TC (1995) The human immunodeficiency virus epidemic in India: Current magnitude and future projections. *Medicine*, 74(2):97–106.

Joint United Nations Programme on HIV/AIDS, World Health Organization (1998) *Epidemiology fact sheet on HIV/AIDS and sexually transmitted diseases: India.* Geneva, UNAIDS/WHO Working Group on Global HIV/AIDS and STD Surveillance.

Kant L (1992) HIV infection: Current dimensions and future implications. *Council of Medical Research Bulletin,* 22:113–126.

Ramasubban R (1995) Patriarchy and the risks of STD and HIV transmission to women. In: Das Gupta M, Chen L, Krishnan TN, eds. *Women's Health in India.* Oxford, Oxford University Press:212–239.

Further reading

Jejeebhoy SJ (1998) Adolescent sexual and reproductive behavior: A review of the evidence from India. *Social Science and Medicine,* 46(10):1275–1290.

Khanna N, Nadkarni V, Bhutani L (1998) India. In: Plummer D et al., eds. *Sexually Transmitted Diseases in Asia and the Pacific.* New South Wales, Australia, Venerology Publishing:115–137.

Nichter M, Nichter M (1996) Education by appropriate analogy. In: Nichter M, Nichter M, eds. *Anthropology and International Health: Asian Case Studies*. New York, Gordon and Breach:401–426.

Watsa MC (1993) Premarital sexual behaviour in urban educated youth in India. Paper presented at the *Workshop on Sexual Aspects of AIDS/STD Prevention in India, Bombay, 23–27 November.*

Dr. Shally Awasthi
Professor
Department of Pediatrics and Clinical Epidemiology Unit
King George's Medical College
Lucknow University
Lucknow, Uttar Pradesh
India

Sexual health services for adolescents at sex clinics in Rawalpindi, Pakistan

Shahid Maqsood Ranjha and Anusheh Hussain

Background

In Pakistan, like many countries in South Asia, talking about sexuality is perceived as taboo or immoral, and sex outside of marriage is strongly condemned. As a result, many people, including health providers, lack the vocabulary to address issues related to sexual and reproductive health. Sexually active unmarried adolescents are often afraid to access reproductive health services, and services that are available to adolescents often reinforce myths and misinformation. Adolescents (defined in this presentation as the age group 12–21 years) make up nearly one-fourth of the Pakistani population (Pakistan Integrated Household Survey, 1995). However, the lack of adequate national policies has led to the neglect of adolescents' reproductive health needs. Several non-governmental organizations (such as PAVHNA, FPAP and ROZAN) provide adolescent reproductive health services, but they are not sufficient to meet the need given the population size and the barriers to access that adolescents face.

Among the few providers of sexual and reproductive health services in Pakistan are the *Hakim Sahibs,* who practise herbal medicine in "sex clinics", which have been present in the subcontinent since herbal medicine began. These practitioners often claim to be specialists in sexual or other health matters, and they typically use the Ayurvedic or homoeopathic system of medication. They have generally learned this skill from their forefathers, and usually have no degree or certificate from any university or medical college. In the 1960s, the Government of Pakistan legalized and registered herbal clinics, including sex clinics. Some *Hakim Sahibs* are legally registered as practitioners of homoeopathic or Greek systems of medicine, but the majority are unregistered and work illegally.

At least two reasons explain the popularity of sex clinics in Pakistan. First, much of the Pakistani population lives in rural areas where basic health services are either unavailable or inaccessible to most of the population. Sex clinics, on the other hand, are abundant in both rural and urban areas, and can be found in every other street and *mohalla* (community). In many places, there are no obvious alternatives. Second, many people prefer the kind of herbal medicine practised in the sex clinics to allopathic medicine available elsewhere.

SAHIL[1], a registered voluntary organization,

[1] SAHIL is the only major organization in Pakistan that focuses on child sexual abuse (CSA) and child prostitution in Pakistan. Our work includes sensitizing the media, conducting research on issues surrounding CSA, developing educational materials for schools on prevention of CSA, and providing a healing centre for adult survivors who were sexually abused as children or were forced into child prostitution.

counsels children and adolescents on a broad range of topics, including issues related to sexuality. As many as 80% of adolescents attending SAHIL's counselling programme seek help for issues related to sexual health, including masturbation, nocturnal emissions, menstrual bleeding and the condition of the hymen. Male and female homosexuality have also emerged as serious concerns. These concerns are exacerbated by myths and misconceptions, guilt and perceived associations with abnormality. SAHIL found that, among the adolescents with sexual health concerns, almost 50% had sought care from *Hakim Sahibs* in local sex clinics before coming to SAHIL. To gain a better understanding of adolescents' experiences at these sex clinics, SAHIL sought to investigate the services provided by the *Hakim Sahibs*, including their knowledge, attitudes and practices, the information they provide, the terminology they use, and the medications they prescribe.

Methods

The study was carried out in Rawalpindi, the twin city of Islamabad. SAHIL is based in Islamabad, but most clients come from Rawalpindi. SAHIL researchers conducted an inventory of sex clinics operating in Rawalpindi. We visited 15 sex clinics where we interviewed 15 *Hakims* and five male clients about their knowledge, attitudes and practices. In addition, we conducted seven case studies using a "mystery client" methodology. SAHIL researchers (five men and two women) sought services from *Hakim Sahibs*, based on the most frequently heard concerns in our counselling programme. These concerns included: (1) hymen rupture; (2) masturbation; (3) nocturnal emission; (4) impotence; (5) premature ejaculation; and (6) homosexuality. Because no *Hakim* was willing to give us samples of their medicines, we used the case studies to obtain samples and conducted laboratory tests to determine the contents.

Key findings

SAHIL found that Rawalpindi, a city of over 10 *lakhs* (one million people), had over 250 herbal clinics, of which over 50 were specifically sex clinics advertising services for sexual health problems, and over 200 others offered sexual health services among a range of other services. The majority of *Hakims* interviewed claimed to have passed their matriculation equivalent to Class 10. Most said that they were in the business because their fathers and forefathers had done the same thing. The study found that the *Hakims*' knowledge about reproductive health, HIV, hepatitis C and other sexually transmitted infections (STIs) was insufficient and myth-ridden. For example, they generally believed that all reproductive and sexual health problems could be fixed by medicines, that semen is a major source of energy, that the direction of the penis plays a major role in sexual health issues, and that masturbation can cause infertility, impotence and premature ejaculation. The majority reported that the hymen could be reconstructed by taking oral medicines, that the absence of a hymen means "sexual corruption", and that homosexuality could cause a decrease in sperm count, leading to permanent infertility.

During the case studies, four out of seven *Hakims* touched or spoke to our male and female researchers in ways that were sexually suggestive or harassing. For example, during check-ups of female clients they said things such as: "you are so young", "your wrists are very beautiful", "you are a pretty girl", etc. Physical check-ups involved attempts to massage the penis or in another case to caress a woman's wrist while pretending to check her pulse. (The latter case was for hymen reconstruction, so it was not clear why the *Hakim* wanted to take a pulse.) On the other hand, we found that *Hakims* were uncomfortable with the language of sexuality. Just like the general public, they used words that were indirect and obscure. For example, they asked women and men if pain was felt in the "lower area", meaning the vagina or penis.

The instruments used during the check-ups seemed to be plastic toys and were mostly self-made. Some *Hakims* took urine samples, even though they had no laboratory equipment. To analyse the urine, they looked at it and prescribed a combination of medicines based on this visual assessment. All *Hakims* demanded their fee before the check-up, and they generally charged Rs 200, not including the cost of medicines.

When asked about the ingredients of the medication they dispensed, all *Hakims* claimed that they used bear testicles, lioness fat, monkey brains, sparrows' kidneys, exotic herbs, beasts' organs, gold and silver. After conducting laboratory test of these medicines, we found that they included appetite stimulants such as *Carmina*, as well as spices, steroids and narcotics, such as opium and synthetic morphine. Additional laboratory tests found testosterone and progesterone (male and female hormones) in five out of seven samples. The cost of medicines varied between Rs 500 and Rs 60 000, but the majority of *Hakims* demanded over Rs 12 000. Our researchers were told that the reason that the medicines were so expensive was that they contained costly ingredients such as "beasts'" organs, gold and silver.

The five adolescent clients interviewed had visited *Hakims* for reproductive health problems or perceived sexual problems, such as premature ejaculation, impotence and nocturnal emission. We found that the clients lacked the same kinds of knowledge as *Hakims* regarding sexual health and sexual diseases. Our major finding, however, was that every adolescent client said that after using medicines they felt better than before visiting the *Hakim*. We can only speculate about why they felt improvement, but perhaps the narcotics used in these medicines reduce anxiety, fear or stress, thereby enhancing sexual activities. In addition, opiates and other narcotics block the senses and thereby help control premature ejaculation. Or, the medicine may lead to perceived improvement by inducing a placebo effect that makes clients feel that they have been treated.

Conclusions

In conclusion, the study found that both *Hakims* and clients reported misconceptions and myths about sexual and reproductive health. Many of the *Hakims* used sexually harassing language and touch. Although clients reported feeling some improvement after taking the costly medicines dispensed by *Hakims*, such medicines contained ingredients such as narcotics and hormones that could be dangerous for their health. These study findings illustrate how denying adolescents sexual health services and basic information about reproductive health has created even more misinformation, trauma, and suffering for them. Quacks continue to thrive, while health professionals turn their backs to the sexual health needs of adolescents. The choice between dogma and adolescent safety and health is clear. This research demonstrates the need to change the behaviour of service providers, as well as the need for adolescents to adopt safe health behaviours.

References

Government of Pakistan (1998) *National Survey of Pakistan* [Unpublished Census data, available from the Government of Pakistan, Statistics Division].

Pakistan Integrated Household Survey (1995) Pakistan Institute of Development Economics. [Available at: www.pide.org.pk/serv04.html]

SAHIL
#13, First Floor
Al Babar Centre, F-8 Markaz
Islamabad
Pakistan

IX

Communication between adolescents and adults about sexual and reproductive health

Access to reproductive health information in Punjab and Sindh, Pakistan: the perspectives of adolescents and parents

Minhaj ul Haque and Azeema Faizunnisa

Background

Pakistan has an adolescent population of nearly 30 million, two-thirds (66%) of whom live in urban areas and one-third (34%) in rural areas (Government of Pakistan, 1998). Pakistani adolescents can be categorized into a number of broad groups—those who are employed, those in school, those married, those in one or none of the above groups (Durrant, 2001). Large gender differences exist within these groups. Fifty-two per cent of adolescent boys are in school compared with only 31% of girls, for example, and 45% of girls are neither married, nor employed nor in school, compared with only 13% of boys.

To obtain more information about the perspectives of young unmarried adolescents, the Population Council carried out a qualitative study using focus group discussions (FGDs) with adolescents and parents. The FGDs covered education, employment, skill-building, autonomy, marriage and health. This paper presents findings related to reproductive health knowledge, practice and determinants, from the perspectives of both adolescents and parents.

Methods

Researchers carried out the study in two stages. In the first stage, they held 13 FGDs with adolescent girls and boys from Punjab. In the second stage, they conducted an additional 12 FGDs with adolescent girls and boys and 12 FGDs with parents from Punjab and Sindh. Adolescent respondents ranged in age from 10 to 19 years; separate FGDs were held for girls and boys. Respondents came from rural and periurban areas, including Sargodha, Rawalpindi, Bahawlapur, Sialkot and Chakwal districts in Punjab, and Khairpur, Hyderabad and Karachi districts in Sindh. The study included only unmarried adolescents and their parents.

Key findings

Through FGDs, researchers explored the channels and mechanisms that young people and their parents use to seek and share reproductive health information. Respondents discussed their preferred sources of information and the ways in which parents and adolescents interact with each other about these issues.

Findings from FGDs with parents suggested that parents, especially fathers, shied away from discussing reproductive health issues with their children. Most parents thought that adolescents would learn about puberty and other reproductive health issues by themselves when the time came.

Reflecting a cultural tendency to seek curative care for an ailment after it strikes rather than take preventive measures, parents described a general apathy towards discussing reproductive health issues with their children before there was a clear need. Parents were aware of the media as an influential source of information and expressed concerns about its negative impact on young people. Parents considered schools and skill development centres as "safe" places for adolescents to learn about reproductive health issues.

Researchers asked young people about their information networks related to reproductive health. FGDs with girls and boys suggested that girls had better personal networks of information among their families than boys. Girls' sources of knowledge included mothers, elder sisters and relatives. In contrast, boys said that they tended to rely on television, films, videos, books, *hakims* and friends as primary sources of information about reproductive health, rather than family members. Boys described their reluctance to talk to parents about puberty, saying for example, *"Boys are too embarrassed to discuss these matters with their fathers. We mostly talk about these things with a close friend or older brother"* (Boys' FGD, rural Punjab).

Nevertheless, both girls and boys felt that there was a need for more information, especially regarding puberty. For example, girls said that they were not given enough information about menstruation. As one respondent described, *"No one tells us, it just happens, and then either an older sister or the mother tells us to take proper measures during the 4–5 days"* (Girls' FGD, rural Punjab). Both girls and boys felt that teachers should provide reproductive health information. In general, adolescents said that they wanted more parental guidance to help prepare them for adulthood.

Girls generally felt that they faced more problems during adolescence than boys, because of limits on their freedom of movement, lack of say in major life decisions, early marriage, lack of education and lack of health care. In FGDs, parents acknowledged that there are gender differences in health-seeking behaviour because of poor access and social barriers. For example, fathers described barriers to taking their daughters to health care facilities saying:

> *People ask embarrassing questions and draw unnecessary conclusions if a young girl falls sick. Therefore, we avoid taking her to the health facility, unless there is a dire need. (*Fathers' FGD, rural Punjab).

Researchers asked adolescents about issues related to marriage. As in much of South Asia, marriage occurs relatively early, and adolescents have almost no say about whom and when to marry. FGD participants discussed this practice and identified early marriage as a problem for many adolescents, particularly rural girls. In FGDs, both girls and boys said that they would like more say in choosing their life partner. Most girls and boys considered 20–25 to be the ideal age for marriage.

Conclusions

In conclusion, girls seem to have better personal information networks, but they also have less access to health services and face greater social constraints. The results of this study suggest that adolescents need more information about reproductive health, including physiological changes during puberty, sex and reproduction. Both young people and parents consider parents, teachers and school textbooks as "safe" and dependable sources of reproductive health information. Most parents say they prefer that others, such as relatives, teachers or elders, discuss reproductive health issues with their children. Parents also suggest that school programmes should provide this information, pointing to a critical opportunity for reproductive health education programmes that want to reach adolescents.

These research findings raise a number of implications for research, policies and programmes. Given that data on adolescents are paltry and often anecdotal, Pakistan needs more in-depth and representative data on the situation of adolescents in various strata of society. Programmes for youth need to evolve at the community level involving local people and need to be integrated with life-skills development. Finally, because the influence of media is so strong, print, electronic and digital media need to address these issues in a culturally sensitive way.

References

Durrant V (2001) *Adolescent Girls and Boys in Pakistan: Opportunities and Constraints in the Transition to Adulthood, Research Report No. 12.* Islamabad, Population Council.

Government of Pakistan (1998) *Population and Housing Census 1998: Advance Tabulation on Sex, Age Group, Marital Status, Literacy and Educational Attainment (Bulletin 6)*. Islamabad, Government of Pakistan, Statistics Division.

Azeema Faizunnisa
Chief, Information Services
Population Council
7, Street 62
Sector F 6/3, Islamabad
Pakistan

Building a supportive environment for adolescent reproductive health programmes in India: essential programme components

Rekha Masilamani

Background

Pathfinder and its partner organizations have launched adolescent reproductive health programmes in several Indian states. One objective of these programmes is to influence parents, families and teachers of adolescents as a way to improve the general environment in which adolescents enter into sexual activity and marriage. This presentation describes these programmes and the barriers they must overcome in order to improve adolescent sexual and reproductive health.

Programme description

Community-based programmes are under way in three slum areas of Delhi, one rural block in Tamil Nadu and nine villages in Rajasthan. These programmes involve community outreach and education, building of referral linkages to services and training of service providers. In Delhi, they also carry out school-based sexuality education programmes that include efforts to sensitize parents and teachers. These programmes focus on adolescent boys and girls, including young married couples.

Their overall intent is to enable young people to choose responsible and healthy behaviours as they enter into sexual activity and marriage. They specifically aim to help young people delay sexual debut, to increase the age at marriage for girls, to encourage young couples to delay first births and to space subsequent births, and to increase the use of spacing methods of contraception. Finally, they aim to prevent sexually transmitted infections and to lower rates of unsafe abortion.

To win over gatekeepers such as parents and teachers, programme staff emphasize the scope, importance and benefits of their efforts. To do this, the programmes have invested resources in strengthening the skills that field staff need in order to communicate with and persuade these groups. In addition, the programmes try to empower parents and adolescents to communicate with each other, by increasing their knowledge, understanding, vocabulary and general comfort level related to sexual and reproductive health.

Barriers to improving sexual and reproductive health

Programme experiences suggest that several barriers impede efforts to help adolescents postpone their sexual debut. Boys describe numerous factors that push them into early sexual activity, including simple curiosity or adventurism, what they call "uncontrollable urges", peer pressure, parental attitudes disapproving interaction between young females and males and favouring early marriage for sons and especially daughters, what boys believe to be tacit "permission" from society, and the common belief that masturbation is harmful. In contrast, girls cite coercion and abuse as the main barriers to delaying sexual debut.

Efforts to increase the age at marriage for girls must overcome parents' fears about the sexual security of their daughters. That is to say, parents fear that until daughters are safely married, they remain at risk of rape, coercion, or elopement—any of which could spell ruin for both the girl and her family.

Programme experiences suggest that efforts to encourage young couples to delay the first birth and space subsequent births using spacing contraception must overcome a number of barriers. First, young couples often feel pressure to have a child soon after marriage in order to prove that they are fertile. In addition, many young people lack adequate knowledge about spacing methods of contraception. Many have concerns about contraceptive safety, diminished pleasure or diminished sexual performance that outweigh the desire to delay pregnancy. Many feel uncomfortable speaking about such issues, lack the vocabulary to discuss them, or feel too shy to initiate such discussions. Many girls believe that boys should initiate discussions about contraception, while many boys believe that responsibility for contraception belongs to girls. Other issues that prevent young people from delaying or spacing pregnancies include the desire to please families and in-laws, as well as age differences between husbands and wives that make it difficult for them to discuss sensitive issues.

Programme experience shows that several barriers hamper efforts to prevent sexually transmitted infections among young people. First, young men often use condoms incorrectly or inconsistently. Second, many object to condoms because they say that they interfere with pleasure or sexual performance. Finally, the common belief that masturbation is harmful may make some boys and young men more likely to have sex with girls or women under circumstances that put them at risk for infection.

Adolescents often feel guilt and shame about sexual matters and say that discussing these topics with parents is taboo. At the same time, many adolescents believe that their families know what is best for sons and daughters, and they therefore entrust their families with responsibility for important life decisions. They generally express a strong desire to please and consult their parents.

Parents and family members say that boys and girls prefer to talk to peers rather than parents. They describe feeling acutely embarrassed at the thought of discussing sexual matters with their children. They also lack the vocabulary and the basic information about sexuality that would help them talk about these matters with their adolescent children. Furthermore, they express concern that discussing such matters might appear to give tacit "permission" to engage in sex. They associate knowledge of sexual matters with promiscuity and a loss of parental control. They are generally concerned for the sexual security of their daughters, but indifferent about their sons' behaviour.

Conclusions

These barriers have important implications for adolescent reproductive health programmes. As gatekeepers, parents, families and teachers have a strong influence on adolescents' behaviour. Together they comprise the social environment in which adolescents make decisions and in which reproductive health programmes must work. Adolescents are not independent adults, but are heavily dependent upon family guidance and approval. For all these reasons, programmes must address the parents, families and teachers who influence adolescents.

Rekha Masilamani
Country Representative
Pathfinder International
102 Adishwar Apartments
34 Feroze Shah Road
New Delhi
India

Experience of family violence: reflections from adolescents in Uttar Pradesh, India

Bella Patel Uttekar, M.E. Khan, Nayan Kumar, Sandhya Barge and Hemlata Sadhwani

Background

It is increasingly being recognized that violence has adverse effects on the physical and mental health of adolescents. In addition, exposure to violence can have implications for their subsequent behaviour (Jejeebhoy, 1998; Centre for Operations Research and Training, 2000). Violence against adolescents is an area that has not been adequately addressed in the existing literature, policies or programmes. To address this gap in knowledge, researchers at the Centre for Operations Research and Training (CORT) in Baroda, India, carried out a study that aimed to understand forms of violence and perpetrators as perceived by adolescents, the actual reported experiences of violence against adolescents and their mothers, the determinants of violence, the consequences and the coping mechanisms that adolescents adopt.

Methods

These data were collected as part of a study carried out in slum areas of Allahabad, Uttar Pradesh, using both qualitative and quantitative research methods. Researchers interviewed 382 adolescents aged 10–18 years (178 boys and 204 girls) using semi-structured questionnaires. During these interviews, the adolescents were asked about quarrels among their parents and about violence that they may have experienced directly. Fourteen respondents (seven boys and seven girls) had lost one parent and hence could not reflect on their parents' behaviour. Researchers also conducted in-depth interviews and a free-listing exercise among a subsample of 42 randomly selected respondents (32 boys and 10 girls).

Key findings

During the free-listing exercise, researchers asked adolescents to list different forms of violence. Male adolescents mentioned: "verbal abuse" (16), beating (7), asking someone to leave the house (3), domestic violence, slapping, throwing out the food plate, tearing clothes and physical fighting. When researchers asked 10 girls to do the same, they reported examples such as arguments and beatings. Girls reported more examples of verbal abuse rather than physical violence when compared with the boys. For example, girls reported scolding, arguments and withholding of food, while boys were more likely to report being slapped or beaten, having objects thrown at them and other forms of physical abuse. Adolescents did not mention sexual harassment during the free-listing exercise, but the topic did come up during in-depth interviews.

About 39% of adolescents living with both parents reported violence (including physical violence and verbal abuse) by their fathers against their mothers. A greater proportion of boys (32%) than girls (20%) reported having witnessed their fathers beating their mothers. Though it is not clear what accounts for the difference, one possibility is that girls were more reluctant to report violence than boys out of concern for their family's *izzat* (honour) (Table 1).

When asked about the frequency of verbal abuse and physical violence against their mothers, 8% of adolescents with two parents reported that such abuse occurred "always", 79% said "sometimes" and 12% said "rarely".

Adolescents were also asked whether they had ever been beaten by their father. Nearly one-third of adolescents reported having been beaten by their fathers, including 49% of boys and 16% of girls. Among those 157 (41%) adolescents who reported either verbal abuse or physical violence, about half (49%) said that they had experienced such abuse one to three times during the past year. About 19% said they had experienced such abuse four to six times during the year. About 18% of boys and 27% of girls reported experiencing violence seven times or more during the year.

Researchers asked adolescents about the kinds of situations that led to violence. Boys mentioned teasing or taunting girls, not attending school, resource problems such as lack of water, conflicts about being forced to go to work, poor academic performance, quarrels with friends, consumption of alcohol, borrowing money to buy tobacco, not attending work, not repaying loans, getting involved in parents' fights, watching girls bathe and gossiping. Girls reported not complying with their gender roles, not attending to household chores, talking with boys, coming home late or going out of the house as the main reasons for violence against them.

Adolescents were asked how they felt about and coped with violent situations. Both boys and girls mentioned that they sometimes stopped talking or eating. Some reported feeling like crying or being alone. Some boys said that they stopped meeting friends who irritated their father, started studying, or left the house for some time. Others said that they accepted their father's beatings. For example, one 17 year-old boy said:

> *What can I do if I do not get a job. My father taunts me and even beats me. I go out of the house early in the morning, look for a job and return home very late in the night. Sometimes I eat, sometimes not. I have no alternative but to tolerate all this till I start earning.*

Other boys said that they got angry with their father. For example, one 16 year-old boy expressed his anger saying:

Table 1. Per cent of adolescents reporting violence by fathers against mother or self

	Boys		Girls		All	
	Number	Per cent	Number	Per cent	Number	Per cent
Among entire sample	178	100	204	100	382	100
Violence against self						
Beats self	87	48.9	32	15.7	119	31.2
Among those with two parents*	171	100	197	100	368	100
Violence against mother						
Beats mother	55	32.2	39	19.8	94	25.5
Pattern of beating						
Beats both mother and self	34	19.9	11	5.6	45	12.2
Beats mother not self	21	12.3	28	14.2	49	13.3
Beats self not mother	49	28.7	20	10.2	69	18.8

* Note: excludes seven boys and seven girls who had lost one parent.

My father beats me, my sister and my mother. He comes home after drinking and abuses us for no reason. I feel he should die so that we can have some peace in our lives.

Conclusions

This study provides a glimpse into the violence witnessed and experienced by adolescents in the slum areas of Uttar Pradesh. There is a need for a deeper understanding of the dynamics and consequences of violence, including sexual violence, which may have both short-term and long-term implications for both victims and perpetrators. In addition, an in-depth understanding of the factors that lead to violent behaviour could help point to strategies to curb such violence. To achieve this, more in-depth research is needed in various settings.

References

Centre for Operations Research and Training (CORT) (2000) *Baseline Survey for Action for Slum Dwellers' Reproductive Health Project.* (Monograph). Baroda, CORT.

Jejeebhoy S (1998) Association between wife-beating and fetal and infant death: Impressions from a survey in rural India. *Studies in Family Planning,* 29(3):300–308.

Bella Patel Utterkar
CORT
402 Woodland Apt
Race Course
Baroda 390 007
India

X

Family life and sex education

Population education in formal and non-formal sectors in India

Vandana Chakrabarti

Background

Since 1980, the United Nations Population Fund (UNFPA) has supported the National Population Education Project (NPEP) in India, which has been implemented in three sectors: school education, higher education and adult education. The programme began with a focus on demographic issues but shifted its concern following the 1994 Cairo International Conference on Population and Development. The project now concentrates on gender equity, women's empowerment, reproductive health and rights, adolescent sexual behaviour, health education, family life education, drug addiction, HIV/AIDS and sustainable development. This paper describes the project and makes a number of recommendations for the future, which may be relevant not only to this project, but to other adolescent programmes as well.

Programme description

In 1980, the project began working in schools, and now reaches 154 million students all over the country in grades I to XII, as well as 4.2 million teachers. It is believed that an effective population education programme in the formal school system will produce a generation of adults capable of making informed and responsible decisions regarding population and development issues. The NPEP was implemented in the higher education sector in 1986 and now reaches 6.7 million students enrolled in more than 225 universities and 400 colleges. This part of the project is designed for unmarried students of reproductive age. In 1986 the NPEP was also implemented in the non-formal adult education sector. It aims to reach 150 million students aged 9–35, of whom about 62% are women or girls. The project is implemented in the adult education sector with technical support from 18 State Resource Centres for Adult Literacy and the National Population Education Resource Centre.

In all three sectors, the project aims to increase awareness, build positive attitudes and change behaviour, through strategies such as integrating population education into the school curriculum, carrying out non-curricular activities, developing materials, conducting advocacy, training and orientation, extension activities, research and evaluation. Because of its scale, the programme has enormous potential for impact; however the scale may also impose certain limits on quality. Everyone from the top manager to the grass-roots volunteer must be inspired in order for the project to achieve its potential.

Recommendations for improving programmes for adolescents

An evaluation of NPEP was conducted at the end of each phase by external agencies. Their recommendations have helped redefine priorities and revise strategies to attain the expected outcomes. On the basis of discussions with the implementers of NPEP in different sectors and with experts who conducted the mid-term review of the current phase, this paper offers the following suggestions for making the project more useful in the future.

1. Unlike in most other countries, adolescent fertility in India occurs largely within marriage. About half of all young women are sexually active before they reach age 18. Presently, age at marriage is discussed only in the primers used by adult learners. Efforts are needed in the school and higher education sectors to educate people about the need to marry later.

2. Although millions of teachers have been trained on population issues, it is unclear how much reproductive health information has actually been imparted to students. Adolescent boys and girls need more education on topics such as anatomy and physiology, changes in puberty, menstruation, conception, infections, sexuality, contraception and sexually transmitted infections.

3. The project needs to include activities focused on increasing the self-esteem and confidence of young women and girls, given that they often feel powerless, particularly when they are married early and sent to live with in-laws. Often they have no say in reproductive matters.

4. The project should also work to develop life skills among adolescents, such as thinking skills (problem-solving, examining choices, decision- making and goal-setting), social skills (building positive relationships, listening and communicating effectively, taking responsibility and coping with stress) and negotiating skills, which require both thinking and social skills. These skills are important in all areas of life, but especially in the area of sexuality and reproductive health.

In terms of recommended strategies, school teachers, college teachers and literacy workers who implement the project need to be involved from the planning stage to ensure that they feel ownership over the programme. The project could strengthen or expand a number of areas, including counselling services in formal education sectors, telephone counselling services, peer education and health camps. The project should help parents and in-laws to understand adolescents better and to work more closely with teachers and literacy workers in order to educate adolescents about reproductive health issues. In addition, adolescent programmes must be supported by research. Only when relevant research is communicated to policy-makers, administrators and project functionaries will more meaningful programmes for adolescents and young adults be developed. Finally, it is important to mention that a project of this magnitude needs to engage in frequent dialogue with stakeholders and to build in monitoring and evaluation systems.

Further reading

Government of India (1997) *Population and Development Education in Schools, Project Agreement between the Government of India and the UNFPA*. New Delhi, Ministry of Human Resource Development, Government of India.

Government of India (1998) *Population and Development Education in Higher Education System, Project Agreement between the Government of India and the UNFPA*. New Delhi, University Grants Commission, Ministry of Human Resource Development, Government of India.

Mohankumar V (1999) Population education in the adult education sector. *Indian Journal of Population Education*. April–September (9):338.

Shirur RR (1999) Reproductive and sexual health education for adolescents—a survey report. *Indian*

Journal of Population Education. New Delhi, October–March (8):48–55.

United Nations Population Fund (1999) *Population and Development Education—Inter-sectoral Research Consultation Report*. New Delhi, UNFPA.

Dr Vandana Chakrabarti
Director
Population Education Resource Centre
SNDT Women's University
New Marine Lines
Mumbai 400 020
India

Communicating with rural adolescents about sex education: experiences from BRAC, Bangladesh

Sabina Faiz Rashid

Background

Despite conservative values in Bangladesh that condemn sexual activity outside of marriage, research indicates that about half of all young men in rural areas have had premarital sex. The figures are lower for women, who are subject to greater social control (Aziz & Maloney, 1985, cited in Caldwell & Pieris, 1999). Overall discussion and knowledge of sexual and reproductive health (SRH) remains at a low level, however, and inadequate education exacerbates an environment of misperceptions (Nahar et al., 1999a). Friends, older cousins, brothers and sisters are adolescents' main sources of information, and they themselves are often ignorant about reproductive health matters. As a result, adolescents lack adequate knowledge and many engage in behaviour that put their SRH at risk.

In 1995, the Bangladesh Rural Advancement Committee (BRAC)[1] set up an Adolescent Reproductive Health Education (ARHE) programme. BRAC provides ARHE classes through its *Kishor Kishori* (KK) schools, which are three-year schools for boys and girls over age 12 who have never before enrolled in school. Pupils come from poor socioeconomic backgrounds, and almost all have illiterate parents. BRAC also provides ARHE through *pathaghars* (community libraries) and government secondary schools. Separate classes for girls and boys are taught for an hour fortnightly in KK schools, and once a month in the *pathaghars*. Currently 803 schools and *pathaghars* teach ARHE to approximately 27 175 rural adolescents. The ARHE curriculum includes physical and mental changes during adolescence, physiology, pregnancy and childbearing, guidance about age at marriage, sexually transmitted infections (STIs), family planning, substance abuse, gender issues, male and female roles in reproduction, and violence against women and girls. In 1999, BRAC evaluated the impact of the ARHE programme in Nilphamari district. This article explores the perceptions of adolescents as they faced psychological and social changes, the programme results of ARHE, and the factors that influenced community acceptance of the programme.

Methods

To evaluate the programme, researchers gathered qualitative data in three KK schools and two *pathaghars* in Nilphamari district. They selected

1 BRAC is one of the world's largest indigenous NGOs. Established in 1972, it has three main integrated but distinct programme areas: education, micro-credit and health.

this site because it had one of the longest-running ARHE programmes, having begun in 1995, and because it was one of the first to implement both phase 1 and phase 2 of the ARHE programme.[2] Respondents included young unmarried students aged 13–15, parents, guardians and teachers.

Researchers held eight focus group discussions (FGDs) with students—five FGDs with a total of 46 girls, and three FGDs with a total of 18 boys. The two extra FGDs for girls were needed as *pathaghars* have only female students in their ARHE classes. Researchers then conducted semi-structured, open-ended interviews with 10 female students and 8 male students. The interview guide allowed various topics to emerge and be pursued. Male researchers interviewed the boys, and female researchers interviewed the girls. Interviewers were young since it was felt that girls and boys would be more likely to open up to someone closer to their age than they would to older interviewers. They carried out the interviews privately and individually to allow respondents to speak freely on sensitive topics.

Researchers interviewed 18 parents and guardians, including mothers and in some cases aunts. They also held four FGDs with a total of 21 mothers and guardians, who had not previously been interviewed. Researchers held informal discussions with seven teachers and 16 programme staff. In addition, one researcher attended ARHE classes in order to observe the teaching style and the level of interaction between teachers and students.

Key findings

Adolescent girls felt that menstruation was the most significant topic covered in the ARHE classes. In Bangladesh, menstruation is associated with sexuality, fertility and "pollution". It is considered a shameful subject that girls rarely discuss, even with their mothers. A recent study found that the majority of girls did not know about menstruation before it began (Nahar et al., 1999b). Interviews confirmed that the onset of menstruation could be traumatic for girls. One girl said, "*I had my menses when I was 12 years old… I was really very scared. I thought I was dying.*"

Family planning was another popular topic with both girls and boys. Family planning is a sensitive subject that is rarely discussed between older women and unmarried girls in the traditional rural culture (Mita & Simmons, 1995). Boys said they particularly wanted information related to sex, including sexually transmitted infections (STIs)/ AIDS and family planning.

Interviews suggested that those who attended ARHE classes became an important source of basic health knowledge for peers and family members. Girls shared their new knowledge with other girls in the village, after school and in the community library. One girl explained:

> *We usually sit and talk together with the other girls in the village. That is when they ask me about what I am learning in class. One girl came…and I told her what I know—use a clean cloth, wash it, and don't worry, it is natural—it is nothing to be scared of.*

Some girls also shared newly acquired knowledge on hygiene during menstruation with their mothers. One mother remarked, "*I am learning from her now.*" Other mothers knew about their daughters' new knowledge without discussing it openly. One mother explained, "*I buy her soap as she said she needs to wash her things with it…but I don't say anything to her…what is there to say? As long as she is learning all this, it is less worry for me.*" Girls tended to share family planning information with sisters-in-law and close friends. They said they had discussed STIs among themselves, but had not generally talked about the issue with adults.

2 In the first phase the curricula emphasized primary health care education; this changed to an emphasis on reproductive health matters in phase 2.

Adolescent boys also reported sharing what they had learned in ARHE classes with friends and male cousins. One boy described the eagerness of other boys who approached him for answers saying:

> *When my friends found out I was learning all of this in the school they came and asked me a lot of questions like, "how does a girl get pregnant?" and "why does menses* [period] *happen?" ... I answered some of the questions, not all, as I don't know many of the answers.*

In general, the ARHE programme seems to have generated a new consciousness about reproductive health matters and broken the shame and silence surrounding girls' and boys' bodies. Nevertheless, the evaluation found that many adolescents who participated in ARHE still lacked knowledge of STIs, including HIV/AIDS. During FGDs it appeared that some adolescents saw AIDS as a potential threat to the community, but not to themselves. Almost all were aware of the link between unprotected sexual intercourse and STIs/AIDS, and almost all knew that condoms were an effective means of prevention. However, a majority of girls and boys appeared confused about transmission routes and symptoms of HIV/AIDS and other STIs. Both adolescents and teachers said that if a person were infected with HIV, she/he would show signs of illness. Adolescents reported that teachers preferred to focus on topics such as menstruation, early marriage and family planning, while skimming over STIs/HIV/AIDS. In part, this may reflect the shame that persists around reproductive health matters. More importantly, teachers acknowledged that their own knowledge was weak, and they blamed lack of detailed information in the curriculum.

One important topic addressed during ARHE is early marriage. Although some adolescents said they wanted to choose their own marriage partners, many admitted that parents were the main decision-makers. In Nilphamari district, many girls are married at age 11–13 or younger. In one school, six out of 14 girls in the ARHE programme were already married, with two expecting their first child. According to the mothers, the main reason for early marriage is fear that their daughters would be raped, fall pregnant or elope. Knowledge that a girl has had premarital sex affects the social status of her entire family. Thus, families continue to practise early marriage, despite awareness of its detrimental effects on the health of girls and their babies.

Many girls who participated in ARHE used their new knowledge to argue against early marriage. One girl implored her mother, "*See—they are BRAC people and they say early marriage is bad.*" Some attitudes may be changing as parents realize the advantages of more schooling and the dangers of early pregnancy, but some mothers confided that they faced derogatory comments from community elders who said, "*your girl has become big now, you should get her married... You are poor. What will she do with all this education?*"

In this context, ARHE classes provide an opportunity for girls and boys to share feelings about 'love' and 'romance' that would have been considered unthinkable for previous generations. A common remark by girls was, "*Prem* [love] *is impure and we should marry who our parents have chosen for us. Doing prem is bad!*" Nonetheless, a number of adolescents said they had "fallen in love" secretly, in the hope of finding a partner to marry. However, these statements were always accompanied by remarks such as, "*There is nothing wrong with the* prem *as long as it is not bad prem* [involving sex]." Good love was defined as leading to marriage, while "impure" love was defined as involving sex before marriage or a relationship that does not lead to marriage (even if it is "pure"). Though social norms are more relaxed for boys, they were still reluctant to share personal stories of romance with researchers.

Some adolescents said that boys initiate relationships with girls through letters, and many described encounters influenced by films and television. As Pelto (1999) argues, since adolescents have few opportunities to practise heterosexual conversations, popular films provide inspiration. A few boys and girls went beyond letters and shared a kiss; one couple went into town to have a photograph taken of themselves; and another went to the cinema together. Most couples resorted to meeting secretly in the evenings, when it was dark and their families were asleep.

Only a few girls and boys mentioned cases of *prem* with happy endings. Girls are particularly vulnerable to coercive and unsafe sexual intimacy. Many girls' narratives centred on betrayal and punishment from village elders, jail and unmarried girls getting pregnant. Some centred on revenge, in which the girl was gang-raped, or had acid thrown on her face. Parents' stories mirrored those of adolescents and were tinged with anxiety. As one parent said, "*What to do if they run off and do bad work? How will we show our face in the village? We worry about our girls!*"

Adolescent girls spoke to researchers about their sexual desires, displaying unusual openness in a society that views women as good and pure if they are sexually passive and considers overt expressions of sexuality as shameful. One girl said, "*Both men and women have equal rights in the sexual relationship. If one wants to mix* [have sex] *then she can have pleasure from it, but if it is forced then one cannot enjoy it.*" Much of the language used by adolescents implied that young people are not fully responsible for their actions because they are driven by "too much desire/ needs". Both girls and boys described "uncontrollable urges" that lead to extramarital activities, saying for example, "*Boys and girls get involved in sexual relations to meet their sexual needs.*"

A number of boys admitted to masturbating regularly and saw it as something for "*jonno mithano*" (satisfying one's needs), in contrast to another study that found that boys considered masturbation a sin (Hashima-e-Nasreen et al., 1998). Some boys mentioned watching pornographic films with friends, saying, "*We feel good, and we sit and masturbate to satisfy our desires.*" Boys said that they would often rent a video player and watch the movies in the privacy of a cousin's or a friend's room, or in village recreation centres. Interviews with boys suggested that this is quite a common practice. Some mothers complained about this practice in FGDs, but said they could not control their sons' behaviour. In one FGD, a mother mentioned that she suspected that her son watched blue films with friends, saying, "*Sometimes I get angry and then they listen, but most of the time they do what they want.*" It appears from the FGDs that these women knew what their sons were up to but largely chose to ignore it. When asked whether her daughter watched blue films, the women looked horrified and the mother stated, "*They would never do such things.*"

Boys appear aware that they have more sexual freedom than girls. While some felt that their behaviour was justified as they had "*more desires*", many boys and girls said that girls share similar feelings, but due to social pressures "*...even if she is bursting to say or do something, she will not do it.*"

Researchers explored parents', teachers' and community members' acceptance of the ARHE programme. With increasing exposure to outside influences, many mothers worried that they were unable to control their adolescent boys and girls, and they felt that life skills and 'health education' were important for their children. However, some mothers were unaware of the details of the ARHE curriculum. A majority thought that their children were being taught *proiyojon* (necessary) life skills to prepare them for the future, but did not know what these supposed life skills were. Boys tended to be too embarrassed to discuss sensitive subjects with their mothers, and a majority of girls discussed only the "safer" topics with their mothers. One adolescent explained, "*My parents don't really know in detail what we are being taught. We remain careful about what we say to them.*" Power relations also play a role. Most families of ARHE participants depend on BRAC to educate their children. One boy explained why his mother did not protest saying, "*She is scared—what if they ask me to leave the school?... She doesn't want to anger the programme staff.*" Furthermore, some teachers come from rich families, with links to village authority figures. Many poor people feel uncomfortable questioning the authority of teachers, who are educated and have a higher social status.

While female teachers said they have gradually become comfortable teaching ARHE to girls (saying it feels like a duty of an older sister), some are still uncomfortable about teaching boys. As a result, some teachers have held classes less frequently than BRAC guidelines require. When researchers raised this issue with two teachers, they admitted to having reservations about teaching sensitive subjects to boys. One commented, "*I cannot teach the boys all these things. I feel ashamed. And what will the community say if they find out?*"

Conclusions

In a strongly conservative environment, the ARHE programme provides adolescents with basic information on sexuality and reproductive health—a major achievement. Community acceptance of the ARHE classes may reflect the growing urbanization of rural areas, the influence of electronic media, and increasing exposure to nongovernmental organizations such as BRAC. In addition, community involvement in the schools, power relations, uneven awareness of course content and the fact that ARHE teachers come from the community may also have helped build acceptance of ARHE by rural communities.

Overall, this research highlights the importance and feasibility of ARHE in rural areas. The programme not only provides information to participating girls and boys, but also indirectly to other adolescents and adults in the villages. ARHE has broken the silence on sensitive topics. Future research needs to focus on what happens to programme participants when they marry. Will husband and wife decide on contraceptive methods together? To what extent will knowledge of reproductive health have a positive effect on their lives?

This summary has been excerpted from an article that first appeared under the title "Providing sex education to rural adolescents in Bangladesh: Experiences from BRAC", published in *Gender and Development*, 2000 (July) 8(2).

Acknowledgements: I would like to thank my colleagues for their assistance during project design and data collection. I am grateful to my research colleague Nusrat Chowdhury and my husband Safi Rahman Khan for their useful comments and critical feedback. I would also like to thank my field researcher assistants, BRAC field office staff and the participants in the research for their time and patience.

References

Caldwell BK, Pieris I (1999) Continued high-risk behaviour among Bangladeshi males. In: Caldwell JC, Caldwell P, Anarfi J, Awusabo-Asare K, Ntozi J, March J et al., eds. *Resistances to Behavioural Change to Reduce HIV/AIDS in Predominantly Heterosexual Epidemics in Third World Countries.* Canberra, Health Transition Centre.

Hashima-e-Nasreen, Chowdhury M, Bhuiya A, Chowdhury S, Ahmed SM (1998) *Integrating Reproductive and Sexual Health into a Grassroot Development Programme.* Dhaka, Bangladesh Rural Advancement Committee—International Centre for Diarrhoeal Diseases Research, Bangladesh.

Mita R, Simmons R (1995) Diffusion of the culture of contraception: programme effects on young women in rural Bangladesh. *Studies in Family Planning*, 26(1):1–13.

Nahar Q, Amin S, Sultan R, Nazrul H, Islam M, Kane TT et al. (1999a) *Strategies to Meet the Health Needs of Adolescents: A Review.* Operations Research Project, Health and Population Extension Division, Special Publications No. 91. Dhaka, International Centre for Diarrhoeal Diseases Research, Bangladesh.

Nahar Q, Huq NL, Reza, M, Ahmed, F (1999b) *Perceptions of Adolescents on Physical Changes During Puberty, ICDDR,B Working Paper*. Dhaka, International Centre for Diarrhoeal Diseases Research, Bangladesh and Concerned Women for Family Development.

Pelto PJ (1999) Sexuality and sexual behaviour: the current discourse. In: Pachauri S, Subramanian S, eds. *Implementing a Reproductive Health Agenda in India: The Beginning*. New Delhi, Population Council.

Sabina Faiz Rashid
Research and Evaluation Division
BRAC (Bangladesh Rural Advancement Committee)

Mailing address:
A23 Century Estate
Bara Maghbazaar
Dhaka 1217
Bangladesh

Reproductive health education: experiences of Parivar Seva Sanstha in communicating with youth in India

Sudha Tewari and Sumita Taneja

Background

Parivar Seva Sanstha (PSS), a nongovernmental organization (NGO), is an affiliate of Marie Stopes International and has provided reproductive health care in India since 1978. The mission of PSS is to enable couples to have "Children by Choice not Chance", through clinic-based services, social marketing of reproductive health products and other outreach programmes. In the course of its work at the clinics in the mid-1980s, PSS observed that young adults were seeking abortion services and lacked accurate information on important aspects of life such as health, nutrition, hygiene, reproduction, motherhood, maturation and family planning.

To address young people's needs, PSS has designed a series of reproductive health education (RHE) programmes for boys and girls between the ages of 10 and 24, adopting a definition of youth that extends from puberty to early adulthood. PSS offers multifaceted programmes for youth that provide sexual and reproductive health (SRH) information and services. Recognizing the important role played by peers and other service providers, such as auxiliary nurse midwives and *anganwari* workers at the village level, PSS trains peer educators and providers to address young people's needs in acceptable and affordable ways. Because subgroups—such as out-of-school youth, young people about to be married and those who are physically or mentally challenged—have different needs, PSS offers programmes that are specifically tailored for these groups. This paper describes different strategies that PSS has used when working with youth.

Description of reproductive health education programmes

PSS programmes address rural and urban youth in school and out of school, including street children, volunteers of Bharat Scouts and Guides and Nehru Yuva Kendra, college students, those who are married or about to be married, as well as those who are mentally or physically challenged. PSS is currently undertaking RHE interventions in schools and colleges in Bhubaneshwar, Balasore, Cuttock, Bangalore, Calcutta, Lucknow and Delhi. A new 6.5-year project funded by the Buffett Foundation in the United States of America has also been launched covering 10 districts in the state of Rajasthan. A team of young educators are being trained to undertake RHE sessions in a sensitive and friendly manner. A curriculum developed by PSS in Hindi and English serves as a broad guideline that educators adapt based on local needs and type of audience. Educators cover a six-session curriculum using participatory teaching techniques and special audiovisual and print materials. Recognizing the importance of addressing gatekeepers and sensitizing them about the need for such education, PSS also involves parents, school authorities and community leaders in its RHE programmes.

During the sessions, educators encourage students to ask questions either orally or by writing them on pieces of paper (to maintain confidentiality). Girls often ask about menstruation, how babies are made, pregnancy, childbirth and personal grooming. For example, a typical set of questions includes: "*We have periods, what do boys have?*" "*Can I ride a bicycle or bathe in a pond during my periods?*" "*Why are girls asked to sit separately during menstruation?*" "*What happens on the wedding night?*" "*What are test-tube babies?*" "*How are twins born?*" "*If only one sperm is needed for conception, what happens to all the others that enter the body?*" Boys often ask about attraction to the opposite sex, masturbation, ejaculation, nocturnal emissions, anatomy and physiology. Typical questions include: "*Do girls also have the same amount of interest in boys?*" "*Being attracted to one girl is okay, but why do I find all girls attractive?*" "*I have read somewhere that one drop of semen is equal to a 100 drops of blood, is it true?*" "*Do girls also masturbate and how?*" "*What should be the size of a normal penis?*" "*Do pregnancies occur without intercourse?*"

In addition, PSS provides medical services in school settings, usually linked with education sessions. Through its existing network of Marie Stopes clinics, PSS organizes health camps in schools, which, besides providing general health check-ups, doctors and counsellors, address adolescents' psychosexual problems, such as concerns about menstruation and masturbation. To control anaemia, staff promote iron supplementation among adolescent girls.

Initially PSS had planned to undertake a longitudinal survey to measure the impact of RHE interventions in schools and colleges over a five-year period, but it proved difficult to follow up students once they left school for further studies or marriage. As an alternative, PSS carries out assessments before and after they follow the curriculum. When groups are illiterate, PSS organizes focus group discussions. While limited as research tools, these tests measure improvement in students' knowledge and allow PSS to gather practical feedback on course content and methodology. An analysis of test results from selected schools in Bhubaneshwar shows a wide range of scores (Table 1).

PSS also conducts programmes for out-of-school youth and those who are mentally or physically challenged. To address the needs of these groups, PSS has developed special teaching and learning techniques, such as clay models, body mapping and exercises. Educators adapt the curriculum for each group and sometimes bring in specialists such as psychologists, nutritionists, doctors and other resource persons.

Training educators and service providers

To expand outreach and reinforce messages, PSS works with peer educators and conducts "training of trainers" programmes for school teachers and counsellors. PSS selects 4 or 5 volunteer youth (often National Service Scheme volunteers) from each school or college for a 3-day training course. Once trained, these peer educators organize

Table 1. Selected pre- and post-intervention test scores among students aged 16–18

Name of school	Batch	No. of students	Stream	Pre-intervention (%) Lowest	Pre-intervention (%) Highest	Post-intervention (%) Lowest	Post-intervention (%) Highest
City Women's College	+2 (girls)	30	Arts	0	42	78	100
Kamala Nehru Women's College	+2 (girls)	30	Science	15	55	90	100
Acharya Harihar College	+2 (boys)	30	Arts	0	38	27	85
Patia College	+2 (boys)	30	Science	20	58	43	90

programmes during events such as World AIDS Day, Women's Day and Independence Day. PSS also trains teachers and counsellors so that there is a trained cadre of persons available on school premises to answer adolescents' queries.

PSS realized that a significant number of adolescents could not be reached through educational institutions, since many children drop out of school because they marry or become pregnant, particularly girls in rural areas. To reach these marginalized groups, PSS identifies and trains other NGO staff and other grass-roots service providers who have access to these adolescents. For example, in four districts of Uttar Pradesh, PSS reached rural adolescent girls and women by training *anganwari* workers on issues related to adolescent sexuality. *Anganwari* workers are community-based, village level workers who provide education and nutritional supplements to preschool children and lactating and pregnant mothers. Once trained, these workers helped mobilize adolescents for community education programmes, which were jointly conducted by the PSS RHE team and the *anganwari* workers.

Because the demand for reproductive health information exceeds what PSS can handle alone, it continues to provide training to those working in schools, health services and NGOs. For example, PSS initiated a "training of trainers" programme with Bharat Scouts and Guides, Volunteers of the National Service Scheme, Teachers Training Institutes and other NGOs. To achieve financial sustainability, PSS charges a token fee to the schools and colleges that can afford to pay.

Some innovative initiatives of PSS

Because so many young people enter marriage without any knowledge of sexuality or contraception, PSS launched an effort to reach young people who were about to be married. In this programme, called *Adhaar* (meaning foundation for marriage), educators covered topics such as courtship, emotional, psychological and physical preparation for marriage, sexuality and contraception, personal grooming, legal issues related to marriage, home management, banking and finance, first aid and crisis management.

In an effort to reach a broad range of youth and adults who are difficult to reach through conventional channels, PSS established a telephone hotline service in Delhi in 1993. This hotline, called "*Sparsh*" or "sensitive touch", answers questions on delicate issues ranging from contraception and sexually transmitted infections to drug and alcohol problems. In addition, the hotline provided counselling to those in distress and referred callers to appropriately qualified professionals. This service received an overwhelming response from the general public (receiving 17 074 phone calls in one year) and the media. When PSS first introduced *Sparsh*, there was no dearth of questions such as: "*Can kissing make me pregnant?*" "*Will using my boyfriend's handkerchief frequently lead to AIDS?*" "*What is a condom?*"

During the course of PSS's work with youth, a need for a Distance Learning Course in Family Life Education (FLE) was expressed by many NGO representatives, doctors, counsellors, school teachers and principals. PSS therefore introduced a one-year Distance Learning Course in FLE. In addition to sending course modules on RH to students against which they submitted assignments, PSS held personal contact programmes twice a year and asked students to work on projects under PSS guidance. Certificates were awarded to students who were successful in the written examination and interview held at the end of the course.

Future strategies

PSS has gained considerable experience in designing innovative programmes to communicate with youth and proposes to adapt the lessons learned to programmes for larger audiences. For example, PSS programmes that addressed adolescents who had just married or were about to do so (i.e. *Adhaar*) focused on urban adolescents. These could be adapted to meet the needs of adolescents in rural areas as well, where marriage continues to occur at an early age. PSS feels that if the programme were packaged as "preparing your girls for marriage", it would face less resistance at the community level and would be widely accepted. In addition, PSS has recognized an unmet need for distance learning courses on SRH that target grass-roots government functionaries and NGO staff such as auxiliary nurse midwives and *anganwari* workers, as well as other NGO functionaries. PSS is considering developing short courses of up to three months instead of one year.

PSS consciously tries to build sustainability into all its projects. However, since RHE programmes are targeted at youth who have little ability to pay, particularly in rural areas, partial cost recovery alone cannot make the programme self-sustaining.

Realizing the importance of investing in adolescents today to create responsible adults of tomorrow, PSS stands committed to addressing the needs of youth by integrating adolescent health interventions in all its ongoing reproductive health projects.

Sudha Tewari
Managing Director
Parivar Seva Sanstha
C374 Defence Colony
New Delhi 110024
India

Counselling young people on sexual and reproductive health: individual and peer programmes

Raj Brahmbhatt

Background

Adolescents, who constitute over one-fifth of India's population (International Institute for Population Sciences, 2000), have limited access to vital information and services pertaining to sexual and reproductive health (SRH). Cultural taboos surrounding communication about sexual matters persist in the parent–child relationship, and young people have few opportunities outside their peer group to talk about their feelings and anxieties.

Founded in 1949, the Family Planning Association of India (FPAI) is the country's largest nongovernmental organization (NGO) providing family planning and other reproductive health services. In addition to clinical services, training and research, FPAI carries out extensive information, education and communications programmes throughout India. The FPAI has experimented with numerous programmes to meet the needs of both urban and rural youth, including campaigns to increase the age at marriage, sexuality and reproductive health education programmes, and counselling services. This paper describes a selection of these programmes.

Selected programme activities for youth

In the late 1960s, FPAI began educating young people in schools, colleges and non-formal educational institutions on issues related to population and family life. These programmes provide an orientation for young people regarding sexuality, reproductive health, the prevention of unplanned pregnancies and sexually transmitted infections (STIs). In designing these programmes, the FPAI kept in view that adolescents have needs that are distinct from those of adults. These education programmes do not merely provide information, but also aim to enhance young people's communication skills, clarify values, change attitudes and prevent risky behaviour.

In 1978, FPAI established Sexuality Education Counselling Research Therapy/Training (SECRT) centres, which provide sexuality education and counselling. Today 37 SECRT centres have reached over 120 000 young people. SECRT centres offer counselling services to both married and unmarried adults and adolescents, on a range of topics, including premarital counselling, family planning, and marital and infertility counselling. FPAI offers these services individually, in groups, by correspondence and over the telephone.

FPAI has developed several innovative approaches in partnership with young people to promote sexual and reproductive health. The organization works through youth clubs in many settings to provide accurate information on family life and adolescent health matters, including the prevention of sexually transmitted infections, including human immmunodeficiency virus infection (STIs/HIV). In addition, FPAI branches have developed peer educator initiatives in collaboration with other youth programmes, such as Youth Parliament, Young Women Information Centres and thespian programmes. In addition, FPAI has developed "Young Inspirers Clubs" in rural and urban areas. These clubs use folk media to raise awareness about STIs/HIV/AIDS, to eradicate myths and misconceptions related to sexuality, and to promote reproductive health. The "Young Inspirers" publish a Hindi newsletter, called YASH (Youth and Sexual Health), to spread life-planning information among their peers. In 1997, FPAI-SECRT initiated "Spearhead Youth Health Leadership Training Programme". This programme has trained nearly 1000 youth leaders, many of whom have served as peer counsellors in the FPAI Young Inspirers Clubs.

In 1999, the FPAI implemented a project on "Enhancing Sexual and Reproductive Health of Young Persons". This project aimed to extend information and counselling on issues related to human sexuality, preparation for marriage, responsible parenthood, gender issues, contraception and prevention of STIs/HIV/AIDS. As part of the project, the six FPAI branches carried out sensitization programmes, organized medical check-up camps and provided counselling and training for teachers and peer educators. The project reached out to rural and urban youth, and the response was overwhelming. For example, the STI/HIV prevention programme reached 7065 young people, including 3391 out-of-school, illiterate youth. In Dharwad (Karnataka), the project established a strong network of young people trained to impart knowledge on sexuality and STIs/HIV/AIDS. Its peer group leaders' training led to the establishment of eight community counselling centres in six villages where four to five peer group leaders provide counselling on a regular basis.

Conclusions

From our experience we have learned many lessons regarding adolescent SRH programmes, a few of which are highlighted below. First, young people are not a homogeneous group, and programmes need to consider economic, social, cultural and religious differences. Cultural sensitivity is essential, and for this reason, no single programme can work for all India. Second, in the absence of other information and services, quacks have taken advantage of adolescents' sexual concerns throughout India. On every street corner, such people advertise services for sexual problems. Young people need services and counselling that do not perpetuate misconceptions. Third, adolescents are more concerned about sex than about reproduction. Programmes need to go beyond limited kinds of "sex education" that focus primarily on anatomy, to "sexuality education" which addresses broader dimensions. Humour and fun are essential elements in gaining a rapport with young people.

Finally, in addition to elements of youth-friendly services such as convenient hours, convenient locations, affordable fees and specially trained staff, FPAI has found that anonymity and drop-in hours are particularly important. FPAI centres use numbers instead of names to identify clinic records, so that young people do not have to reveal their identity. Welcoming drop-in clients is essential, because many young people have few opportunities to come to the clinic. Allowing them the freedom to drop into the clinic without a prearranged appointment has proven to be an important way to increase access. It is these kinds of counselling and awareness-building strategies that can help young people get the education, health care and skills that they need early in life to ensure their well-being as adults.

Reference

International Institute for Population Sciences (2000) *National Family Health Survey (NFHS-2), India 1998–1999, Health and Family Welfare Wallchart.* Mumbai, International Institute for Population Sciences, and Washington, DC, Population Reference Bureau.

Dr Raj Brahmbhatt
FPAI
Baja Bhavan
Nariman Point
Mumbai 400 020
India

The Healthy Adolescent Project in India (HAPI)

Matthew Tiedemann and Shakuntala DasGupta

Background

As in many Asian countries, there is an urgent need to improve reproductive health knowledge and behaviour among adolescents and young adults in India. Over 20% of the population in India is between the ages of 10 and 19. Young people tend to marry early, and experience high fertility rates, low levels of contraceptive use, high abortion rates, and high levels of violence and sexual coercion (International Institute for Population Sciences, 2000). To address these issues, Family Health International (FHI), the World Association of Girl Guides and Girls Scouts (WAGGGS) and the Bharat Scouts and Guides Association (BSG), the largest youth organization in India, have collaborated on a two-year project called the Healthy Adolescent Project in India (HAPI), with funding from the David and Lucile Packard Foundation. The purpose of HAPI is to address gaps in reproductive health knowledge and services for adolescents and young adults by enhancing young people's knowledge and skills, using a life-skills approach. The project also aims to help participants develop healthy values and attitudes, and to establish links between Scouts and Guides and local health providers. The Family Planning Association of India/Calcutta Branch (FPAI) selected and supervises a team of community health workers who are charged with establishing this link with local health providers.

The project has its headquarters in Kolkata and focuses on West Bengal, where the Guide and Scout associations have a strong presence and have expressed considerable interest in activities intended to enhance adolescent sexual and reproductive health.

Project description

To improve the reproductive health of adolescents, the project incorporates a reproductive and general health curriculum into girl guide and boy scout programmes in seven project communities in West Bengal along the Eastern and South-Eastern Railways. Through a series of health education activities, guides and scouts learn basic facts about their health and how to convey this information to their peers. By aiming to train 900 peer educators, each of whom would make 25 contacts, the project hopes to reach as many as 22 500 young people. The HAPI project relies on the BSG's existing volunteer structure. The project has three coordinators (the only full-time paid staff), 12 BSG trainers and 17 FPAI health workers, all of whom work with leaders of 30 BSG units, evenly split between boy scouts and girl guides.

The collaborating organizations have developed a curriculum that the scouts and guides will follow to earn their HAPI merit badges. Merit badges are a key motivational tool in scouting and guiding. After completing a series of activities on a particular topic, as outlined in the BSG curriculum, the scout or guide earns a badge symbolizing the skill acquired. This badge is worn on the uniform and is a public sign of the young person's accomplishments. The HAPI badge is larger than the typical BSG badge, in recognition of the fact that the curriculum is much more demanding than others, and as a way to enhance awareness of the project. After earning the badge, the scouts and guides earn peer education achievement certificates.

The HAPI curriculum draws on other adolescent curricula adapted for the specific conditions in India. In addition, the project has developed an accompanying handbook for unit leaders, which provides detailed instructions for leading scouts and guides through each part of the badge curriculum. The project has also supplied a range of other resource and reference materials for the trainers, unit leaders and adolescents.

The project curriculum takes a holistic approach to adolescent health, covering reproductive health topics as well as broader health and other issues related to the transition to adulthood. This approach tries to put sensitive reproductive health information into a positive, non-threatening context, by emphasizing the effects on the adolescents' overall health. Specifically, the project addresses topics such as the human body and physical changes, female and male reproductive systems, sexually transmitted infections (STIs), contraception, pregnancy, gender roles, self-esteem, hygiene, nutrition, disease prevention and healthy relationships. The curriculum is divided into two levels, for ages 10–13 and ages 14–25. HAPI uses a participatory, interactive training methodology, both for adult trainers and for adolescent scouts and guides. The approach emphasizes "learning by doing", or experiential learning. Participants work in small groups and learn by taking part in activities rather than passively receiving information through lectures or reading. Such activities include skits, dance, drama and games. The curriculum provides age-specific information, and topics progress from basic to more challenging.

One strength of the project is that it links educational programmes with locally available clinical services. To earn their HAPI badge, adolescents must meet with the community health worker assigned to their unit and visit local health clinics. To build links with health care providers, the FPAI community health workers arrange talks by local physicians and other health care providers. Health workers lead sessions that cover reproductive health topics. In addition, the project plans to hold special events at health centres, clinics and hospitals to introduce adolescents to the health providers in their area. In this way, health providers become familiar with adolescents' needs, while young people learn about what services are available. We anticipate that this interaction between adolescents and local clinics will make young people more familiar and comfortable with the services provided, and thereby increase their use of the services. We also anticipate that, as clinicians become more familiar with adolescent clients, their services will become more sensitive to adolescents' needs.

Project evaluation

At the beginning of the project, FHI, WAGGGS and BSG conducted a needs assessment in each area to determine local needs and to identify what others have done in the area of adolescent reproductive health. This information was used to adapt the project to the local context. BSG, WAGGGS and FHI have been regularly monitoring the project's progress, by collecting process indicators and conducting two formal monitoring visits. In addition, the project has contracted with a research firm to collaborate with FHI on a quantitative pre- and post-intervention survey using a quasi-experimental design. Evaluators will conduct the survey among scouts and guides in 30 experimental units that participated in the project and 30 control units that did not, matched as closely as possible. In this way it is hoped to assess the impact of the project on participants in terms of reproductive health knowledge and behaviours, perceptions of the future and self-image. Because the effects of the intervention may be mediated by variables such as the level of project participation (e.g., levels of achievement, number of meetings attended, etc.), sex, age, unit and BSG branch, these variables will be included in the multivariate analyses comparing BSG units that did and did not participate in the HAPI project.

FHI and WAGGGS have provided the initial training for coordinators, community health workers, trainers who are responsible for training adult scout and guide leaders, and members of the support committee. The project is also in the process of organizing an awareness camp for personnel. Coordinators are working with schools and local institutions to gain their support for the project, and to gain parental consent for adolescents to take part. In addition, a baseline survey is under way to assess the knowledge, skills, values and attitudes of both intervention and control groups.

Conclusions

The project faces a number of challenges. These challenges include the need to gain the support of parents, communities, and schools, as well as the need to address the very low knowledge levels of younger participants. Given the sensitivity of some of the topics addressed, the project cannot take place without the support of communities, parents, schools and other local institutions. The project has great potential, however. Because the number of young people participating in guiding and scouting activities totals nearly 20 000 in West Bengal and over three million across all of India (figures from BSG Annual Report 1998/1999), if the HAPI project is successful, it could be expanded in the future to reach a large number of adolescents.

Reference

International Institute for Population Sciences (IIPS) (2000) *National Family Health Survey (NFHS-2), 1998–1999*. Mumbai, International Institute for Population Sciences and ORC Macro.

Matthew Tiedemann
Family Health International
PO Box 13950
Research Triangle Park, NC 27709
USA

XI

Building self-efficacy among adolescents

Adolescent girls in India choose a better future: an impact assessment of an educational programme

Marta Levitt-Dayal, Renuka Motihar, Shubhada Kanani and Arundhati Mishra

Background

Over the last decade, the Centre for Development and Population Activities (CEDPA) has been working to challenge gender inequities, expand life options and empower girls aged 12–20 through an integrated programme called the "Better Life Options Program" (BLP). The programme provides courses for girls in non-formal education, vocational skills, personality development, and family life education, and teaches them basic skills for living, such as how to use the post office, bank and transport system. The programme also provides opportunities for recreation and focuses on developing leadership skills. To carry out these activities, CEDPA has used the centre-based approach and has established village training centres run by local literate women. In addition, it trains alumni girls as peer educators and motivates them to open their own learning centres.

As part of an evaluation, CEDPA carried out a study to assess the impact of the BLP on the lives of girls who participated between 1996 and 1999. The study objectives were to compare BLP alumni with a similar control group of girls who had not participated in the programme, in terms of educational attainment, income generation, decision-making, mobility, self-esteem, fertility, age at marriage, child-spacing, use of contraceptives and health-seeking behaviours. This paper presents the study findings and discusses CEDPA's future strategies.

Methods

A comparative cross-sectional design was used in three intervention areas—periurban Delhi, rural Madhya Pradesh, and rural Gujarat—where the projects had been implemented by the three partner organizations, Prerana, Bharatiya Grameen Mahila Sangh (BGMS) and Gujarat State Crime Prevention Trust (GSCPT). A random sample of 1693 young women aged 15–26 was surveyed, including 858 controls and 835 BLP alumni. Respondents included both married and unmarried women. Control areas were similar to intervention sites in terms of access to health facilities and ethnic groups. Researchers adapted survey questions from the Demographic and Health Survey, and included questions about education, economic empowerment, health-seeking behaviour and related topics.

The study had limitations. First, many alumni had married and moved away and were not available to participate in the survey. Second, the programme did not collect baseline data; therefore, researchers selected a post-test-only control group experimental design. Since participation was voluntary, it is possible that self-selection bias may have accounted for some differences between the alumni and control groups. To reduce this, we controlled for two critical variables—girls' education and parents' education. Finally, there may be a gap between reported and actual behaviour.

Key findings

The study found significant differences between the controls and BLP alumni in terms of education, vocational skills, economic empowerment, autonomy, self-confidence, reproductive behaviour and health-seeking behaviour. BLP alumni were significantly more likely to be literate, to have completed secondary education, to be employed and to have learned a vocational skill. They were more likely to have travelled outside their village and to have gone to a health centre alone in the previous six months. In addition, BLP alumni were more likely to have the autonomy to make their own decisions about going to the market, spending what they earned and deciding when to marry. These differences in autonomy were significant even after controlling for education of girls and their parents (Table 1).

In terms of reproductive health-seeking behaviour, married alumni (*N*=292) reported significantly more positive behaviours than married controls (*N*=269) in a number of indicators related to reproductive health and child survival. BLP alumni were significantly more likely to have married at age 18 or above and to use contraception. Among respondents who had experienced a pregnancy, alumni (*N*=179) were more likely than controls (*N*=223) to have received prenatal and postnatal care and to have delivered their baby in a health institution. Girls' education seemed to be the critical factor in many of these positive reproductive health behaviours. However, receiving prenatal care, two doses of tetanus toxoid (TT2) and postnatal care remained significant when we controlled for the girls' education (Figure 1).

In terms of child survival practices among married respondents with children, BLP alumni reported higher rates of complete primary vaccinations among children over one year old compared with controls (63% versus 32%), and higher rates of having given oral rehydration solution during bouts of diarrhoea (42% versus 12%). These practices remained highly significant even after controlling for girls' education.

Conclusions

This programme evaluation found significant differences between girls who had participated in the "Better Life Options Program" and girls from the control group, in terms of economic empowerment and health. Though differences between these groups may reflect a certain amount of self-selection, survey findings suggest that the BLP integrated model can have a significant impact on participants' economic empowerment, self-esteem, autonomous decision-making, reproductive health and child survival practices. Two additional lessons learned from the programme

Table 1. Selected indicators of education, autonomy, and mobility among alumni and controls

Indicator	Control group (%) (*N* = 858)	BLP alumni (%) (*N* = 835)
Illiterate	32	5
Completed secondary education	46	66
Had learned a vocational skill	22	99
Employed/self-employed	8	35
Could decide when to marry	7	25
Could decide how to spend money earned	12	42
Could decide to go to market	27	52
Travelled alone to health centre in past six months	6	25
Travelled alone outside village in past six months	21	68

Figure 1. Per cent of BLP alumni and controls reporting selected reproductive health behaviours

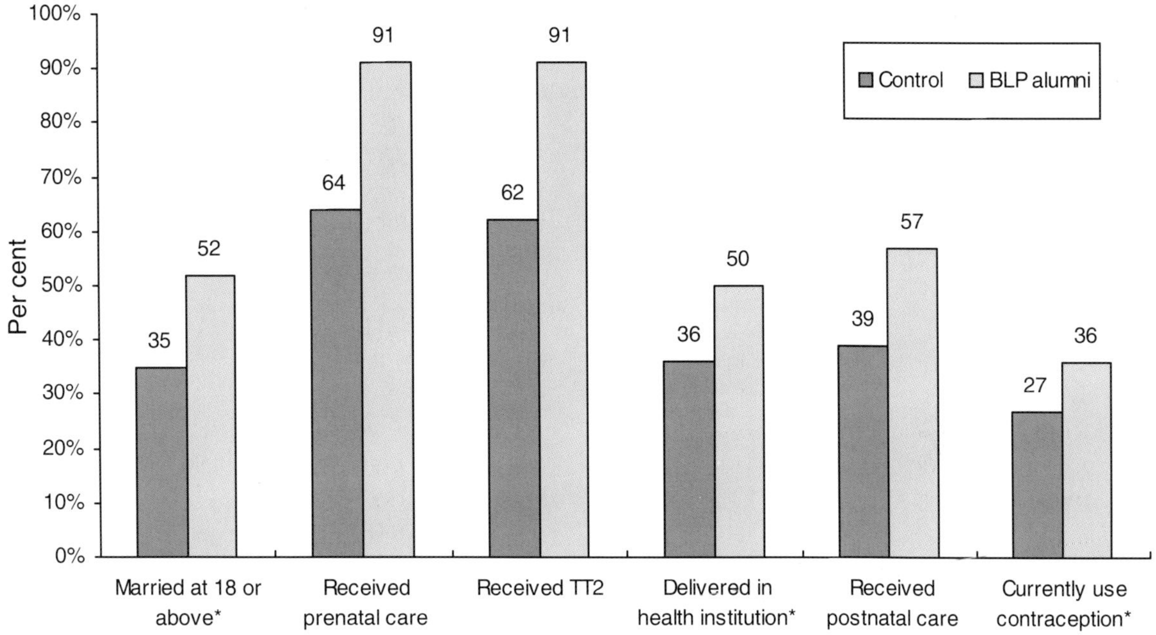

* Becomes non-significant when girls' education is controlled.

were that using vocational skills as an entry point increased girls' participation in the programme, and involving the family and community helped to increase acceptance of girls' newly acquired skills and empowerment. The assessment has also reinforced the importance of an integrated model for youth development, linking livelihoods and reproductive health. In the future, CEDPA plans to strengthen the adolescent-friendly reproductive health component, including adding iron supplementation and tetanus immunization for adolescent girls. The organization also plans to increase its promotion efforts to keep girls in school and help them complete secondary education. Finally, CEDPA plans to initiate a "Better Life Options Program" for boys.

Acknowledgements: The authors would like to acknowledge the efforts of the research team at Aarogya, Baroda—Dr P.V. Kotecha, Smita Maniar and Vaishali Zararia—and The Bill and Melinda Gates Foundation for their support of this study.

Marta Levitt-Dayal
Country Director
Centre for Development and Population Activities (CEDPA)
50M Shanti Path
Gate No. 3, Niti Marg
Chanakyapuri
New Delhi 110021
India

Training school teachers to pass on life skills to adolescents

Mridula Seth

Background

The education and health needs of adolescents in remote villages of Rajasthan are not adequately served through the existing government system. Moreover, reaching these adolescents directly is difficult since many are not part of the formal education system. As a result, programmes need to explore alternative strategies for reaching this population.

The Shiksha Karma project is currently pursuing one such strategy to reach rural youth. The Shiksha Karmi project works to expand primary school education in rural villages of Rajasthan. Men and women selected as Shiksha Karmis (SKs) have few educational qualifications and no teaching experience when they begin, but they undergo extensive training and preparation to become primary school teachers. As primary school teachers, they do not work directly with adolescents. Nonetheless, they represent a potential channel for spreading information and serving as change agents in areas that generally lack other organized groups or educated persons. As a result, the Shiksha Karmi Board and the United Nations Population Fund (UNFPA) identified the SKs as an important resource to improve the skills and the health—particularly the reproductive health—of rural youth. To achieve this, UNFPA and the Shiksha Karmi Board have undertaken a pilot project to introduce health education and "life skills" into the SK training.

The World Health Organization (WHO) (1993) defines "life skills" as "the abilities for adaptive and positive behaviour that enable individuals to deal effectively with the demands and challenges of everyday life". WHO (1994) identified a core set of life skills that included problem-solving, decision-making, goal-setting, critical thinking, communication skills, assertiveness, self-awareness and skills for coping with stress. In terms of reproductive health, for example, such skills can influence women's fertility even without formal education, by helping them make informed decisions and negotiate with their families.

In this paper, life skills have been conceptualized in terms of thinking, social and negotiation skills. Self-awareness and social awareness, planning and problem-solving are considered to be thinking skills. Establishing relationships and communicating effectively are considered social skills. Negotiation skills are an outcome of thinking and social skills. This paper describes the preliminary experiences with life skills education from the Shiksha Karmi project and discusses some preliminary lessons learned.

Project description

The project provided training in life skills education to women preparing to become SKs. The aim was to build the life skills of the SK trainees and simultaneously prepare them to build such skills among members of the communities in which they would work. The project developed a framework to address a number of issues, including: (a) self-awareness; (b) social awareness such as social norms, gender discrimination and values; (c) problem-solving; (d) working with others; (e) communication skills; and (f) negotiation skills, including how to be assertive and how to resist peer pressure. In terms of health concepts, the framework addressed topics such as physical and emotional changes during adolescence, locally available services, and information related to sex determination, abortion, infertility, HIV/AIDS, reproductive tract infections (RTIs)/sexually transmitted infections (STIs), menstrual hygiene, fertility awareness and other health issues.

The project developed and field-tested a training manual using participatory methods such as body mapping, role-plays, questions boxes, case studies, brainstorming, games and songs (United Nations Population Fund, 2000). To enhance long-term sustainability, the project trained 13 resource persons, who trained as many as 185 SKs in seven districts during 2000.

Programme evaluation

Life skills education has become an integral part of the residential training of SKs. Assessing the effectiveness of life skills interventions poses a challenge, however. While measuring gains in knowledge is difficult enough, it is even more difficult to measure changes in thinking, social and negotiation skills. The project has received feedback through group discussions, case studies and the "critical incidence technique". The critical incidence technique allows information to be collected about an incident that had a marked influence on a respondent's life. By analysing the incident, the researcher can draw inferences about the impact or effectiveness of an intervention on the respondent's personal, social and/or professional life.

This feedback clearly suggested a positive impact on participants, particularly among those selected as "Master Trainers". In general, SK trainees reported a greater ability to resist peer pressure, to convince their husbands and mothers-in-law to support family planning, and to share information on sex discrimination with others. In terms of health issues, SK trainees reported that the most relevant content of training included information about RTIs/STIs, contraceptives and menstrual hygiene. At the time of reporting, SKs had not yet had a chance to hold sessions with adolescents in their villages, but they had reported sharing information with village women. Trainees also reported giving more importance to their own health and having fewer inhibitions about discussing sexual and reproductive health issues.

Conclusions

Many lessons were learned from the pilot project about life skills interventions, a few of which are highlighted below. First, each group must choose which life skills are relevant to its own needs and situation. It is essential to identify the skills and resources that already exist among those who receive training. Second, teachers need to enhance their own life skills before they can effectively develop such skills in their students. Third, life skills interventions need to use experiential, participatory methods, and they are not effective if participants simply sit passively taking in information. Finally, there is a need for better indicators to evaluate life skills interventions.

References

World Health Organization (1993) *Increasing the Relevance of Education for Health Professionals.* Geneva, World Health Organization (WHO Technical Report Series No. 838).

World Health Organization (1994) *The Development and Dissemination of Life Skills Education: An Overview.* Geneva, MNH/PSF, World Health Organization.

United Nations Population Fund (2000) *Building life skills for better health—the Rajasthan experience.* Delhi, UNFPA (unpublished report available from the UNFPA Delhi office: http://www.unfpa.org.in)

Mridula Seth
UNFPA
55 Lodi Estate
New Delhi 110013
India

XII

Access to and quality of reproductive health services

Adolescent-friendly health services

V. Chandra Mouli

Background

Adolescence, the second decade of life, is a period in which an individual undergoes major physical and psychological changes. Alongside this, there are enormous changes in the person's social interactions and relationships. It is more of a phase in an individual's life than a fixed time period; a phase in which the individual is no longer a child but is not yet an adult; a time of both opportunity and risk.

Adolescence presents a window of opportunity in several ways. Health problems "carried over" from childhood could be addressed during this period. Actions could be taken to set the stage for healthy adulthood and reduce the likelihood of problems (such as heart disease) in the years that lie ahead. At the same time, it is a period of risk, often marked by such health problems as too early and unwanted pregnancies, and such behaviours as smoking that have serious immediate or longer-term consequences.

The World Health Organization (WHO), in conjunction with the United Nations Children's Fund (UNICEF) and the United Nations Population Fund (UNFPA) has developed a common agenda for action in adolescent health and development. This common agenda is aimed at providing a safe and supportive environment, health and counselling services (World Health Organization, United Nations Children's Fund & United Nations Population Fund, 1997)

In examining the different elements of this comprehensive approach, a useful analogy is that of a 7 year old child who needs to cross the road every day to get to school. She needs information and skills—where to look, what to look for, when to walk across and when not to do so. She needs a safe and supportive environment—a pedestrian crossing, traffic lights that work or a traffic warden in position, drivers who respect traffic rules or are punished if they do not do so. She may also need health and counselling services, if she stumbles and falls, or is struck by a vehicle.

Many individuals and institutions have important contributions to make to the health and development of adolescents. It may be useful to think of them in concentric circles of contact and influence. At the centre is the adolescent himself or herself. Parents, siblings and some other family members are in immediate contact with the adolescent and constitute the first circle. The second circle includes people in regular contact with them such as personal friends, family friends, teachers, religious leaders and others. The third circle includes musicians, film stars and sports figures, who can have a tremendous influence on them from afar. Finally in the fourth circle, politicians, journalists and bureaucrats (within the government and private sectors) affect their lives in small and big ways, through their words and deeds.

Health workers and facilities fit within the second circle in this scheme. Clearly, they play an important role in helping ill adolescents get back to good health (by diagnosing health problems, detecting problem behaviours and managing or referring them elsewhere). They also play an important role in helping healthy adolescents stay well and develop into healthy adults, by providing information, advice and preventive services (or products). Services are provided in a range of health facilities or recognized institutions that provide health services. For example, facilities include small clinics providing a limited range of (primary level) health services to large hospital complexes providing a wide range of (tertiary level) health and social services. Health facilities may be operated by the public, private (profit-seeking) or non-profit, nongovernmental sector. They may exist as independent entities or be located within institutions providing other services to adolescents, including schools, correctional institutions and residential institutions such as youth hostels. They may also be established through social marketing programmes in shops, or provided in the community by outreach programmes. And they may be provided on a temporary basis in sites where large numbers of people are forced to live in camp-like conditions, for example in the aftermath of a natural disaster, civil strife or war.

Obstacles adolescents face in seeking care

Generally speaking, adolescents tend to be healthy and make the transition into adulthood in good health. Although they may develop some of the health problems of children, such as intestinal and respiratory infections, and others that are more prevalent in adulthood, such as anaemia and sexually transmitted infections (STIs), by and large, the illnesses of childhood have been overcome and left behind, and the diseases and disorders of older years appear far away. The feeling of invulnerability that their general good health engenders may, however, lead them to ignore or underestimate health threats, such as the adverse consequences of risky sexual activity or drug use.

Adolescents are a diverse group. For example, a boy of 12 is at a very different stage of personal development than a boy of 18. Similarly, he is different in psychological and social terms from a girl of 12, in addition to obvious physical differences. Social circumstances can also influence personal development, so that the health and development of a boy of 12 who is part of a caring middle class family are likely to be very different from those of a boy of the same age who is fending for himself on the street. Finally, even two boys of the same age, growing up in very similar circumstances may proceed through adolescence in different ways, and at different "speeds".

The sexual and reproductive health service needs of adolescents are correspondingly heterogeneous. Adolescents who are not yet sexually active have different needs from those who are; sexually active adolescents in stable, monogamous relationships may have different needs from those in more casual relationships. A different set of needs characterizes those faced with unwanted pregnancy or infection, or those who have been coerced into sex. It is important therefore for health providers to be aware of the diversity of sexual and reproductive health needs of adolescents. It is also important for them to be aware of the fact that adolescents are indeed at risk of developing health problems prevalent among adults, such as anaemia and STIs, and in some cases, may be more vulnerable than adults. For example, adolescent girls may be more susceptible than adult women to STIs for both biological and social reasons. When they acquire an infection, they are also more likely to develop long-term complications (Brabin et al., 2001). Finally, it is important to note that many health problems and problem behaviours are interlinked, such as drug use and depression, alcohol use and injuries resulting from road traffic accidents, and undernutrition and complications in pregnancy and childbirth (World Health Organization, 1999).

Adolescents who perceive themselves to be well are unlikely to seek health care. They may seek health care at hospitals and clinics only if they are injured or suffer from conditions that are not related to sexual or reproductive health. In many cases they do not recognize that they are ill (e.g. many STIs are asymptomatic). Those who do recognize the need may not want to draw attention to themselves and may try to solve the problem themselves or turn to their friends, siblings or parents (especially girls) for help.

Even when adolescents choose to seek care, in many parts of the world, there are important barriers preventing access to care. First, in many places, health services such as emergency contraception and safe abortion are not available, either to adolescents or to adults. In many other places, where these health services are available, restrictive laws and policies may prevent them from being provided to some groups, such as unmarried adolescents. Even when laws and policies are not an obstacle, judgemental health workers may withhold services from unmarried adolescents. This means that for all practical purposes, some of the health services that adolescents need are not *available* to them.

Second, even where they are available, adolescents may not be able to obtain the health services they need for several reasons. For example, they may not know where to go; facilities may be located a long distance away from where they live, study or work, or in places that are difficult to reach; and facilities may not be open at times of the day when they can get away from their study/work. In short, health services are not *accessible* to them.

Third, health services may be delivered in ways that adolescents perceive to be threatening or of poor quality (see for example, Senderowitz, 2000). Experience suggests that adolescents are reluctant to use available services for fear that they may be: observed by acquaintances also awaiting services; required to go through a long bureaucratic procedure before they get to see a health worker; or obliged to wait for lengthy periods before they see a health worker or obtain the health services they need. Of greater concern are their fears concerning interaction with health workers. For example, adolescents may fear that they will be humiliated by health workers who ask awkward questions or subject them to unpleasant and painful procedures, that health workers will demand the consent of parents or guardians or will not respect confidentiality. Finally, lack of affordability poses yet another obstacle to access. In short, health services are not *acceptable* to adolescents.

In summary, adolescents face a number of obstacles relating to availability, accessibility and acceptability of services.

Adolescent-friendly services

There is a growing recognition of the pressing need to overcome these obstacles, and a number of initiatives are under way in both developed and developing countries that focus on making existing health facilities more "adolescent-friendly". Based on these initiatives, there is growing evidence of what constitutes the essential elements of adolescent-friendly health services (World Health Organization, 1999). These include:

- policies that guarantee confidentiality, do not require parental consent and do not withhold services and products from adolescents;
- procedures that allow simple registration or retrieval processes, short waiting times, facilities to "drop in" without prior appointment, strong linkages to other health and social service providers, affordable services with flexible payment requirements, etc.;
- staff who are technically competent, willing to devote adequate time to clients, interested in, understanding of and considerate of adolescent

needs, able to relate to adolescents and perceived as trustworthy; a mechanism whereby adolescents may see a particular provider at repeat visits;

- an environment that is physically appealing and accessible, offering convenient working hours and location, as well as privacy in the examination or consultation room, as well as in the waiting room and entrance, and one that is not perceived as stigmatizing—for example labelled or identified as an STI clinic.

Adolescent-friendly services also require inputs from the community and from adolescent. Communities need to be well informed about and supportive of the work that is under way. At the same time, adolescents must be well informed about available services and their quality, and must be able to participate actively in the design of appropriate services.

Conclusion

Priorities in adolescent-friendly health services will undoubtedly vary according to the nature of the health services provided and the population group to be reached. For example, privacy is likely to be high on the list of concerns for an adolescent seeking treatment for a sexually transmitted infection, but it may not be an issue at all for an adolescent seeking treatment for a twisted ankle. Further, approaches that make services friendly to one group of adolescents (such as adolescent males) may not make them any friendlier—or may even make them less friendly—to another group (such as girls in their early adolescent years). In other words, although the elements listed above must be considered, the priority assigned to each will have to be tailored to meet the special needs of adolescents who are being addressed. They will also need to offer these services in ways that respect social and cultural sensitivities, yet are feasible and sustainable. Providing adolescents with services that are of good quality and are provided in a client-centred manner is an enormous and difficult task, yet one that has huge public health implications for the prevention of health problems of adolescents and their prompt detection and management.

References

Brabin L, Chandra Mouli V, Ferguson J, Ndowa F (2001) Tailoring clinical management practices to meet the special needs of adolescents: Sexually transmitted infections. *International Journal of Gynaecology and Obstetrics*, 75(2):123–136.

Senderowitz J (2000) *A Review of Programme Approaches to Adolescent Reproductive Health.* Paper prepared for the US Agency for International Development. Washington, DC, USAID.

World Health Organization (1999) *Programming for adolescent health and development.* Geneva, World Health Organization.

World Health Organization (2000) *Synthesis of the findings of the assessment phase of action research projects aimed at improving the access of school-going adolescents to the health services they need* (unpublished draft). Geneva, World Health Organization.

World Health Organization, United Nations Children's Fund and United Nations Population Fund (1997) *Action for adolescent health. Towards a common agenda. Recommendations from a joint study group.* Geneva, World Health Organization.

V. Chandra Mouli
Department of Child and Adolescent Health and Development
World Health Organization
1211 Geneva 27
Switzerland

Making nongovernmental organization initiatives "youth-friendly"

Sharon Epstein

Background

In recent years, there has been heightened interest in adolescent reproductive health (ARH) around the world, including South Asia. This interest stems in part from the large numbers of young people already in or due to enter the 10–24 year age group, as well as growing concern about the impact of HIV/AIDS. In addition, relatively small studies in South Asia indicate the number of boys and girls who have sex before marriage may be underestimated or increasing. Lacking accurate information and adequate services, young people face the risk of early, frequent, or unwanted pregnancies, increased morbidity, both personally and in their children, and the spread of sexually transmitted infections (STIs) including HIV/AIDS.

Over the past ten years, the number and types of strategies for influencing adolescent behaviours and reproductive health outcomes have rapidly increased. The Focus on Young Adults (FOCUS) programme reviewed and synthesized evaluation data from hundreds of ARH programmes and studies from around the world. As FOCUS concluded its work in 2001, the programme put out a summary of findings containing practical and actionable policy and programme recommendations. Because ARH studies have mainly focused on small populations and interventions without comparisons or controls, it has sometimes been difficult to determine whether an outcome is valid or whether a finding has programme or policy implications. Nevertheless, many common findings have emerged. This paper discusses the characteristics that make a reproductive health programme "youth-friendly", the results of research and evaluation data from ARH programmes, and the comparative advantages that nongovernmental organizations (NGOs) and governments have in working with youth.

Adolescent reproductive health programme experience: results of research and evaluation

Senderowitz (1999) reviewed the literature and found that young people typically cite the following characteristics of "youth-friendly" reproductive health services: special hours or settings for adolescents; convenient access; a place that does not look like a clinic; a place used by their peers; empathetic, knowledgeable and trustworthy counsellors; good humane treatment that is non-judgemental and non-punitive; and counselling linked to services designed with young people's needs and interests in mind. In most studies, the characteristics of providers ranked among the most important factors determining use of services.

Nevertheless, it is difficult to get adolescents to use clinics. In some cases young people lack the ability to access services apart from their family. In other cases they are concerned that a family or community member will discover their visit to a clinic. Protecting privacy and confidentiality is therefore of the utmost importance for both married and unmarried youth. Because adolescents do not go to clinics, reproductive health programmes need to reach out to them where they congregate. In some cases, programmes have to create opportunities foryoung people to gather together, with or without adults present.

Many reproductive health programmes have tried to reach out to adolescents by working through the school system. This remains difficult in many South Asian countries, however, because many young people drop out of school at an early age or do not attend regularly, and the schools may not be open regularly or fully functioning. Teachers are often uncomfortable with the topic of sexuality and reproductive health. In some cases, conservative opposition prevents sexuality and reproductive health education in schools, although health professionals can counter this by using their influence to stimulate open and informed discussion of ARH.

Ample evidence suggests that neither information nor services alone are enough to produce changes in young people's behaviour. For example, even where both are available, non-use, variable use or ineffective use of contraceptives remain problems. One reason for this may be that young people are not as free as adults to make and carry through independent decisions. Young people cite a need for counselling and support in managing friendships, and partner and family relationships. Programmes need to commit time and resources to this kind of counselling. Many organizations have set up peer counselling programmes, although such programmes require careful planning, adult supervision and operational support. They can also be quite costly, as young people who have been trained grow out of adolescence or lose interest.

Young people have requested programmes that use the "life skills approach", which includes but also goes beyond reproductive health to help young people develop practical and applied skills in other areas of life. Other examples of innovative programmes include efforts to train service providers in the private, for-profit sector (such as pharmacies or private doctors) to serve adolescents, provide counselling and contraceptive services at workplace or military sites where adolescents are employed or serve as recruits, set up emergency drop-in centres, offer special hours or facilities for boys, develop long-term adult/adolescent mentoring programmes, and provide discussion opportunities for young unmarried couples and newly-weds on marriage and parenthood.

The public–private partnership

In many cases, young people do not identify reproductive health as a need, much less as their only or most important need. A multisectoral approach to adolescent interests seems most likely to convince young people that adults care about them as "whole persons", and are ready to address the full range of issues in their lives. ARH programmes, therefore, have to build closer relationships with other parts of the health system, as well as with programmes that offer youth other services such as basic literacy and numeracy, education, employment training, job counselling and placement, and housing.

Because adolescents' needs go beyond reproductive health and even health in general, no one organization—be it public or private—should attempt to serve all their needs. Health organizations are not terribly good at providing non-health services. Public and private organizations need to recognize their distinct comparative advantages and collaborate more closely. While governments in principle have the ability to deploy resources for ARH on a long-term and national basis, the public sector may not be the best entity to deliver such tailored services. Public services tend to be clinic-based, which have the limitations mentioned earlier. The funding that would be needed to make government clinics "youth-friendly" may be more effectively used in outsourcing to and commissioning NGOs to scale-up ARH services at the community level. Also, NGOs excel in serving married and unmarried adolescents who are "outside the system" and are likely to remain fearful and suspicious of government officials. For sensitive issues such as homosexuality, divorce, abuse and violence, rape, bride-burning and incest, which can present threats to young people from family and community authorities, NGOs have a distinct advantage in responding to quickly and maintaining privacy.

There is a tremendous need for more cross-referral, joint planning and complementary delivery of services among organizations that want to meet young people's needs. For example, if counselling is offered through a hotline in one location, the hotline needs to establish formal agreements with other services, such as pharmacies, private physicians, abuse/violence crisis centres, mental health counsellors, lawyers and legal services centres, micro credit facilities, or job training programmes. To build this kind of collaboration and develop and implement mutually acceptable service standards, NGOs need to overcome their historical competitiveness with one another. They need to find ways to do joint planning, facilitate cross-referrals, and submit collaborative proposals for funding. Governments and donors that support reproductive health services should consider funding "ARH consortia" of private and public organizations, rather than individual organizations.

The literature points to a series of strategies that have ***not*** worked well for NGOs or governments, including programmes that have focused only on "family planning", making no allowances for the different needs of adults and adolescents. Some programmes fail to involve young people in planning, implementation and evaluation. Some focus solely on negative reproductive health behaviours and outcomes, as if every adolescent is dangerous, antisocial and ill-intentioned. Some programmes have failed to address young people's physical and emotional concerns about sexuality and development compared with peers. Others have not understood or acknowledged violent situations within families and communities that put adolescents at great risk. Programmes have tried to change too many behaviours at once. They have assumed (without gathering data) that unmarried young people and married women are not sexually active outside the bounds of marriage. Issues of same-sex relationships are generally not acknowledged. Programmes have focused only on the adolescent/parent relationship and failed to consider adolescents' relationships within the extended family structure, particularly those of married adolescents. Programmes have overestimated the contribution that youth centres can make in the area of reproductive health, and have underestimated how much youth centres cost to establish and operate. Finally, programmes have failed to pay enough attention to building coalitions or alliances with other organizations.

Given the limitations of past efforts to evaluate ARH programmes, it is important to ensure that rigorous evaluation is built into all stages of ARH programmes. Ideally, cost-effective, methodologically sound evaluation designs should be built into projects before they begin. Programme staff can draw on the services of evaluation and research experts in their own countries or refer directly to new evaluation workbooks and tools that have recently become available (for example, see Nelson, MacLaren & Magnani, 2000; Adamchak et al., 2000).

Conclusions

More research and evaluation on some issues related to ARH are no doubt genuinely needed. However, as this paper has attempted to illustrate, there is a substantial and growing body of evidence from developing countries that indicates the directions that programmes and resource allocation should take. It is time for all of us working in reproductive health to expand youth-friendly programmes on the basis of what we ***already*** know.

This is equally true for national-level and other government decision-makers, reproductive health programme managers and reproductive health donors.

References

Adamchak S, Bond K, MacLaren L, Magnani R, Nelson K and Seltzer J (2000) *A Guide to Monitoring and Evaluating Adolescent Reproductive Health Programs.* Washington, DC, FOCUS on Young Adults. [Available from the FOCUS Web site: http://www.pathfind.org/focus.htm]

Nelson K, MacLaren L, Magnani R (2000) *Assessing and Planning for Youth Friendly Reproductive Health Services.* FOCUS on Young Adults Tool Series (4 Workbooks). [Available from the FOCUS Web site: http://www.pathfind.org/focus.htm]

Senderowitz J (1999) *Making Reproductive Health Services Youth Friendly.* Washington, DC, FOCUS on Young Adults. [Available from the FOCUS Web site: http://www.pathfind.org/focus.htm]

Further reading

Alauddin M, MacLaren L (1999) *Reaching Newlywed and Married Adolescents*. In FOCUS Series. Washington, DC, FOCUS on Young Adults.

Dickson-Tetteh K and the University Research Corporation (2000) *National Adolescent Friendly Clinic Initiative (NAFCI) of South Africa: Standards and Criteria*. Washington, DC, University Research Corporation.

Population Reference Bureau (2000) *The World's Youth 2000*. Washington, DC, Population Reference Bureau.

Population Reports (1998) *New GATHER Guide to Counselling.* The Population Information Program, Center for Communication Programs, The Johns Hopkins University School of Public Health.

Stewart L (2000) *Presentation on Adolescent Reproductive Health at Tulane University, School of Public Health and Tropical Medicine*. New Orleans, Louisiana, Focus on Young Adults.

United Nations Population Fund (1999) *Implementing the Reproductive Health Vision—Progress and Future Challenges for UNFPA: Adolescents and Youth. UNFPA Evaluation Findings*. New York, UNFPA. [Available from the UNFPA Country Office or from Delia Barcelona, Youth RH Task Force Leader, UNFPA Headquarters, New York, USA]

Sharon Epstein, MA, MPH
Programme Director
FOCUS on Young Adults
1201 Connecticut Avenue, NW, Suite 501
Washington, DC 20036
USA

Reproductive health services for adolescents: recent experiences from a pilot project in Bangladesh

Ismat Bhuiya, Ubaidur Rob, M.E. Khan and Ahmed Al Kabir

Background

Adolescents represent approximately one-fourth of the Bangladesh population. This large group is not adequately prepared for reproductive and sexual life, since its members lack basic information about their bodies, sexuality, contraception and sexually transmitted infections (STIs) including HIV/AIDS. Despite the persistence of early marriage among women in Bangladesh, the gap between age at menarche and age at marriage is growing (Mitra et al., 1997). Though social customs discourage premarital sexual relationships, small-scale studies suggest that, by age 19, a considerable proportion of young men have experienced premarital sex, and such experience is not unknown among girls (Haider et al., 1997; Nahar et al., 1999).

Adolescents in Bangladesh have limited access to reproductive health (RH) services, and the services that do exist are often unresponsive to the broader needs of adolescents, especially those who are unmarried (Nahar et al., 1999). Knowledge about sexuality and reproductive health is generally low. For example, one study (Rob et al., 2001) found that the majority of adolescents had no idea about changes associated with puberty, such as menstruation or wet dreams, until they occurred. Other studies have found that adolescents have inadequate knowledge about STIs including HIV/AIDS (Bhuiya et al., 2000). In a national survey (Haider et al., 1997), few female adolescents could answer questions about STIs correctly, and only 5% could identify any symptom of an STI.

To address these issues, the Population Council designed a multicountry operations research project to determine the feasibility, effectiveness and cost of creating sustainable 'adolescent-friendly' reproductive health care services through a package of interventions. In collaboration with the Urban Family Health Partnership (UFHP), the Population Council is implementing this project in north-western areas—Pabna and Dinajpur are experimental, while Rangpur is a control area. Participating clinics are open to married and unmarried adolescents, but the project focuses mainly on the needs of unmarried adolescents. In preparation for the intervention, the Population Council conducted a baseline survey on adolescents' knowledge, attitudes and practices related to sexual and reproductive health. Though the project is ongoing, this paper describes the baseline survey results and preliminary experiences from the project intervention.

Methods

To evaluate the intervention, researchers are using a quasi-experimental, pre-post design in two study sites and one control area. Prior to the intervention, researchers carried out a baseline survey among 2971 unmarried and married adolescents aged 13–19 and their parents. The sample was designed to include roughly equal numbers of adolescents in school and out of school, boys and girls. Within each of the four strata, researchers used systematic random sampling. In addition, researchers interviewed every second parent or guardian, for a total of 1531 parents. In each case they selected the parent of the same sex as the adolescent respondent. Approximately 12% of the respondents were married, but because the planned intervention mainly focuses on unmarried adolescents, married adolescents were excluded from the subsequent analysis.

Key findings

Few adolescents (less than 1% of girls and 2% of boys) reported discussing reproductive health issues with their father. In contrast, more than two-thirds (68%) of girls reported discussing such issues with their mother, compared with 3% of boys. Approximately 48% of girls and 58% of boys reported that they had received RH information from sources other than a parent or guardian. Of that group, girls were more likely than boys to have received RH information from family members other than parents (64% compared with 6%); and nearly all boys (96%) and half of the girls (45%) reported receiving RH information from friends.

A total of 127 unmarried boys and three unmarried girls reported having had had premarital sex, with a mean age at first sexual experience of 15. Of these, 57 adolescents said they had sexual intercourse within the past six months. Relatively few used condoms or any other contraceptive. Only 22% and 27% of the 127 adolescents had used a condom at first and last intercourse respectively. Of the127 adolescent boys, 52 reported having sex with commercial sex workers (CSWs), of whom 10 had used a condom. Fifteen male adolescents (out of 127) had experienced signs and symptoms of STIs, but only nine had sought treatment (Figure 1).

Figure 1. Numbers of unmarried adolescents reporting selected behaviours, out of 1462 boys and 1164 girls

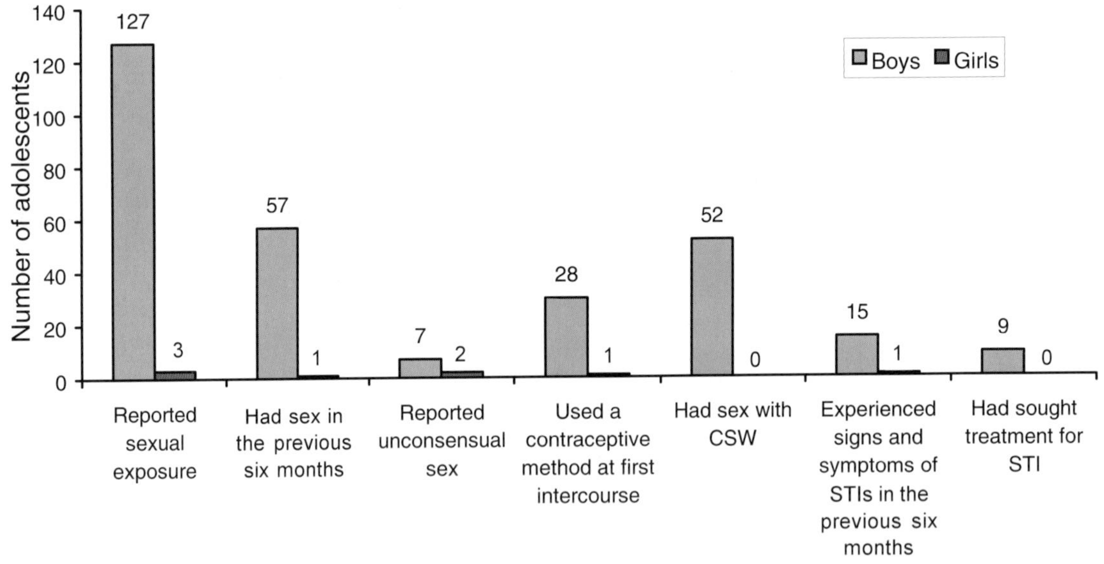

To assess the extent to which young people used services, researchers asked unmarried adolescents whether they had visited health facilities for RH services in relation to any problems of menstruation, discharge from penis or vagina, itching in the genital area, or ulcer in the genital area in the previous six months. Over 90% of adolescents reported that they had not. Of the 22 adolescents who had visited a health facility (15 girls and 7 boys), girls visited government facilities more than boys, and boys visited private facilities more than girls. Researchers asked all unmarried adolescents whether they thought they would be treated in a respectful manner if they visited clinics or pharmacies for family planning services. Most (85%) felt that they would not be treated respectfully. A larger proportion of boys than girls (15% versus 1%) thought that they would be treated well if they visited a family planning clinic. When asked about STI services, only 26% of boys and 7% of girls thought that they would be treated well if they visited a clinic, and a similarly low proportion (24% and 6%) thought that they would be treated well if they visited a pharmacy.

Programme description

Using the findings from the baseline survey, the project is trying to modify existing services at UFHP clinics to be more "adolescent-friendly" by introducing several interventions. These include: training staff to treat adolescent clients with respect, introducing designated hours specifically for adolescent clients, and increasing privacy and confidentiality by ensuring that doctors who take clinical histories and perform physical examinations also provide counselling. The participating clinics offer reproductive health services, treatment for general adolescent health issues, prevention and treatment of RTIs and STIs, including HIV/AIDS, family planning services, antenatal care, postnatal care, treatment for anxiety and depression, counselling and referrals.

To increase access, UFHP introduced a special pre-paid health card for adolescents, which costs Taka 20 (US$ 0.27). Young people can use this card to consult doctors at UFHP clinics without paying fees for one year. Adolescents who participate in the project's reproductive health education sessions receive a free health card. In addition, the project has established a telephone hotline and post-box facilities for adolescents who are not comfortable visiting the clinic. Counsellors answer all queries over the phone without asking callers to identify themselves. To answer queries received at the post-box, staff print answers in the adolescents' column of a local newspaper. To create an enabling environment for these interventions, the project distributed educational materials and undertook sensitization meetings to discuss adolescents' RH needs with gatekeepers such as parents, teachers, religious leaders, community leaders, health providers, political leaders and government officials.

In addition, the project developed a 20-hour reproductive health education curriculum for adolescents that addresses personal hygiene, nutrition, sanitation, changes during adolescence, child health and immunizations, marriage and legal rights, gender roles, drug abuse, sexual relationships, sexual abuse, STIs including HIV/AIDS, childbirth process, antenatal care, postnatal care, population growth and family planning. The project designed the curriculum with simple language, stories and case studies.

To reach adolescents who are no longer in school with the RH curriculum, the project used household listings to identify out-of-school girls and boys aged 13–19, whom they formed into groups of 12 to 15 adolescents, grouped by age, sex, employment status and marital status. To teach these groups, the project selected facilitators among young adults aged 21–28, who had at least 14 years of education. Facilitators received a five-day training course on adolescent reproductive health issues and facilitation skills.

The project has also used the school system to reach adolescents. Seven secondary schools agreed to introduce RH courses in classes 8 and

9. From each school, the project selected two teachers to receive a four-day training on the RH curriculum. The teachers prepared a lesson plan based on the RH curriculum for conducting sessions. They also planned to meet once a month to share their experiences. During training sessions and monthly meetings, teachers said that they were comfortable with the curriculum, although they expressed reservations about promoting condoms.

Conclusions

The baseline study found evidence of sexual activity among unmarried adolescents, particularly among boys. However, sexually active, unmarried adolescents reported that they did not feel comfortable seeking advice or buying condoms from nearby clinics or pharmacies and few had actually sought a service. In addition, they perceived providers to be judgemental and unfriendly. Preliminary findings from the survey and initial project experiences suggest the following. First, health services in Bangladesh should provide reproductive health services for both married and unmarried young people. Second, to increase access to services, it is important to address the social environment and increase community support for information and services for adolescents. Finally, organizations that provide services should introduce special hours for adolescent clients and train their providers to receive, counsel and provide care for adolescents.

References

Bhuiya I, Rob U, Khan ME, Al Kabir A (2000) Reproductive health related KAPB of adolescents. Paper presented in a *Workshop in Dinajpur.*

Haider SJ, Saleh N, Kamal N, Gray A (1997) *Study of Adolescents: Dynamics of Perception, Attitude, Knowledge and Use of Reproductive Health Care.* Dhaka, Population Council.

Mitra SN, Al-Sabir A, Cross AR, Jamil K (1997) *Bangladesh Demographic and Health Survey 1996–1997.* Dhaka and Calverton, Maryland: National Institute of Population Research and Training (NIPORT), Mitra and Associates and Macro International Inc.

Nahar et al. (1999) *Strategies to Meet the Health Needs of Adolescents: A Review.* Dhaka, International Centre for Diarrhoeal Diseases Research, Bangladesh. .

Rob U, Khan ME, Bhuiya I, Kabir M (2001) Factors influencing adolescent sexual activity and contraception in Bangladesh. Paper presented at the *Population Association of America, Washington, DC, March 2001.*

Ismat Bhuiya
FRONTIERS in Reproductive Health Program
Population Council
House CES(B) 21, Road 118
Gulshan, Dhaka
Bangladesh

Attitudes of family planning workers towards providing contraceptive services for unmarried young adults in eight centres in China

Gao Ersheng, Tu Xiaowen and Lou Chaohua

Background

With the opening of the system and general socioeconomic development in China, attitudes towards premarital sexual behaviour have changed, especially among adolescents. Sexual activity among young unmarried men and women has increased rapidly during the past decade. A survey conducted in seven Chinese provinces found that the proportion of married women who had had a premarital pregnancy was 16.8% in urban areas and 12.2% in rural areas. The proportions of urban and rural married women who had premarital induced abortions were 2.4% and 1.9%, respectively, between 1987 and 1991. The study also found that rates of premarital pregnancy among this group had increased between 1987 and 1991 (Xu, 1998). Surveys conducted among unmarried women visiting maternal and child health centres in Shanghai, Nanjing and other cities in the 1990s for the required premarital physical examination showed that about 70% of women were sexually experienced (Gao, Tu & Yuan, 1997; Dai et al., 1996). Many of these sexually experienced women were younger than 24 years at the time of first intercourse (Gao, 1997).

Although the proportion of sexually active unmarried young adults is high, their contraceptive use rate is low, which places them at high risk of unplanned pregnancy and induced abortion (Xu, 1998; Sun, 1994; Li et al., 1998; Liu et al., 1992). Lack of information about fertility and contraception and lack of access to contraceptive methods, are two important reasons for low contraceptive use among young unmarried people in China (Gao, Tu & Yuan, 1997). Their lack of knowledge about sex and reproductive health combined with increased premarital sex has also put unmarried youth at increased risk of sexually transmitted infections (STIs). Studies have found that between 25% and 35% of STI patients are young and unmarried (Hu, 1996; Xia, 1995; Li et al., 1997; Xu, 1997).

There is an urgent need to provide sex education to raise awareness about self-protection as well as to promote use of contraceptive services among unmarried young adults in China. However, current family planning (FP) services in China are mainly for married couples and pay little attention to the needs of the unmarried. Meeting the reproductive health needs of young unmarried people has become a challenge for the Chinese government and relevant departments.

This paper describes a multicentre study that was designed to determine the attitudes toward providing contraceptive and sexual/reproductive health services to sexually active unmarried young adults, among different groups. Respondents included sexually active, unmarried young adults, their parents, service providers and policy-makers in different areas in China. The purpose of the study was: 1) to identify unmet needs and barriers to provision of contraceptive, sexual and reproductive health services; 2) to find acceptable and feasible ways to provide services for young adults; and 3) to ascertain the views of policy-makers and others on providing services. This paper focuses on attitudes of family planning workers towards contraceptive services for sexually active, unmarried young adults.

Methods

This study was carried out in eight cities, namely Shanghai, Fujian, Henan, Hebei, Jiangsu, Zhejiang, Sichuan and Chongqing. From May to December 1998, researchers recruited 1927 family planning workers to participate in a survey, including 965 contraceptive providers and 962 contraceptive distributors.[1] In addition, they conducted focus group discussions with family planning staff and contraceptive providers in eight centres.

Key findings

Attitudes towards providing contraceptive and sexual/reproductive health services to unmarried young adults vary between areas and population groups. About 60% of respondents approved of the idea that the Government should provide contraceptive services for unmarried young adults, a figure that ranged from 28.3% to 80% among the eight centres. Thirty-six per cent of respondents disapproved, and another 4% said that they did not have an opinion. Family planning workers from urban areas were more likely to oppose providing such services. One important reason why some FP workers objected to actively providing contraceptive services for young unmarried people was that they did not consider them to be their target population.

The results of logistic regression indicated that where respondents came from, their income, and their awareness of the magnitude and consequences of sexual intercourse among unmarried young adults were significantly related to their attitudes towards active government provision of contraceptive services for unmarried young adults. Whether the respondents were contraceptive providers or distributors had no significant relation to their attitudes towards active government provision of contraceptive services for unmarried young adults.

Family planning workers' suggestions for acceptable and feasible ways to provide contraceptive services varied from one centre to another. Generally speaking, however, FP workers from all eight centres considered drug stores the most acceptable place to provide contraceptive services for unmarried young adults, especially in urban areas. In rural areas, respondents also considered the FP network among the most acceptable ways to provide contraceptive services for unmarried young adults, because the custom of engagement before marriage is common in some rural areas, and because there are fewer drug stores in rural areas than in urban areas. Respondents recommended doctors or FP workers as the most suitable people for providing contraceptive services for unmarried young adults, and they recommended condoms as the most suitable contraceptive method for this group.

Conclusions

The study findings point to a number of policy recommendations, including the following:

- The study highlighted the urgent need to change the attitudes of FP workers towards provision of contraceptive services for unmarried young adults, especially in some areas in China.

[1] Contraceptive providers are defined as family planning staff in stations of contraceptive services and family planning offices, while contraceptive distributors are defined as family planning workers in residential areas and work units.

- The Government should develop clear policies to include young unmarried people in family planning programmes.
- It is important to find acceptable and feasible ways to serve different target populations in different provinces and cities, in particular, to explore ways suited to urban and rural areas. It is also important to consider strengthening the supervision of drug stores, training drug store clerks and setting up condom vending machines in public places to increase access for unmarried young adults.

Acknowledgements: This study was supported by WHO. The institutes that participated in the study and the principal investigators of each institute were: Shanghai Institute of Planned Parenthood Research (SIPPR): Tu XW, Lou CH; Hebei Family Planning Research Institute (FPRI): Yu JR; Henan FPRI: Gan SX; Jiangsu FPRI: Ding JH; Zhejiang Academy of Medical Sciences FPRI: Sun DL; Fujian FPRI: Zhang YL; Sichuan FPRI: Cui N; Chongqing FPRI: Li H. SIPPR was the coordinating centre and Dr Gao E the coordinator of this multicentre study.

References

Dai MJ et al. (1996) The relationship between attitudes towards premarital sexual behavior and premarital sexual behavior among adolescents, *School Medicine of China,* 17(1):17–19.

Gao ES (1997) *Study on the needs and unmet needs for newly married women in Shanghai. Final report.*

Gao ES, Tu XW, Yuan W (1997) Factors influencing premarital contraceptive use at time of first intercourse among women in Shanghai. *Chinese Population Science*, 61(4):57–64.

Hu XG (1996) The study of STDs among 429 unmarried adolescents. *Chinese Journal of Prevention and Therapy of STDs/AIDS,* 2(5):206–207.

Li CL et al. (1997) STDs epidemic of Shandong province in 1996. *Chinese Journal of Prevention and Therapy of STDs/AIDS,* 3(4):152.

Li DM et al. (1998) The survey of 1010 induced abortions among unmarried women in Shanghai. *Population Studies*, 22(3):31–34.

Liu YR et al. (1992) The analysis of family background among unmarried female youth who had induced abortion. *Reproduction and Contraception*, 12(5):82–83.

Sun RD (1994) Survey on premarital pregnancies. *Population and Eugenics,* 1:4–5.

Xia ZL (1995) Epidemiology analysis of 9687 STD patients from 1989 to 1993 in Yunnan province. *Chinese Journal of Prevention and Therapy of STDs/AIDS*, 1(2):17–18.

Xu L (1998) Trends, outcomes and influences of premarital pregnancy in seven Chinese provinces. *Population Studies*, 21(1):51–54.

Xu YP (1997) Epidemiology analysis of syphilis between 1991 and 1995 in Zhejiang province. *Chinese Journal of Prevention and Therapy of STDs/AIDS,* 3(2):58–59.

Dr Gao Ersheng
Shanghai Institute of Planned Parenthood Research
2140 Xie Tu Road
Shanghai 200030
China

Providing adolescent-friendly reproductive health services: the Thai experience

Yupa Poonkhum

Background

Evidence suggests that many Thai youth have premarital sex. The first sexual experience is often unprotected, which can lead to sexually transmitted infections (STIs), including HIV/AIDS, unwanted pregnancies and illegal abortion. Although the Government has a policy to promote family life/sex education in schools, adolescents face many barriers to obtaining information and services related to sexual and reproductive health. To address this situation, the Thai Department of Health began a project in 1997 entitled "Development Model to Improve Adolescent Reproductive Health Services for Thai Adolescents", supported by the World Health Organization Regional Office for South-East Asia (WHO/SEARO). This paper describes the project and presents preliminary findings and lessons learned.

Methods

The first phase of this project was to assess the status of adolescents' reproductive health (RH) in Thailand and to identify their needs for reproductive health services. This situation analysis included a review of the existing research literature and focus group discussions (FGDs) with adolescents in schools. In addition, the Department of Health held a "grid workshop" with experts in adolescent programmes. During this workshop, experts were asked to brainstorm ideas that could contribute to guidelines and recommendations for policy-makers and relevant stakeholders. Information obtained from this first phase was used to design the second phase of the project, which aims to improve the accessibility and quality of RH services for adolescents, and to increase RH knowledge and life skills among adolescents.

Key findings

The situation analysis highlighted the need for "adolescent-friendly" counselling and health services. During focus group discussions, adolescents expressed preferences regarding the delivery of RH services, including a preference for providers of the same sex, who are friendly, generous and know how to communicate with adolescents. In terms of atmosphere, FGD respondents emphasized a private, relaxed atmosphere that protects confidentiality, is decorated in an "adolescent style" and is not called a clinic. They suggested that such services be conveniently located in towns and near destinations such as cinemas, discotheques, shopping malls and department stores. When asked about preferred hours and days of operation, adolescents suggested that services be available every day,

24 hours a day, but especially after office hours. They mentioned a need for both face-to-face and telephone counselling, preferably free of cost. Finally, they recommended that the services be promoted through radio programmes, as well as posters, leaflets and stickers.

Project design

This pilot project targeted in-school adolescents, as more than 60% of Thai adolescents are in the school system. The second phase of the project promotes four main strategies, namely RH life skills education in schools, peer education, training of parents and counselling services at selected health sites. The Department of Health is carrying out this phase in two districts of Nakorn Sri-Thammarat Province, in southern Thailand. The four participating organizations are: 1) the Provincial Public Health Office, an administrative and implementing agency in the areas of health promotion, health prevention, surveillance and basic medical treatment; 2) the Maharaj Provincial Hospital; 3) the Pakpanung District Hospital; and 4) the Buddhists Association, a provincial nongovernmental organization whose mission is to promote good mental health among all age groups.

The first three of these organizations have established "adolescent-friendly rooms" in which they provide counselling services. The Department of Health installed telephones in each of the "rooms" so that staff could also counsel adolescents over the phone. The first adolescent-friendly room at the Provincial Hospital is near the outpatient department. The second adolescent-friendly room is located at the Provincial Public Health Office, which stands apart from the clinic building. The last adolescent-friendly room is behind the outpatient department at the District Hospital. The Buddhists Association provides only telephone counselling during the evening (18:00–21:00)

To ensure the quality of services, a working group was created to monitor the project and provide ongoing training in counselling skills to the staff. To promote the services, participants met with disc jockeys from local radio programmes and asked them to help advertise the services. They also produced training materials, such as manuals on frequently asked questions and on how to provide counselling, as well as promotional material such as posters, stickers, calendar cards and signboards, which were disseminated in schools and public places. The final component of this project was to train peers, teachers and parents to help increase RH knowledge and life skills among adolescents.

The project has incorporated many of the findings from the focus group discussions. For example, training in counselling skills was a centrepiece of the project. Services are not offered in a "clinic", but in an adolescent-friendly "room". Efforts are made to protect confidentiality through anonymous record-keeping. In three sites, telephone services are offered from 09:00 to 21:00, while the Buddhists Association provides telephone counselling during the evening. Counselling and family planning methods are offered free of charge. The project has followed the recommendation that the services be promoted by radio.

However, the project has not been able to incorporate all of the adolescents' suggestions. For example, it did not set up adolescent-friendly rooms in commercial areas, because it tried to use existing government resources in an effort to keep costs low. Moreover, it has been impossible to ensure that all counsellors are the same sex as the clients, as most counsellors are women.

Lessons learned

The Department of Health has not yet undertaken the final evaluation, but several preliminary lessons have been learned, based on client records, discussions and observations during supervision and monitoring activities. First, the project demonstrated that establishing adolescent-friendly services at government hospitals is feasible and sustainable. Using their government budgets, these hospitals managed to set up adolescent-friendly services and to support counsellors through overtime payments. Second, in the process of conducting the focus group discussions, health providers began to realize the magnitude and severity of RH problems among adolescents in their provincial area, and most expressed a new willingness to devote themselves to prevention of adolescent RH problems.

However, the project has found that hospitals may not be the best location for adolescent-friendly rooms because of low acceptability among adolescents. The majority of adolescent clients have preferred telephone counselling to face-to-face counselling, probably because it gives them more privacy and confidentiality. Most call after office hours or around noon. Few adolescents have come for face-to-face counselling services. As a result, the project may need to find more acceptable sites that will attract adolescents.

Finally, the project experience suggests that, despite training, not all staff can be good counsellors. Some have not followed counselling procedures, have tried to dominate clients' decision-making, or conversely, have lacked confidence in their skills. Refresher courses, case conferences, supervision and back-up have proven essential to ensuring quality services.

The project found that a variety of means is needed to communicate with adolescents. Client records revealed that radio programmes, friends, teachers and other advertising efforts such as posters, stickers and signboards played a significant role in promoting the services among adolescents. Radio broadcasting is the most expensive means, but it seems to reach the majority of adolescents.

Conclusions

Based on experiences gained from this project, the relevant research, as well as a recognition of the magnitude of RH problems among Thai adolescents, the Director General of the Department of Health has declared that adolescent-friendly services are the Department's top priority. He aims to improve the accessibility, availability and quality of counselling and health services for Thai adolescents, with an emphasis on outreach services. To achieve these objectives, the Department of Health will collaborate with health promoting centres, provincial public health offices, provincial hospitals, district hospitals and other relevant governmental and nongovernmental organizations to gain more experience with adolescent-friendly services in various settings. The plan is to establish at least 24 adolescent-friendly corners"(called "Friend Corners") in the year 2001, and 51 more by the year 2002, at attractive locations such as department stores, youth centres, colleges and universities.

Yupa Poonkhum, MPH
Senior Public Health Technical Officer
Family Planning and Population Division
Department of Health
Ministry of Public Health
Nonthaburi 11000
Thailand

Establishing adolescent health services in a general health facility

Rajesh Mehta

Background

It has increasingly been recognized that adolescents form a specific group in society and have their own specific needs. Adolescence has become a more clearly defined developmental stage in human life, and there is currently a greater recognition of this group's biological, psychosocial and health needs than before (Senderowitz, 1999). Exploration and experimentation, the hallmark of adolescent behaviour (Sigel & Emans, 1997), often propel adolescents towards risk-taking and exposure to unwanted pregnancy, HIV/AIDS and other sexually transmitted infections, substance abuse and unintended injuries. At the same time, adolescents often face constraints in seeking services, including misperceptions about their own needs, fear of disclosure and service provider's negative attitudes (Senderowitz, 1999). To overcome these constraints, it is imperative to develop specifically designated services for adolescents.

Adolescent-friendly services should be able to attract young people, meet their needs comfortably and with sensitivity, and retain young clients for continuing care. The most important attributes of adolescent-friendly services are specially trained staff whose attitudes respect privacy and confidentiality, and a comfortable clinic environment. Ideally, the holistic package of services should include reproductive health services, nutrition counselling, counselling to promote responsible sexual behaviour and prevent substance abuse, and services such as immunizations and life skills education. Although outreach services such as school-linked clinics, workplace clinics, satellite clinics and mobile clinics have proven to be more successful and cost-effective, services for adolescents can be provided from fixed sites such as hospitals and clinics (Advocates for Youth, 1995; Action Health Incorporated, 1998a, 1998b; Association for Reproductive and Family Health, 1998; Johns Hopkins University/Population Communication Services, 1998).

Safdarjang Hospital is a government hospital in New Delhi that has 1500 beds and provides services free of cost to the public. Until now, no specific services have existed for adolescents. Children up to 12 years of age are seen in the Paediatrics Outpatient Department, and those above 12 years of age are seen in the Medical Outpatient Department or other specialty clinics. However, with the increased recognition of adolescents' needs, the Safdarjang Hospital is planning to implement a specially designed set of services for adolescents. This paper describes the effort that is under way.

Project description

To achieve the objectives of the project, the hospital will take the following steps. First, it will assess the felt needs of adolescents. Second, it will advocate for adolescent health care and work to generate demand in the community for adolescent services. Third, it will establish an Adolescent Clinic that will provide clinic-based preventive, promotive and curative services. Finally, the hospital plans to build linkages with schools, colleges and nongovernmental organizations (NGOs).

To assess the health care needs of adolescents, researchers will carry out a survey of health awareness and health care needs among school and college students using a self-administered questionnaire. This will give us an idea about the needs as perceived by adolescents themselves. We then plan to develop IEC (information, education and communication) materials, including fact sheets on relevant issues to provide information to adolescents. This material will be available at the clinic, where clients can read it while they wait or take copies home with them to read later.

The hospital will also build networks with local schools and colleges in the vicinity, and develop a training curriculum for school and college teachers. Two teachers from each partner school and college will be trained as school counsellors so that they can deal with day-to-day problems of their students and refer students to the hospital clinic when needed.

In preparation for the opening of the Adolescent Clinic, doctors and other clinic staff will receive training in counselling skills and adolescent-friendly characteristics. Once the clinic opens, staff will provide the following services: (i) curative services provided by a multi-specialty team consisting of a paediatrician, an obstetrician, a psychiatrist and counsellors; (ii) referrals to other specialty services, by providing referral cards that entitle them to preferential services the next morning; and (iii) preventive and promotive services, including growth and development monitoring, vaccinations, nutrition counselling and counselling to prevent risk-taking behaviour and encourage healthy behaviour.

The Adolescent Clinic will aim to provide services that respect young people, honour their privacy, allow adequate time for client–provider interactions, and are convenient in terms of hours and location. The hospital will monitor the quality of services provided at the Adolescent Clinic through the use of exit-interviews among a random sample of clients attending the clinic. The "mystery client" method will also be applied periodically.

Finally, the hospital will develop linkages and partnerships with NGOs that provide services to out-of-school adolescents. A two-way arrangement will be developed whereby adolescents who need specialist services will be referred to the hospital, and clinic clients who need social support will be referred to the NGOs. To accomplish this, the hospital will provide training to NGO personnel.

References

Action Health Incorporated (1998a) Mobile clinic goes to school. *Growing Up*, March, vol. 6, No. 1.

Action Health Incorporated (1998b) The youth clinic. *Growing Up*, June, vol. 6 No. 2

Advocates for Youth (1995) *School Based and School-Linked Health Center: The Facts.* Washington, DC, Advocates for Youth.

Association for Reproductive and Family Health (1998) *ARFH and Youth Friendly Services: The Satellite Experience.* Ibadan, Nigeria, ARFH.

Johns Hopkins University/Population Communication Services (1998) *"Your Electronic Counselor" makes Sex Education accessible to Young People in Peru.* Baltimore, Maryland, JHU/PCS.

Senderowitz J (1999) *Making Reproductive Health Services Youth Friendly: Research, Program and Policy Series.* Washington, DC, FOCUS on Young Adults. [Available from the FOCUS Website: http://www.pathfind.org/focus.htm]

Sigel EJ, Emans SJ (1997) In: Gellis Kagan, eds. *Current Pediatric Therapy*:856–861.

Dr Rajesh Mehta
Senior Paediatrician and Coordinator
SHAHN (Safdarjang Hospital Adolescent Healthcare Network)
Department of Paediatrics
Safdarjang Hospital
New Delhi 110029
India

XIII

Panel discussions: views of young people, governments and interested agencies

Putting reproductive health within the wider context of adolescent lives: challenges and experiences

Five young people from South Asia participated in the panel discussion entitled "Putting Reproductive Health within the Wider Context of Adolescent Lives: Challenges and Experiences". Panellists presented their perceptions and experiences of adolescents' reproductive and sexual health needs, drawing from both their work and their personal lives. They discussed the challenges they face, and identified areas for further work. Ms Poonam Muttreja moderated the session and stressed the importance of listening to young people and learning from their insights. The panellists had a variety of experiences and backgrounds, including those of a peer educator, a law student/volunteer, a high school student/volunteer, a trainer/puppeteer and a social science researcher who presented the perspectives of rural adolescents. Four of the five presenters were from India, and one was from Bangladesh.[1]

Each of the five presenters had been involved in adolescent sexual and reproductive health (ASRH) programmes, and each spoke from both their professional and personal experience. While they had diverse backgrounds and experiences, their presentations emphasized similar themes. All panellists argued that it is essential to consider the "young people behind the numbers" (Namit Kapoor—FPAI, Jabalpur, India) and to recognize the diverse sociocultural milieus within South Asia, which shape young people's perceptions and behaviours (Priyanka Debnath—FPAB, Dhaka, Bangladesh). All panellists expressed concern about unsafe and unwanted sexual activity among South Asian adolescents. They argued that many young people's sexual and reproductive health needs remain unmet, and they identified a range of innovative strategies for meeting those needs in ways that would be acceptable to youth.

Issues and concerns

Panellists highlighted a range of factors that undermine sexual and reproductive health in the region, including the following. Premarital sexual relations among young people are not rare, but they tend to occur secretly, without full information and without protection. Meanwhile, traditional norms make it nearly impossible for many young people to talk with their parents or teachers about sex or puberty. Panellists argued that although adolescents represent a large segment of the population, they remain invisible in many ways—unable to speak out about their intimate concerns and unable to get adults to recognize or meet their

[1] The lack of representation of other countries was noted by the Chair and was attributed to the inability of young people to attend due to other commitments, largely academic examinations.

reproductive health needs. Panellists lamented the tendency of policy-makers to perceive young people as a homogeneous group, a perception that may obscure the unique needs of different groups—for example, girls versus boys, or those from poorer versus more affluent economic backgrounds.

Panellists presented many examples of young people who lack even the most basic information about bodily changes during puberty or the risks of unprotected sexual behaviour. They suggested that myths, misconceptions and a lack of awareness about ASRH are widespread among South Asian youth—irrespective of socioeconomic status, religion, sex and residence. Panellists expressed concern that this situation has serious adverse consequences for the mental, physical and emotional health of adolescent girls and boys. One panellist narrated the experience of a young, educated, urban girl who feared that she had developed cancer when she experienced her first menstrual period (Priyanka Debnath—FPAB, Dhaka, Bangladesh). Another panellist described how misconceptions about pregnancy, conception and pubertal changes exacerbated risk-taking behaviours among rural youth (Laboni Jana—CINI, West Bengal, India).

Panellists argued that because young people lack reliable sources of information and counselling on sex and reproduction, they rely instead on media, peers and pornographic material for information. One panellist pointed out that young people turn to these sources not out of choice, but because they lack other options (Imran Haidar—IFSHA, New Delhi, India). Not only do these sources often provide misleading and inaccurate information, they often promote gender stereotypes, inequality and misconceptions. Many young people would prefer to get their information from parents and teachers; however, many parents and teachers are too embarrassed to discuss these issues with adolescents. Furthermore, many parents, teachers, service providers and even health trainers are themselves poorly informed. In some cases, these adults perpetuate old myths and misconceptions. For example, one panel member narrated an incident in which a health trainer conducting an information session for adolescents expressed the view that masturbation was wrong and should not be practised (Imran Haidar—IFSHA, New Delhi, India). Panellists suggested that the lack of sensitive, trusted and knowledgeable adults is a major concern for adolescents.

Panellists also discussed adolescents' inability to access health services. They described a range of concerns—including the general lack of services, providers' judgemental attitudes and young people's fears about confidentiality. Panellists noted that young people generally perceive service providers to be unresponsive to their physical and emotional needs, unwilling to provide relevant and sensitive information, and lacking the practical skills and knowledge necessary to help young people make informed decisions (Namit Kapoor—FPAI, Jabalpur, India; Laboni Jana—CINI, West Bengal, India).

Panellists also highlighted the failure of governments to address young people's needs. They argued that while governments generally recognize that adolescents constitute a significant proportion of national populations, they neglect to "look beyond the numbers". It is imperative, panellists argued, that South Asian governments recognize the varied needs of young people, break the silence around those needs and provide information and services in a sensitive, confidential and respectful manner. Panellists made the important point that many programmes designed to provide information or services to adolescents have not adopted priorities or approaches acceptable to youth. Panellists urged governments to listen to youth when designing programmes intended to serve young people. They argued that programmes must be flexible and take into consideration the fact that young people are a heterogeneous group with concerns that vary by residence, marital status, age and sex, as well as sexual lifestyle.

Finally, panellists argued that programmes and policies must consider sexual and reproductive health in the context of adolescent development more generally and address young people's needs in a holistic and comprehensive manner (Priyanka Debnath—FPAB, Dhaka, Bangladesh). Panellists also discussed the issue of adolescents' rights. They pointed out that their rights remain poorly understood and poorly articulated in government programmes in South Asia.

Strategies

Panellists identified a host of strategies that programmes can use to address adolescent sexual and reproductive health—at the level of families, communities and governments. Many of their comments reflected their personal experiences. Above all, panellists argued, programmes must treat adolescents as active and equal partners rather than passive recipients of services. Once again, they argued that young people must participate in programme planning and implementation (Priyanka Debnath—FPAB, Dhaka, Bangladesh).

At the family level, panellists pointed out that close interaction with parents has a protective influence on young people (Laboni Jana – CINI, West Bengal, India). Reflecting on her personal experience, one panellist highlighted her close and open relationship with her mother including communication about sexual health issues. She attributed her self-confidence, her overall feeling of security and her ability to communicate with other young people in her work and personal life to this close parental involvement (Urvashi Gupta – FPAI, Bhopal, India). More generally, panellists underscored the need for communication between a range of trusted adults and young people.

Panellists called for the development of innovative ways of raising young people's awareness of their health and their rights. They strongly supported the idea of providing information on sexuality from a young age, building appropriately on this education from childhood all the way through adolescence. Panellists suggested that there is no magic age at which society should initiate sexuality education, since young people's needs vary throughout their life. Rather, they argued, messages need to be tailored to young people's concerns as they arise. Child sexual abuse illustrates the need to educate children from an early age—for example, by making children understand appropriate behaviour, their own rights and how to deal with abuse when it occurs (Imran Haidar—IFSHA, New Delhi, India). Others in the audience concurred with this view.

With regard to strategies for imparting information and delivering services, panellists made several suggestions. They repeatedly mentioned the need to present information to adolescents in creative ways that open safe avenues for discussion and respect confidentiality. Specifically, they mentioned the following examples:

- The "Young Inspirers" Programme in Lucknow forms youth groups that participate in programme planning and implementation; young people have found these activities highly acceptable as evidenced by high rates of youth participation (Namit Kapoor—FPAI, Jabalpur, India).

- A talk show entitled "Interaction" provides accurate information to urban girls. This example illustrates the positive role that media can play in disseminating sexual and reproductive health messages to adolescents as well as to the larger community (Priyanka Debnath—FPAB, Dhaka, Bangladesh).

- One panellist discussed puppets and theatre as a way to demystify sensitive topics and provide information to adolescents in a captivating and non-threatening way (Imran Haidar—IFSHA, New Delhi, India).

- Another panellist shared her experience of providing confidential information using a letterbox approach. Adolescents "posted" their questions anonymously in a box after a workshop session, and workshop facilitators provided the answers to the whole group (Urvashi Gupta—FPAI, Bhopal, India).

- Panellists also mentioned talks, street plays and periodic bulletins as ways to create informal fora for discussion and information provision (Namit Kapoor—FPAI, Jabalpur, India).

- Panellists argued that mixed-sex training sessions with peer educators and adolescents have helped reduce levels of sexual harassment among both rural and urban participants (Laboni Jana—CINI, West Bengal, India; Namit Kapoor —FPAI, Jabalpur, India).

Panellists suggested that interaction between young people and adult researchers, programme managers, trainers and service providers can provide important new directions for adolescent sexual and reproductive health programmes. They repeatedly stressed peer educators and youth involvement as necessary components of youth programmes, and they recommended expanding the pool of peer educators and building networks of young people to exchange ideas and design new programmes. Whatever strategy a programme uses, panellists argued that success ultimately depends on the skills of the educator or provider — including their gender sensitivity, knowledge, training and communication skills. There is no substitute for skilled educators, whether they are teachers, service providers or peers.

Finally, panellists were acutely aware of the cultural and programmatic milieu in which South Asian adolescents are socialized and the implications of this context for adolescent sexual and reproductive health. They argued that strategies must be both realistic and acceptable—realistic in that they must consider sociocultural sensitivities at the community level, and acceptable in that they must respond to adolescents' needs, raise awareness and enhance young people's ability to make informed choices.

The panellists:

Priyanka Debnath
Student/volunteer
Family Planning Association of Bangladesh (FPAB)
Dhaka
Bangladesh

Urvashi Gupta
Peer educator/volunteer
Family Planning Association of India (FPAI)
Bhopal, Madhya Pradesh
India

Imran Haidar
Trainer and puppeteer with Interventions for Support Healing and Awareness (IFSHA)
New Delhi
India

Laboni Jana
Adolescent Resource Center
Child in Need Institute (CINI)
West Bengal
India

Namit Kapoor
Peer educator/volunteer
FPAI
Jabalpur, Madhya Pradesh
India

The session moderator was Ms Poonam Muttreja, Regional Director, MacArthur Foundation, New Delhi, India.

Enhancing adolescents' reproductive health: strategies and challenges

Representatives from governments, non-governmental organizations (NGOs) and international agencies participated in a panel discussion entitled "Enhancing Adolescents' Reproductive Health: Strategies and Challenges", moderated by Dr Iqbal Shah. The objective of this discussion was to share information about adolescent sexual and reproductive health (ASRH) programmes from different sectors and different countries. Panellists were asked to draw from their personal and institutional experiences in discussing strategies and approaches used by ASRH programmes, as well as challenges and opportunities confronting those who work in this area. Panellists included government representatives from India, Nepal and Sri Lanka, as well as NGO representatives from Bangladesh[1] and Pakistan, and representatives from international agencies with a wide regional presence, including UNAIDS (the Joint United Nations Programme on HIV/AIDS) and the World Health Organization Regional Office for South-East Asia (WHO/SEARO).

Despite their different perspectives, all panellists stressed several similar themes, many of which coincided with those expressed by young people themselves in an earlier panel discussion. Every panellist called for youth involvement in the design and implementation of programmes: the need to plan *with* rather than *for* young people. They argued that strategies for youth must be different from those for adults, which requires innovative programming at both the macro and grassroots levels. Panellists also agreed on the need for comprehensive policies for youth at the national level. In terms of programme priorities, all panellists mentioned the need to raise young people's awareness of risks through both school-based sex education and non-formal, community-based programmes. Participants outlined a range of approaches, reflecting different social, cultural and political contexts in the region. Finally, there was a consensus among panel members that operationalizing ASRH policies and programmes presents a major challenge in each of their countries.

Dr Firoza Mehrotra highlighted the Government of India's commitment to issues concerning young people—including their sexual and reproductive health. She described a variety of policies and programmes that address young people's needs—notably the National Population Policy, the National

1 The moderator noted Dr Halida Hanum Akhter's extensive experience and involvement in government committees on reproductive health issues and her current involvement in a quasi-government organization in Bangladesh, and asked her to provide an overview of the Bangladesh Government's programmes and perspectives on adolescent sexual and reproductive health issues.

Youth Policy, the National AIDS Policy, the Ninth Five Year Plan and the Reproductive and Child Health Programme. The National Youth Policy, for example, emphasizes youth participation, empowerment of young people, gender equity and rights. In addition, the policy calls for an intersectoral approach grounded in a realistic needs assessment. Both the National Population Policy and the National AIDS Policy recognize youth as an underserved population and devote considerable attention to strategies for this group. Central tenets of these policies include youth participation and well-being, along with a commitment to address youth in a holistic and comprehensive way. Dr Mehrotra discussed the urgent need to translate macro-level policies to the grassroots level. Finally, she reiterated the Government's commitment to engage youth in programme design and programme implementation. Referring to the Delhi Declaration, a statement by youth made at the South Asia Conference on Adolescents held in New Delhi a year earlier, she highlighted the multifaceted needs of adolescents—for education, employment, and health-related information, counselling and services. She also highlighted their eloquent call for parents, school systems and Governments to address these needs.

Dr Deepthi Perera presented the ways in which the Government of Sri Lanka has addressed young people's sexual and reproductive health. Young people in Sri Lanka face many of the same risks and sociocultural obstacles to sexual and reproductive health as young people in India. An important difference, however, lies in their educational attainment. Because large numbers of young people in Sri Lanka complete secondary education, the Government has taken measures to address sexual and reproductive health needs through schools. Dr Perera described how programmes have taken a multi-pronged approach, including training teachers to deliver appropriate information in friendly and non-threatening ways, and incorporating sex education into the school curriculum. At the same time, the Government has built partnerships with NGOs, universities and civil society for implementing ASRH programmes.

In Nepal, the focus has been somewhat different. Dr Pathak highlighted three ways that the Government of Nepal serves young people's sexual and reproductive health needs. These include: fostering a safe and supportive environment, providing health services and counselling, and providing information. The Government implements a range of interventions in schools and in community settings. Programmes address young people themselves as well as adults who play important roles in the socialization of young people —parents, teachers and others. These programmes use innovative measures to reach youth, including youth groups, telephone counselling, camps and training programmes. Finally, they attempt to address adolescent sexual and reproductive health needs in a comprehensive and integrated way.

In Bangladesh, the Government has incorporated adolescent sexual and reproductive health issues into the health policy and essential services packages programme. Dr Halida Akhter described how the Government of Bangladesh has operationalized its commitment to achieving ICPD[2] goals. The Government has focused on meeting adolescents' needs through the provision of services and information, as well as through education programmes and campaigns to change behaviour. It has implemented programmes in schools as well as in community settings, in partnership with NGOs, bilateral and donor agencies, and civil society. Efforts are currently under way to translate national policy into a set of achievable goals and activities.

In contrast to these experiences, national policies in Pakistan rarely mention young people's sexual and reproductive health, and Government input on

---

2 The objectives outlined at the 1994 International Conference on Population and Development held in Cairo, Egypt (United Nations 1994).

the topic is minimal. Ms Yasmeen Qazi outlined this situation and identified several challenges that confront programmes for young people, including weak commitment at the highest level, limited resources, lack of a national policy and the paucity of research that might indicate how best to move forward. Despite these challenges, Ms Yasmeen Qazi described how networking through media, policy-makers, NGOs and communities has encouraged a shift in Government thinking. As a result, various stakeholders have begun to discuss programme development in the area of adolescent health and development.

Representatives of international agencies engaged in addressing the sexual and reproductive health of young people outlined priorities facing national programmes. Dr Swaroop Sarkar, UNAIDS, New Delhi, highlighted the need for programmes to move forward on several fronts, including mobilizing resources, making existing networks sustainable, forging new partnerships, scaling up programmes and mobilizing gatekeepers. He argued that international agencies can play a pivotal role in fostering networks and dialogue among different sectors. Dr Neena Raina, WHO/SEARO, discussed the need to review existing policies and programmes. She also outlined essential ingredients of successful programmes, including generating a sense of ownership and forging partnerships among stakeholders, developing indicators for evaluation, and most important, involving adolescents at all stages of programme design and implementation.

The discussion was summarized by one panellist (Dr Firoza Mehrotra) who outlined some lessons that Governments could learn from the Conference about programmes for young people:

- Involve young people in the design and implementation of all programmes.
- Gain rapport with, orient and sensitize trusted adults—including parents and teachers—to increase their support for youth programmes.
- Orient parents to communicate better with their children on sensitive issues relating to adolescent sexual and reproductive health.
- Develop materials in consultation with adolescents, and field-test them for feasibility and acceptability.
- Maintain the confidentiality of young clients and offer them services that are accessible, non-threatening, and non-judgemental.
- Take into consideration the suggestion that peer educators can make better teachers than adults.
- Understand that life skills and coping skills are an integral part of adolescents' needs; sexuality education is only one, albeit important component of these needs.
- Influence the media to provide positive role models, address gender stereotypes and provide accurate information on sexual and reproductive health issues.
- Forge partnerships with NGOs and other civil society groups.

Finally, all panellists recognized the familiar challenges facing adolescent sexual and reproductive health programmes, including: balancing priorities *vis-à-vis* resources, scaling up programmes and sustaining them, and building effective partnerships. Despite the diverse contexts and strategies in the region, the panel discussion conveyed a strong message that all countries of the region have made an increased commitment to address the sexual and reproductive health needs of young people.

Reference

United Nations (1994). *Programme of action adopted at the International Conference on Population and Development, Cairo, 5-13*

September, 1994. New York, United Nations (document No. A/CONF. 171/13).

The panellists:

Dr Halida Hanum Akhter
Director
Bangladesh Institute of Research for Promotion of Essential & Reproductive Health and Technologies (BIRPERHT)
Dhaka
Bangladesh

Dr Firoza Mehrotra
Planning Commission
Government of India
New Delhi
India

Dr Laxmi R. Pathak
Ministry of Health
Government of Nepal
Kathmandu
Nepal

Dr Deepthi Perera
Director of Youth, Elderly and Displaced Persons
Dept of Health – Ministry of Health
Government of Sri Lanka
Colombo
Sri Lanka

Ms Yasmeen Qazi
Executive Director
PAVHNA (Pakistan Voluntary Health & Nutrition Association)
Karachi
Pakistan

Dr Neena Raina
WHO/SEARO
New Delhi
India

Dr Swaroop Sarkar
UNAIDS
New Delhi
India

The session moderator was Dr Iqbal Shah, World Health Organization, Geneva, Switzerland.

XIV

Looking forward: recommendations of the conference

Looking forward: recommendations for policies, programmes and research

Sarah Bott, Iqbal Shah and Shireen J. Jejeebhoy

Programme recommendations

This Conference brought together over 250 people from many different disciplines, sectors and countries. A central aim of the Conference was to encourage dialogue among government representatives, researchers, programme managers and service providers. The Conference organizers hoped that after participants shared their perspectives, knowledge and experience, service providers would return to their practices with more sensitivity towards adolescents, researchers would identify future lines of research most likely to benefit young people, and decision-makers would design policies and programmes based on a more informed understanding of adolescents' needs and successful public health strategies. Indeed, in his inaugural speech on the first day of the Conference, Mr Nanda, Secretary of Family Welfare, Government of India, affirmed the Government of India's interest in the Conference recommendations with a view towards incorporating them in strategies currently being formulated for adolescent reproductive health.

In general terms, participants called for governments and nongovernmental organizations (NGOs) in South Asia (and elsewhere) to address young people's sexual and reproductive health needs and concerns, including the spread of HIV/AIDS and other sexually transmitted infections (STIs), high rates of unwanted pregnancy, obstetric complications and unsafe abortion. To accomplish this, they argued for a twofold approach: investment in prevention and services for specific health problems, as well as investment in young people's broader needs—for education, jobs, and supportive families and communities.

As a group, adolescents have diverse life experiences; they include married and unmarried individuals, male and female, those who are not yet sexually active, those who are sexually experienced but have suffered no adverse consequences, and those who have engaged in risky sex and suffered health consequences. Services designed for one group may not be acceptable or appropriate for another. Participants noted that NGOs have been innovators in developing "youth-friendly" services, and their efforts provide important lessons about how to design programmes for youth. In most cases, however, their coverage is limited and their experiences tend to be poorly documented and evaluated. To overcome these challenges, participants called for programmes to forge partnerships among governmental, non-governmental and private sectors, to build on existing systems and to reach beyond the clinic to where young people actually spend their time.

Papers in this collection include many other specific policy and programme recommendations, as summarized in the following pages.

- *Intensify efforts to postpone early marriage and childbearing among adolescent girls*

Papers in this collection highlight the great gender divide that exists with regard to adolescent reproductive health. As many as 1 in 10 adolescent South Asian women (aged 15–19) gives birth each year, often before reaching physical maturity, and often without adequate obstetric care. A number of authors call for efforts to raise awareness among girls, parents, teachers and community leaders about the negative impact of early marriage and pregnancy on the health of women and children. They suggest several ways to address this issue, including community-based education, changing the laws where necessary, holding governments accountable for enforcing the legal age of marriage for girls, and expanding educational and occupational opportunities for young women. Simultaneously, programmes need to find ways to enhance married girls' autonomy within their marital homes, perhaps by encouraging education, strengthening girls' life skills and generating employment opportunities. Given the low status of married adolescent girls in many communities, some authors suggest that programmes must target not only young married women, but also more powerful family decision-makers, such as husbands and mothers-in-law.

- *Train providers to recognize married girls as a high-risk group and to understand the negative health consequences of their social status*

In many parts of South Asia, married adolescent women have little autonomy over their sexual and reproductive lives. As a result, many experience risky pregnancies, forced sex and STIs. The evidence suggests that providers should be trained to recognize married adolescent girls as a high-risk group. Providers need to offer information, counselling and services in ways that consider girls' lack of power within their husbands' families. They should reach out beyond the clinic to encourage young women and families to seek prenatal visits and adequate obstetric care. Under the right circumstances and with careful training, providers could also be encouraged to ask about young women's experiences of coercion and violence, as well as STI symptoms. In general, many providers need to learn how to provide care that takes into consideration the social and economic constraints that young women face.

- *Prioritize public health strategies that prevent the spread of sexually transmitted infections, including HIV/AIDS among young people*

Studies in this collection suggest that premarital sex among young people in South Asia is both more common than generally assumed and increasing. Typically, South Asian societies have placed great value on young women's chastity before marriage, but have not placed strict social controls on the sexual behaviour of young men. As a result, not only are many young men at risk of STI/HIV infection, but young women who abstain from sex before marriage are often exposed to STIs through their husband's behaviour. The growing severity of the HIV/AIDS epidemic in South Asia should compel every sector of society to consider what it can do. Authors in this collection suggest a host of measures, including: (a) increase access to information and particularly risk awareness through education programmes in the schools and through community-based efforts; (b) increase access to quality health care for young people; and (c) carry out targeted campaigns to increase condom use among high-risk groups, such as boys and young men who have sex with commercial sex workers.

- *Enhance young people's ability to make informed choices about their own health and risk behaviour*

As has been observed in many settings, this collection of papers notes that young people need basic knowledge about sex, negotiation skills and the ability to communicate with both peers and adults in order to make informed decisions about sexual and reproductive health. Studies presented at this Conference suggest that relatively few adolescents in South Asia are fortunate enough to experience these protective circumstances. Adolescents across virtually all South Asian countries face barriers to information and services. Adults such as parents, teachers, service providers and government officials have great influence over adolescents' access to information and services, but the attitudes of these groups have often not kept pace with rapid social and economic change. Meanwhile, mass media have an increasingly powerful, but not always positive, role in spreading information and messages about how young people should behave. Programmes that effectively increase young people's knowledge and life skills may offer one way to combat the spread of STIs, including HIV/AIDS among both young women and young men. While there is consensus that adolescents need more (and better quality) sex education, there is often controversy over what content is appropriate for adolescents at different ages, and who can best deliver this information. As a result, programmes must involve a wide constituency—including parents, teachers, peers, religious leaders, community leaders and others. Papers in this collection suggest that such efforts are most likely to succeed when: (a) they address a broad array of topics and skills that young people value; (b) they use a curriculum adapted to local belief systems and behaviour patterns; (c) they collaborate with groups within the community to build support for their work, including parents, community leaders and service providers; and (d) they ensure that staff are well trained and sensitive to the perspectives of young people.

- *Sensitize adults to provide a more supportive environment for youth*

Studies in this collection point out that good rapport and communication with trusted adults—especially parents—may help protect young people from risky or non-consensual sex. Most young people in these studies say that they want more information from adults in their lives, and many specifically say they wish they could discuss sexual and reproductive health matters more openly with their parents. These findings suggest a need to devise, implement and scale up activities that strengthen these ties. Programmes need to give parents, teachers and other trusted adults the skills to understand adolescent development, to discuss sensitive issues without embarrassment, and to provide a supportive environment more generally. Such interventions need to be rigorously evaluated, and strategies that prove effective need to be more widely applied.

- *Increase access to high-quality "youth-friendly" health services drawing from the international experience*

Many studies in this collection describe barriers that prevent young people from gaining access to high quality health services. Many young people do not have money to pay for services, do not want to raise suspicion of sexual activity, or in many cases—particularly in the case of young girls—do not have authority within their families to make decisions about their own health. Other barriers include: inconvenient locations and hours, long waits, high costs and providers whom adolescents perceive to be threatening, judgemental, or unwilling to respect young clients' confidentiality.

Studies suggest that adolescents throughout the world define youth-friendly services in broadly similar ways. For example, young people typically mention special hours or sites for adolescents, convenient locations and hours, drop-in hours, a place that does not look like a clinic, affordable fees and respect for confidentiality. Several authors emphasize the importance of services such as counselling and life skills development that help young people manage their relationships with friends, partners and families. Others highlight the need for providers to understand the physiological differences between adolescents and adults, differences that increase obstetric risk and make certain contraceptive methods more or less appropriate for young people. Perhaps most important, young people say that they want staff to be empathetic, trustworthy and non-judgemental. Evidence from some communities (see Bhuiya et al., this volume) suggests that the perceived unfriendliness of providers deserves responsibility for much of their reluctance to use health services.

There is now sufficient evidence—both from the international literature and from South Asia—to justify widespread efforts to increase access to health care by making services more "youth-friendly" along the lines described here. Experience from existing programmes suggests that to accomplish this objective on a national scale, public sector programmes need to build partnerships with both private and nongovernmental sectors.

Recommendations for research

During the Conference, several participants remarked that just a few years ago, it would have been difficult to predict the wealth of information shared during this Conference. Nevertheless, important knowledge gaps remain. The Conference highlighted many areas that merit additional research. There is much that we still do not know about South Asian adolescents' lives or about effective strategies to address their sexual and reproductive health needs. This section summarizes some key research priorities that Conference participants identified.

- *Investigate sexual and reproductive choice among married youth*

Given that a large proportion of South Asian women continue to marry in adolescence, there is a need for better understanding of areas such as: (a) why parents continue to marry their daughters early; (b) what factors constrain married adolescents' ability to make sexual and reproductive choices; (c) how programmes and policies can ease social pressure on girls to bear children before they are physically mature; (d) what are the experiences and needs of young first-time parents; and (e) what are the circumstances surrounding young married women's exposure to unsafe pregnancy, STIs and sexual coercion more generally. This Conference highlighted the need for both social science and operations research to explore the effectiveness of interventions designed to enhance the autonomy and well-being of married adolescent women.

- *Investigate pre- and extramarital sexual behaviour, awareness and attitudes, including how adolescents form sexual partnerships and what factors increase or protect them from risk*

The severity of HIV/AIDS in South Asia calls for special efforts to understand the levels and patterns of sexual activity, the ways in which sexual partnerships are formed, and the social and cultural factors that facilitate or hinder healthy behaviour. For example, more research on the magnitude and social context of unprotected sex with commercial sex workers could raise awareness about young people's vulnerability and could help identify public health strategies that could protect young people from HIV/AIDS and other STIs. More generally, many settings need a better understanding of premarital behaviour patterns, norms and gender roles among women and men, including how young people form relationships, how they make decisions about sex and how they communicate with adult gatekeepers. Papers presented at this Conference reflect the limitations of the broader research literature from this region; most focus on small samples or particular groups such as college students or street children. To achieve a more complete picture of adolescents' extramarital experiences, we need research that is both more representative and more in-depth.

- *Explore the levels, patterns and context of unwanted pregnancy and abortion among young women*

Studies in this collection suggest that unwanted pregnancy and abortion are observed among disturbingly high proportions of adolescent women. Evidence suggests that sexually active girls are more likely than adult women to have an unmet need for contraception, to experience an unwanted pregnancy, to delay seeking abortion, to seek abortion services from unqualified providers, to lack family support and to experience post-abortion complications. Despite the serious implications of these findings, there is limited information about unwanted pregnancy and abortion among adolescents—in part due to the practical difficulties of studying such a sensitive issue. To address the problem, we need more information about how adolescents deal with unwanted pregnancy, how they make decisions, what factors limit their access to health care, what providers they choose and why, what consequences they experience, and—in the case of abortion-seekers—whether they receive counselling on post-abortion contraception.

- *Explore sexual coercion and rape suffered by adolescent girls and boys, both married and unmarried*

This collection highlights adolescent girls' and boys' vulnerability to sexual harassment, coercion and violence. Such coercion may involve physical force, threats or blackmail, as well as behaviours such as offers of money or favours in exchange for sex. Several authors note that, in some cases, parents curtail educational opportunities for girls precisely because they want to protect their unmarried daughters from such coercion. At the same time, the experience of forced sex within marriage is reported by women in several studies in South Asia, and even considered normal by some. Given the dearth of data on this topic, however, more research is needed to document levels and patterns of sexual coercion and violence, their nature and extent, the factors that protect adolescents or render them more vulnerable to coercion, and the consequences of coercion for contraceptive use, reproductive choices and broad efforts to protect their own health. In particular, authors note that not enough is known about the extent to which adolescents as a group suffer from mental health problems associated with such coercion.

- *Investigate adolescents' access to health care and the quality of that care*

Several papers in this collection call for researchers to help identify ways to increase young people's access to high quality care. First, authors note that those who wish to make services "youth-friendly" need to understand the specific factors in each community that prevent young people from obtaining appropriate information and services. This enables programmes to be adapted to the local social and cultural setting. Second, studies suggest that young people in South Asia often turn to unqualified providers, because of a lack of accessible alternatives. More evidence about inadequate care could build political will to reform the informal health sector and increase access to better-quality services. Third, Conference participants suggested that we need more research on quality of care in "youth-friendly" services. How should evaluators measure quality of care for young people? What approaches have successfully changed provider attitudes? How can programmes increase quality of care and sustain it as they scale up? Are some models of "youth-friendly" services better than others? How much do they cost? Fourth, authors note a number of specific operations research questions that remain unanswered. For example, can programmes that provide services in places where adolescents actually spend their time (e.g. mobile clinics, malls, schools, etc.) attract more clients than traditional clinic facilities? Are drugstores equipped to serve young people's contraceptive needs? What are the strengths and weaknesses of peer counsellors compared with adult counsellors?

- *Investigate the needs and attitudes among different subgroups and settings*

Several Conference participants note the dearth of information about selected subgroups and settings. For example, how can services and programmes reach out-of-school adolescents? What are the particular needs of subgroups within the broad age range of 10 to 19? What do youth aged 13 to 15 need compared to those who are aged 16 to 19? How do attitudes, needs and behaviour vary by setting, by rural and urban residence, by marital status, and socioeconomic situation? Such data could contribute to more effective policies and programmes, at both the local and national levels.

- *Methodological innovations*

This Conference highlighted the need for certain methodological innovations in research on adolescent sexual and reproductive health (ASRH). Researchers must overcome several limitations of existing designs. First, study samples need to be more representative of the populations from which they are drawn. Second, the sensitive nature of adolescent sexuality calls for greater reliance on qualitative methods, either on their own, or to provide more insights into quantitative findings. Third, research questions must be carefully framed and pilot-tested to allow for as much insight as possible. Whatever methodology they use, researchers must go beyond simple descriptions of data to more rigorous analyses of behavioural relationships and the social and cultural correlates of adolescent reproductive health. Researchers should also consider how to ensure informed consent among young people—both in research and in service provision.

- *The need for more rigorous operations research and programme evaluation*

Finally, many papers in this collection argue that we need to invest more resources in operations research and programme evaluation. Most ASRH programmes in South Asia have not had a strong evaluation component. Donors and programme managers need rigorous evidence about the feasibility, effectiveness and acceptability of interventions designed to provide sexual and reproductive health information and services to young people in different settings in order to identify which strategies are effective, and therefore worth scaling up. Too often, however, programmes hesitate to invest money in evaluation, and simply hope that their efforts produced results. Authors identified a number of specific programme evaluation questions that merit attention. For example, to what extent do life skills programmes affect adolescents' decision-making, negotiation and communication skills and (where applicable) sexual and reproductive behaviour? Also, while many have recommended that programmes train providers to deliver "youth-friendly" services, few programmes have evaluated the extent to which such training has actually changed provider attitudes, knowledge, counselling skills, treatment of their clients, or respect for adolescents' confidentiality.

Conclusion

Conference participants described many innovative programmes and approaches from different parts of South Asia, and they suggest that the momentum to address these issues is gaining strength. During the Panel session "Putting Reproductive Health within the Wider Context of Adolescents' Lives: Challenges and Experiences", young panellists from Bangladesh and India shared their recommendations, their vision and their commitment. The young panellists and the papers in this collection emphasize the extent to which adolescents' broader needs—e.g. for education, employment, health care, self-esteem and family support—are inextricably linked to sexual and reproductive health. Society cannot adequately address one set of needs without considering the other.

Finally, although this collection provides a wealth of information about adolescent sexual and reproductive health in South Asia, it also highlights the knowledge gaps that remain. To make informed policy decisions, we need more social science and operations research to understand why adolescents' sexual and reproductive health needs remain unmet and how services should be structured given the social, cultural and economic constraints that adolescents face. At the same time, programmes need to learn from documented successes from other settings. As John Townsend (FRONTIERS Project, Population Council, USA) noted during the Conference, to date there have been more diagnostic studies than interventions research, more experience with information provision than service provision, more resources invested in developing service delivery models than in evaluating programmes, and little research on quality of services for adolescents. Ultimately, developing and sustaining youth-centred programmes require an understanding of what young people need and want, a willingness to innovate and a commitment to adapt to young people instead of expecting young people to use service delivery models intended for either children or older adults.

Papers from this Conference portray adolescence as a complex transition period with great potential and risks. Adolescents differ by age, ethnic group, culture, religion and socioeconomic status. Nonetheless, South Asian adolescents have much in common. Whether urban or rural, whether married or unmarried, whether living in Bangladesh, India, Nepal, Pakistan, or Sri Lanka, adolescents face many sexual and reproductive health problems that are not being adequately addressed by society.

There is an urgent need for programme managers and researcher to act in three related areas:

- At the level of the adolescent, there is a need to enhance young people's awareness, self-efficacy and autonomy to enable informed decision-making and reduce unsafe and unwanted sexual activity.
- At the same time, parents, teachers and the adult community more generally must facilitate this decision-making, whether through free and open communication, or by creating an environment that protects adolescents from abuse, and enables them to access information and services without fear.
- Finally, health services and providers must learn to welcome and serve young people's sexual and reproductive health concerns and needs.

Such actions taken by governments, NGOs and individual communities to promote adolescent sexual and reproductive health will have far-reaching implications for young people, communities and nations.

Annex 1

International Conference on Adolescent Reproductive Health: Evidence and Programme Implications for South Asia

1–4 November 2000, Mumbai, India

CONFERENCE AGENDA

Registration

Inauguration

Perspectives on key issues
Chairperson: *Nirmal K. Ganguly* (Indian Council of Medical Research, New Delhi, India)

On being an adolescent in the 21st century
Paul F.A. Van Look (World Health Organization, Geneva, Switzerland)

Programming for adolescents: Indian perspectives
A.R. Nanda (Ministry of Health and Family Welfare, New Delhi, India)

Key concerns and priorities for action
Ena Singh (United Nations Population Fund, New Delhi, India)

Session 1: Sexual and reproductive health of married adolescents
Chairperson: Gunvanti Goding (Welcome Trust, UK)

Sexual and reproductive health of married adolescents: findings from NFHS-II
Sumati Kulkarni (International Institute for Population Sciences, Mumbai, India)

When marriage occurs in adolescents: the sexual and reproductive health needs of married adolescents in Bangladesh
Syeda Nahid Mukith Chowdhury (Population Council, Bangladesh)

Early marriage and childbearing: risks and consequences
Ramesh K. Adhikari (Institute of Medicine, Kathmandu, Nepal)

Newly married adolescent women: experiences from a case study in urban India
Annie George (University of California, San Francisco, CA, USA)

Reproductive health status of married adolescents
Sandhya Barge (Centre of Operations Research and Training, Vadodara, India)

Analysing adolescent pregnancy and its outcome
*Shivani Sachdev** (JJ Hospital, Mumbai, India)

Discussant's comments
Leela Visaria (New Delhi, India)

* Abstract presentation.

Session 2: Panel discussion—Putting reproductive health within the wider context of adolescents' lives: challenges and experiences
Moderator: *Poonam Muttreja* (MacArthur Foundation, India)

Panellists: *Priyanka Debnath* (Family Planning Association, Dhaka, Bangladesh); *Urvashi Gupta* (Family Planning Association, Bhopal, India); *Imran Haidar* (Interventions for Support, Healing and Awareness (IFSHA), New Delhi, India); *Laboni Jana* (Child In Need Institute, Kolkata, India); *Namit Kapoor* (Family Planning Association, Jabalpur, India).

Session 3: Sexual risk behaviours, perceptions and norms among unmarried adolescents: evidence from case studies
Chairperson: *Padam Singh* (Indian Council for Medical Research, New Delhi, India)

Risk behaviours and misperceptions among low-income college students of Mumbai
Leena Abraham (Tata Institute of Social Sciences, Mumbai, India)

Adolescent reproductive and sexual health: an exploration of trends in Pakistan
Yasmeen Sabeeh Qazi (Pakistan Voluntary Health and Nutrition Association, Karachi, Pakistan)

Youth perspectives on the influence of gender norms on the reproductive health of adolescents in Nepal
Shyam Thapa (Family Health International, Kathmandu, Nepal)

A study of reproductive health awareness and sex behaviour among adolescents in India
Azad S. Kundu (Indian Council of Medical Research, New Delhi, India) (Summary not available)

Youth and sexuality in Sri Lanka
Kalinga Tudor Silva (University of Peradeniya, Peradeniya, Sri Lanka)

Adolescent sexual and reproductive health in Bangladesh: a needs assessment
*Leena Choudhary** (International Planned Parenthood Federation, London, UK)

Discussant's comments
Ravi Verma (International Institute for Population Sciences, Mumbai, India)

Session 4: Meeting adolescents' needs for contraception
Chairperson: Badri Saxena (New Delhi, India)

Adolescence and safety of contraceptives
Olav Meirik (Santiago, Chile)

Contraceptive behaviours among adolescents in Asia: issues and challenges
Saroj Pachauri (Population Council, New Delhi, India)

Constraints to condom use among young men engaged in risky sexual behaviour in border towns of Nepal
Anand Tamang (Centre for Research on Environment, Health and Population Activities, Kathmandu, Nepal)

Attitude of family planning workers towards providing contraceptive services for unmarried young adults in eight provinces/cities of China
Gao Ersheng (Shanghai Institute of Planned Parenthood Research, Shanghai, China)

* Abstract presentation.

Evaluation of reproductive and contraceptive knowledge and sexual behaviour of undergraduate university students
*Lata Dandekar** (Gourai Maternity and Nursing Home, Mumbai, India)

Discussant's comments
Roger Ingham (University of Southampton, Southampton, UK)

Session 5: Reproductive tract and sexually transmitted infections
Chairperson: *Somnath Roy* (India)

The risk of infections: gynaecological problems among young married women in Tamil Nadu
Abraham Joseph (Christian Medical College, Vellore, India)

Impact of STIs and AIDS on adolescents: a global perspective
Purnima Mane (Population Council, Washington, DC, USA)

Developing an interactive STD-prevention programme for youth: lessons from a north Indian slum
Shally Awasthi (King George's Medical College, Lucknow, India)

Adolescents attending STI clinics: case study from Pakistan
Shahid Maqsood Ranjha (SAHIL, Islamabad, Pakistan)

Gynaecological morbidity among teenage mothers: a study based on rural women of Uttar Pradesh
*Sampurna Singh** (International Institute for Population Sciences, Mumbai, India)

Discussant's comments
Radhika Ramasubban (SOCTEC, Mumbai, India)

Session 6: Panel discussion—Sexual and reproductive health of young people: problems and interventions
Moderator: *Mahinder Watsa* (Family Planning Association India, Mumbai)

Panellists: *Halida H. Akhter* (Bangladesh Institute of Research for Promotion of Essential and Reproductive Health and Technologies, Dhaka, Bangladesh); *Daphney Conco* (Addinston Hospital, Durban, South Africa); *Gao Ersheng* (Shanghai Institute of Planned Parenthood Research, Shanghai, China); *Roger Ingham* (University of Southampton, Southampton, UK); *Vijay Kulkarni* (Mumbai, India); *Duru Shah* (Mumbai, India); Vihang Vahia (Pune, India).

Session 7: Emergency contraception and termination of pregnancy
Chairperson: *N.C. Saxena* (ICMR, New Delhi, India)

Menstrual regulation among adolescents in Bangladesh: risks and experiences
Halida H. Akhter (Bangladesh Institute of Research for Promotion of Essential and Reproductive Health and Technologies, Dhaka, Bangladesh)

Induced abortions: decision-making, provider choice and morbidity experience in rural adolescents
Bela Ganatra (Johns Hopkins University, Baltimore, MD, USA)

Terminating unwanted pregnancies among adolescents: magnitude and experiences
Nozer Sheriyar (Family Planning Association India, Mumbai) (Summary not available)

Situation analysis of emergency contraceptive drug use among young people in Thailand: a Bangkok case study
Wanapa Naravage (Program for Appropriate Technology in Health, Bangkok, Thailand)

* Abstract presentation.

Adolescent abortion: a view from rural Bangladesh
*M. Kapil Ahmed** (International Centre for Diarrhoeal Disease Research, Dhaka, Bangladesh)

Abortion among young married women in Colombo district
*P. Hewage** (University of Ruhuna, Colombo, Sri Lanka)

Discussant's comments
Dale Huntington (Population Council, New Delhi, India)

Session 8: Unwanted sex: sexual violence and coercion
Chairperson: *Azeema Faizunnisa* (Population Council, Islamabad, Pakistan)

Adolescents and sexual coercion
Geeta Sodhi (Swaasthya, New Delhi, India)

Experience of sexual coercion among street boys in Bangalore
Jayashree Ramakrishna (National Institute of Mental Health and Neuro Sciences, Bangalore, India)

Prevalence and correlates of abuse in adolescents in higher secondary schools in Goa
Vikram Patel (Sangath Centre for Child Development and Family Guidance, Goa, India)

Experience of violence: Reflections from male adolescents
Bella Patel Uttekar (Centre of Operations Research and Training, Vadodara, India)

Discussant's comments
Surinder Jaswal (Tata Institute of Social Sciences, Mumbai, India)

Session 9: Communicating with adolescents
Chairperson: *Nina Puri* (FPA India)

Educational strategies in family life and sex education: non-formal, school and higher education levels—how far does it go and how much further does it need to go?
Vandana Chakrabarti (SNDT Women's University, Mumbai, India)

Counselling youth on sexual and reproductive health: individual and peer programmes
Raj Brahmbhatt (Family Planning Association of India, Mumbai, India)

Reproductive health education: experiences of Privar Seva Sanstha in communicating with youth
Sudha Tewari (Parivar Seva Sanstha, New Delhi, India)

Providing sex education to rural adolescents in Bangladesh: experiences from BRAC
Sabina Rashid (Bangladesh Rural Advancement Committee, Dhaka, Bangladesh)

The Healthy Adolescent Project in India
Matthew Tiedemann (Family Health International, Research Triangle Park, NC, USA)

Barriers in reproductive health services in school based family life education programmes
*Rama Sivaram** (KEM Hospital Research Centre, Pune, India)

Impact of IEC on AIDS awareness among adolescents in Haryana, India
*Rajesh Kumar** (Post Graduate Institute of Medical Education and Research, Chandigarh, India)

Discussant's comments
Sabiha Syed (United Nations Educational, Scientific and Cultural Organization, Paris, France)

* Abstract presentation.

Session 10: Poster presentations

Session 11: Building a safe and supportive environment
Chairperson: *Sharon Epstein* (FOCUS on Young Adults, Washington, DC, USA)

Adolescent girls in India choose a better future: an impact assessment
Marta Levitt-Dayal (the Centre for Development and Population Activities, New Delhi, India)

Connections with parents, families and teachers: the views from both sides
Rekha Masilamani (Pathfinder International, New Delhi, India)

A gender-sensitive perspective from two generations: motives and seekers of reproductive health knowledge in Pakistan
Minhaj ul Haque (Population Council, Islamabad, Pakistan)

Enabling adolescents to build life skills: capacity building of facilitators
Mridula Seth (United Nations Population Fund, New Delhi, India)

Integrating adolescent reproductive health into public health services in Bawal Block, Haryana
*Sunil Mehra** (Mamta, New Delhi, India)

Adolescent girl's initiative in Mumbai
*Parimala Subramanian** (KEM Hospital, Mumbai, India)

Discussant's comments
Hally Mahler (Family Health International, Research Triangle Park, NC, USA)

Session 12: Access to and quality of reproductive health services: adolescent perspectives
Chairperson: *Meenakshi Datta-Ghosh* (Ministry of Health and Family Welfare, New Delhi, India)

What is adolescent friendly?
V. Chandra Mouli (World Health Organization, Geneva, Switzerland)

Reproductive health services for adolescents: recent experience from a pilot project
Ismat Bhuiya (Population Council, Dhaka, Bangladesh)

Making NGO initiatives youth friendly
Sharon Epstein (FOCUS on Young Adults, Washington, DC, USA)

Establishing adolescent health services in a general health facility
Rajesh Mehta (Safdarjang Hospital, New Delhi, India)

Providing adolescent-friendly health services: the Thai experience
Yupa Poonkhum (Family Planning and Population Division, Ministry of Public Health, Nonthaburi, Thailand)

Adolescent friendly reproductive health services
*A.K.M. Alamgir** (Bangladesh Open University, Gazipur, Bangladesh)

Discussant's comments
John Townsend (FRONTIERS Project, Population Council, Washington, DC, USA)

* Abstract presentation.

Session 13: Panel discussion—Enhancing adolescent reproductive health: strategies and challenges
Moderator: *Iqbal Shah* (World Health Organization, Geneva, Switzerland)

Panellists: *Yasmeen Qazi* (Karachi, Pakistan); *Halida Hanum Akhter* (Bangladesh Institute of Research for Promotion of Essential and Reproductive Health and Technologies, Dhaka, Bangladesh); *Firoza Mehrotra* (Planning Commission, Government of India, New Delhi); *Laxmi R. Pathak* (Family Health Division, HMG of Nepal, Kathmandu); *Deepthi Perera* (Department of Health Services, Ministry of Health, Colombo, Sri Lanka); *Neena Raina* (World Health Organization, New Delhi, India); *Swaroop Sarkar* (UNAIDS, New Delhi).

VALEDICTORY FUNCTION
Chairperson: *Meenakshi Datta-Ghosh*

Iqbal Shah
Harbans S. Juneja
Purnima Mane
V. Chandra Mouli
Padam Singh
Shireen Jejeebhoy
Chander Puri

Note: Institutional affiliations of presenters reflect the situation at the time of the Conference.